Pedodontics
– a clinical approach

Pedodontics
– a clinical approach

Editors

Göran Koch
Thomas Modéer
Sven Poulsen
Per Rasmussen

Munksgaard

Pedodontics - a clinical approach

1st edition, 2nd printing, 1994

Copyright © 1991, Munksgaard, Copenhagen

No part of this publication may be reproduced, stored in a retrieval system, or transmitted in any form or by any means, electronic, mechanical photocopying, recording or otherwise without prior permission by the copyright owner

Drawings, composition and typesetting by Jens L. Kirkegaard

Printed in Denmark, by P. J. Schmidt, Vojens

ISBN 87-16-06812-2

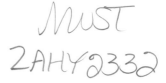

LIST OF CONTRIBUTORS

ALMER NIELSEN, LIS, DDS
Assistant Professor
Department of Pediatric Dentistry, The Royal Dental College, Copenhagen, Denmark

ATTRAMADAL, AUDUN, DDS, Dr.Odont.
Professor
Department of Pedodontics, School of Dentistry, University of Bergen, Norway

DAHLLÖF, GÖRAN, DDS, Odont.Dr.
Associate Professor
Department of Pedodontics, School of Dentistry, Karolinska Institute,
Stockholm, Sweden

EGERMARK-ERIKSSON, INGER, DDS, Odont.Dr.
Chairman
Orthodontic Clinic, Kungsbacka, Sweden

ESPELID, IVAR, DDS, Lic.Odont, Dr.Odont.
Associate Professor
Department of Pedodontics, School of Dentistry, University of Bergen, Norway

FRIIS-HASCHÉ, ERIK,DDS, Dr.Odont., BA
Associate Professor
Department of Pediatric Dentistry, Psychological Clinic, The Royal Dental College,
Copenhagen, Denmark

GRANATH, LARS, LDS, Odont.Dr.
Professor and Chairman
Department of Pedodontics, School of Dentistry, University of Lund, Sweden

HALLONSTEN, ANNA-LENA, DDS, Dr.Med.Sci.
Senior Consultant
Department of Pedodontics, The Institute for Postgraduate Dental Education,
Jönköping, Sweden

HEIDE, SYNNØVE, DDS
Department of Pedodontics and Caries Prophylaxis, School of Dentistry,
University of Oslo, Norway

HOLM, ANNA-KARIN, DDS, Odont.Dr.
Professor and Chairman
Department of Pedodontics, School of Dentistry, University of Umeå, Sweden

HOLST, ANNALENA, DDS, Odont.Dr.
Chairman
Department of Pedodontics, Karlskrona, Sweden

HÄGG, URBAN, DDS, Odont.Dr.
Associate Professor
Department of Orthodontics, School of Dentistry, University of Lund, Sweden

HØLUND, ULLA, DDS, Ph.D.
Assistant Professor
Department of Child Dental Health and Conmunity Dentistry,
The Royal Dental College, Aarhus, Denmark

HÖSKULDSSON, ÓLAFUR, DDS
Assistant Professor and Division Head
Division of Pedodontics, Faculty of Odontology, University of Iceland, Iceland

JACOBSEN, INGEBORG, DDS, Dr.Odont.
Professor
Department of Pedodontics and Caries Prophylaxis, School of Dentistry,
University of Oslo, Norway

JENSEN, BIRGIT LETH, DDS, Lic.Odont.
Assistant professor
Department of Pediatric Dentistry, The Royal Dental College, Copenhagen, Denmark

KOCH, GÖRAN, DDS, Odont.Dr.
Professor and Chairman
Department of Pedodontics, The Institute for Postgraduate Dental Education,
Jönköping, Sweden

KREIBORG, SVEN, DDS, Dr.Odont. Ph.D.
Professor and Chairman
Department of Pediatric Dentistry, The Royal Dental College, Copenhagen, Dennark

KØLSEN PETERSEN, JENS, DDS, M.S.
Associate Professor
Department of Oral and Maxillofacial Surgery, The Royal Dental College,
Aarhus, Denmark

MATSSON, LARS, DDS, Odont.Dr.
Associate Professor
Department of Pedodontics, School of Dentistry, University of Umeå, Sweden

MEJÀRE, INGEGERD, DDS, Odont.Dr.
Associate Professor
Department of Pedodontics, Eastman Dental Institute, Stockholm, Sweden

MODÉER, THOMAS, DDS, Odont.Dr.
Professor and Chairman
Department of Pedodontics, School of Dentistry, Karolinska Institute,
Stockholm, Sweden

NORÉN, JÖRGEN G., DDS, B.Sc., Odont.Dr.
Associate Professor and Chairman
Department of Pedodontics, School of Dentistry, University of Göteborg, Sweden

NYSTRÖM, MARJATTA, DDS, Dr.Odont.
Instructor
Department of Pedodontics and Orthodontics, Institute of Dentistry,
University of Helsinki, Finland

POULSEN, SVEN, DDS, Ph.D., Dr.Odont.
Professor and Chairman
Department of Child Dental Health and Community Dentistry,
The Royal Dental College, Aarhus, Denmark

RAADAL, MAGNE, DDS, Dr.Odont.
Associate Professor
Department of Pedodontics, School of Dentistry, University of Bergen, Norway

RASMUSSEN, PER, DDS, Lic. Odont., Dr.Odont.
Professor and Chairnan
Department of Pedodontics, School of Dentistry, University of Bergen, Norway

RÖLLA, GUNNAR, DDS, Dr.Odont.
Professor and Chairman
Department of Pedodontics and Caries Prophylaxis, School of Dentistry,
University of Oslo, Norway

RØLLING, INGE, DDS, Ph.D., Dr.Odont.
Associate Professor
Department of Child Dental Health and Community Dentistry,
The Royal Dental College, Aarhus, Denmark

SCHRÖDER, ULLA, DDS, Odont.Dr.
Associate Professor
Department of Pedodontics, School of Dentistry, University of Lund, Sweden

STORHAUG, KARI, DDS, Dr.Odont.
Assistant Professor
Institute of Community Dentistry, School of Dentistry, University of Oslo, Norway

SVATUN, BJARNE, DDS, Dr.Odont.
Assistant Professor
Department of Pedodontics and Caries Prophylaxis, School of Dentistry,
University of Oslo, Norway

SVEDIN, CARL-GÖRAN, M.D.
Department of Child and Adolescent, Psychiatry Faculty of Health Sciences,
University of Linköping, Sweden

THESLEFF, IRMA, DDS, Dr.Odont.
Professor and Chairman
Department of Pedodontics and Orthodontics, Institute of Dentistry,
University of Helsinki, Finland

CONTENTS

CHAPTER 1

INTRODUCTION

A high standard of pediatric dental care is the key to achieving good oral health throughout life and should, therefore, be a primary social goal.

In Scandinavia it has for many years been a major ambition to provide all children and adolescents with continuous dental care based on prevention. This has resulted in a tremendous improvement in the oral health of the young and is now evident even in younger adults. This pediatric dental care comprises not only the prevention and management of dental caries and gingivitis, but also all aspects of tooth and occlusal developmental disturbances, traumatic injuries, oral pathological conditions, juvenile prosthodontics, pain control, dental treatment of handicapped and medically compromised children, etc; all adapted to the special conditions of the two dentitions in a growing child.

Good pediatric dental care, thus, implies a wide range of knowledge and skills. This has long been emphasized in Scandinavia and has resulted in a world-renowned standard of pedodontic teaching and training.

Intensive research and development activity in both preventive and clinical pediatric dental care provides the basis for continuous evaluation and improvement of education and treatment.

The aim of this textbook is to give a comprehensive presentation of the scientific background, treatment philosophies and clinical procedures prevailing in pedodontic education in Scandinavia. It is a complete revision of "Pedodontics - a systematic approach" and special emphasis is focused on the clinical aspects of pediatric dentistry. The authors are all active in pediatric dentistry departments of universities and postgraduate dental education centers in Denmark, Finland, Iceland, Norway, and Sweden. Each chapter is written by a group, the first name being the coordinator.

It is our belief that this book can be used not only by students, but also by all dental practitioners wishing to update their knowledge and skill in clinical pedodontics.

The editors

CHAPTER 2

SOMATIC GROWTH AND DEVELOPMENT

Prenatal growth
Disturbances in prenatal development
Normal postnatal growth and maturity assessment
Aberrant postnatal growth
Child health care

Growth is defined as an increase in size and/or weight of a tissue, an organ or an individual. *Development* is defined as any process of continuous changes occurring in a predetermined order. Man uses the first third of his life growing and developing, preparing for adult life and reproduction. The growing period starts at conception and ends a few years after puberty, and is normally divided into two main periods: *prenatal* and *postnatal*. A thorough knowledge of the growth and development of the child is essential to pediatric medicine, but also important in other professions dealing with children, including pedodontics.

PRENATAL GROWTH

Prenatal growth from conception to birth is usually divided into three trimesters, without, however, any clearcut borderlines between them.

First trimester (embryonal period 0-12 weeks) is characterized by differentiation of tissues and formation of organs. The body size and weight is still low at the end of this period (7.5 cm/14 g), water content is high, and mineralization of bones and teeth has not yet started. During the first trimester the embryo is especially vulnerable to teratogenic influences. Manifestations of chromosomal aberrations and inherited disorders also occur at this time, often leading to unnoticed abortions.

Second trimester (12-27 weeks) is characterized by rapid growth and maturation. Of special importance is the development of the internal organs and their preparation for postnatal function.

Third trimester (28-40 weeks) together with the second trimester are named the *fetal period*. Normally the borderline for survival is the 28th week (35 cm, 1,000 g), but modern technique in premature care has lowered that borderline significantly. During the third trimester the increasing weight of the fetus is the dominant factor (Fig. 2-1).

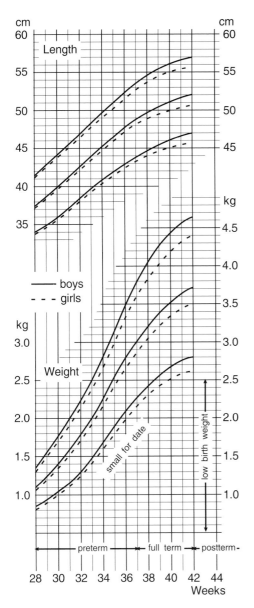

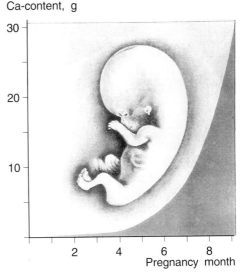

Fig. 2-2. Calcium accumulation in fetal life. Most of the calcium is incorporated during the third trimester.

Fig. 2-1. Prenatal growth chart for length and weight (Means ± 2SD). Adapted from Nordisk lærebog i pædiatri, 1985.

A characteristic feature is the accumulation of subcutaneous fat, increase in muscle mass and reduced water-content. Accumulation of calcium due to the mineralization of bones and teeth is also very important.

Thus, during the third trimester the calcium content of the fetus increases from 5 g to about 30 g (Fig. 2-2). Therefore, in cases of premature birth the body store of calcium may be very low, enhancing the danger of disturbances in calcium metabolism during the neonatal period.

Birth (full term) is from 37 to 42 weeks after postmenstrual gestation (35-40 weeks after conception). Children born earlier than 37 weeks are named *preterm* (premature), and if born later than 42 weeks *postterm*. If a child is born with a low birth weight, it may be premature, or it may be "small for date" (Fig. 2-1). In neonatal medicine it is important to distinguish between the two possibilities, because premature children need special care because of immature organs. Special neurological tests are developed to determine the degree of maturity of the newborn child.

The mechanisms of prenatal growth and its regulation are only partly known. Most

Growth rate - height, cm/year

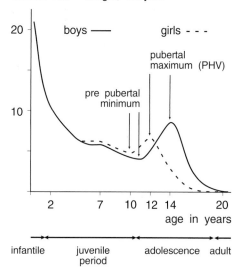

Fig. 2-3. Growth velocity curves for Danish boys and girls. Modified from(1).

of the hormones known to influence postnatal growth seem to have negligible influence on prenatal growth. Insulin, however, influences prenatal growth, as do the factors as the mother's body size and health, placental circulation, intrauterine nutrition, etc.

DISTURBANCES IN PRENATAL DEVELOPMENT

Aberrant development may arise in both the embryonal and the fetal periods, and the causes may be genetic, as well as environmental, factors. The genetic factors may be chromosomal aberrations (e.g. Down's syndrome), polygenic action (e.g. cleft lip/palate), or monogenic action (e.g. enzyme deficiencies, amelogenesis imperfecta, several craniofacial syndromes). A lot of environmental factors (teratogenes) are known to influence prenatal development strongly:

maternal medication (e.g. thalidomide), maternal infections (e.g. rubella, toxoplasmosis) and several others (e.g. X-ray radiation, anoxemia, maternal malnutrition and alcoholism). However, in 65-70% of prenatal malformations no detectable etiological factor is found.

The teratogenic effects will generally depend on the nature of the agent, its intensity, and the period during which the fetus encounters it. Organs in strong development will suffer most. The most vulnerable time is the embryonal period.

The fetus is less vulnerable during the fetal period and aberrations are likely to be growth retardation and minor organ traumas instead of major malformations. Fetal growth impairment may also be caused by placental insufficiency. This is often the case in multiple births, but may also be caused by maternal malnutrition or smoking. These children may be born at full term, but are "small for date".

NORMAL POSTNATAL GROWTH AND MATURITY ASSESSMENT

Postnatal growth and development begin at birth and terminate when adult maturity is attained and/or growth ceases. Maturity is defined as being grown and developed to the point of being fit for any appropriate action, function, or state. It is usually described in relation to the attainment of specific stages (e.g. stages of bone morphology in hand/wrist, sexual features, tooth formation/eruption), and expressed in terms of developmental age (e.g. skeletal and dental age).

Because of great individual variation in somatic maturation at any chronological age, developmental age is often a more suitable measure of development than chronological age, especially in the diagnosis of a patient with a disturbed growth pattern, but also in treatment planning for interceptive orthodontics or dentofacial corrections.

When estimating a child's progress to maturity one is usually comparing its stage with standards obtained from representative samples of a similar population at the same age. Standards of standing height, weight, skeletal development, secondary sexual characteristics, and dental development are used in this context. Thus, it may be possible to estimate if the child is an early, average or late maturer compared with his peers. New standards have to be established regularly due to the *secular trend*, as improved nutrition and better health during the last century has significantly influenced the rate of maturation and final height and weight (Fig. 2-7).

Standing height itself is not an expression of maturity because the final height will differ widely. However, the shape and pattern of the individual curve (accumulated growth) and the velocity curve (growth per year) have a characteristic pattern in all children. The velocity curve (Fig. 2-3) may be divided into three periods: 1) the infantile period characterized by a high growth rate which rapidly declines; 2) the juvenile period with a relatively slow growth which declines until 3) the adolescent period starts, characterized by a marked increase in growth rate, reaching the pubertal maximum of growth, followed by a decline of growth rate until growth terminates and adulthood is reached. The average girl begins the adolescent period at 10 years, reaches her pubertal maximum of growth at 12 years and terminates growth at 17 years. The average boy will experience his adolescent period 2 years later. However, the individual variation is great in both sexes. Thus, an early maturer of both sexes will experience the adolescent period 6 years before a late maturer of the same sex. The growth rate at the pubertal maximum is in girls 8.5 cm/year (SD = 1 cm), and in boys 10.0 cm/year (SD = 1 cm). Thus, men are taller than women due to a longer juvenile period and a higher growth rate at the pubertal maximum.

Longitudinal records of standing height (Figs. 2-4, 2-5) are most often used in pediatric medicine. Data are plotted on charts with curves for mean figures and plus/minus SD (or percentiles), establishing several "growth channels". Normally, a child will stay within a certain channel. If it leaves the channel, it may indicate a growth disturbance disorder. However, during the pubertal growth spurt a temporary change to another growth channel is quite common if the individual has an early or a late onset of puberty.

The proportions of the body also undergo significant changes during postnatal growth. At birth the head and torso are oversized compared with the lower limbs. Thus, the head comprises about one fourth, and in the adult one eighth, of the total body height.

Weight is a widely used measurement, but an unsatisfactory indicator of somatic maturation. An increase in weight may be due to growth, but also to an increase of fat or water in the body. Conversely, adequate growth in height may not be accompanied by increase in weight, if fat is lost at the same time. Weight standards are presented in Figs. 2-4, 2-5.

Skeletal maturity/bone age is a measure of how far the ossification of the bones has progressed towards maturity judged by morphology and mineralization of bones in the hand and wrist (Fig. 2-6). Skeletal maturity may be assessed by comparison with standards(3), by a scoring method(5) or by studying specific individual bones(1). The first two methods are mostly used in pediatric medicine, while the last method is wide-

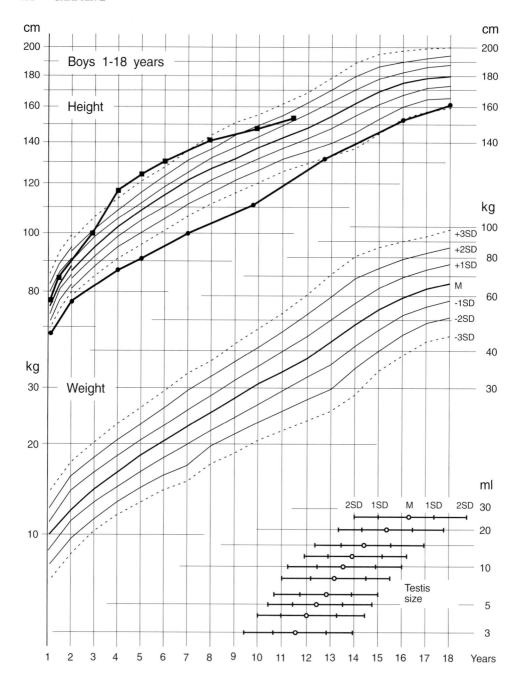

Fig. 2-4. Growth chart for Swedish boys from 1-18 years (mean ± 1,2,3 SD).
■ – ■ is the growth curve for a boy with accelerated growth (pubertas praecox).
• – • is the growth curve for a boy with retarded growth (hypopituitarism).

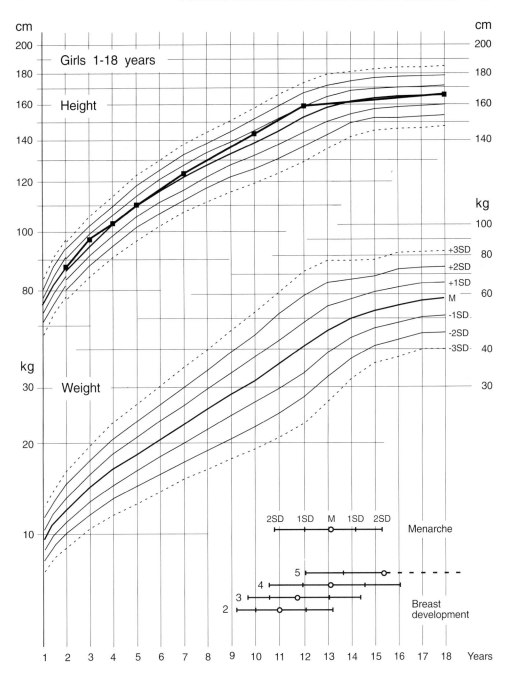

Fig. 2-5. Growth chart for Swedish girls from 1-18 years (means ± 1,2,3 SD).
■ - ■ is the growth curve for a girl with early maturation.

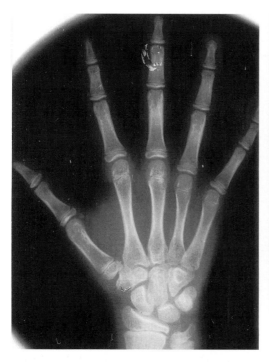
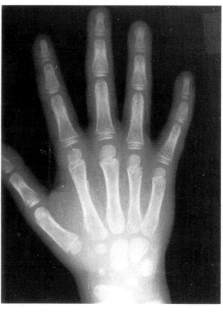

Fig. 2-6. Hand/wrist x-ray of monozygotic twins at 6 years. The twin to the left has pubertas prae-cox and a skeletal age of 13 years. The twin to the right has a skeletal age corresponding to chronological age.

ly used in orthodontic treatment planning to assess, for example, whether a patient is approaching, has attained, or passed his pubertal maximum growth.

Secondary sexual characteristics in boys are: genital development, increase in testicular volume, pubic, axillary and facial hair, and voice changes; and in girls: breast development, pubic and axillary hair and menarche (first menstrual bleeding). The development of secondary sexual characteristics has been divided into a number of stages through which all individuals of the respective sex will pass. The association between pubertal growth maximum and some of these stages is high. Assessment of those stages can thus be used to estimate the individuals position on the growth curve in an indirect way. Reference values for tes-

ticular size, menarche and breast development are indicated in Figs. 2-4, 2-5.

Dental maturity and dental age is a measure of how far the teeth have progressed towards maturity judged from x-rays. The Demirjian system(2) is most used (Chapter 4), but several other systems have been developed with reference to Nordic tooth development schedules. Dental maturity may also be assessed by counting the teeth visible in the mouth, provided that the child is in one of the periods of active eruption.

The association between dental maturity and general growth/skeletal maturity is poor. However, the correlation between dental age and chronological age is somewhat better than that between skeletal and chronological age. Dental maturity is com-

TABLE 2-1

Factors causing disturbances in postnatal growth.

Primary disturbances of growth	Secondary disturbances of growth
Skeletal dysplasias	Malnutrition
Chromosomal aberrations	Systemic and metabolic disorders
Congenital errors of metabolism	Deprivation dwarfism
Intrauterine growth retardation	Endocrine disorders
Miscellaneous syndromes	Constitutional growth delay
Genetic short stature	

monly used in estimating the chronological age of adopted and immigrant children with uncertain birth records (Chapter 4). However, it is little used after the age of 7 years.

ABERRANT POSTNATAL GROWTH

In the Nordic countries most children are seen by their dentist more frequently than by their family doctor. Therefore, the pedo-dontist should have a thorough knowledge of somatic growth and development and, thus, be able to contribute to the diagnosis of infants and children with deviant growth patterns. Normal growth can occur only if the child is healthy and able to produce in its tissues, or absorb from the diet, the factors needed to obtain optimal growth and development.

Evaluation of body height and weight should include several successive measurements recorded on a reference chart. Knowledge of skeletal age is also of great importance in the diagnosis and treatment of children with aberrant growth, to disclose whether a growth retardation is associated with a concomitant change in skeletal maturity.

Growth disturbances may be divided into two main groups (Table 2-1). A distinc-tion between primary and secondary disturbances is necessary as their cause, diagnostic approach, treatment and prognosis differ markedly. Most cases of primary growth disturbances will result in decreased adult stature as possibilities of adequate treatment are scarce. Secondary growth disturbances may often be treated with good results, and normal adult height is often attained if adequate treatment is commenced at an early age.

Primary growth disturbances

Skeletal dysplasia comprises more than 100 disorders which appear either as a result of a genetic defect or of prenatal damage to the skeletal system. It may be exemplified by *achondroplasia,* a monogenic (autosomal dominant) inherited disorder characterized by disproportionate shortening of the limbs, resulting in an adult height of about 130 cm. The maxilla is retrognathic, leaving a relative protrusion of the forehead and the mandible (Fig. 2-10).

Chromosomal aberrations (e.g. Down's syndrome, Turner's syndrome) often include retarded growth.

Congenital errors of metabolism may be exemplified by the mucopolysaccharidoses which are genetically conditioned (autoso-

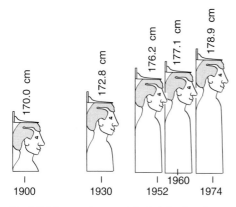

Fig. 2-7. The secular trend in height development. Norwegian military recruits have increased in average height from 170cm to 179cm over the last 75 years.

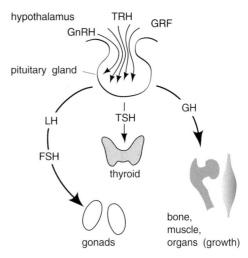

Fig. 2-8. The link between hypothalamus, the pituitary gland and target organs for the most important growth regulating hormones.

mally recessive) failures in the connective tissues' intercellular substance, comprising many different types (Hunter, Hurler, Morquio's syndrome, etc.). In Morquio's syndrome dwarfism is pronounced.

Intrauterine growth retardation may be caused by several factors including placental insufficiencies (p. 18).

Miscellaneous syndromes refer to several syndromes of unknown etiology, but identified because of typical features and impaired growth. The growth retardation will often be recognized at birth.

Genetic short stature. Body height is determined by several genes (polygenic) coming from both parents. Generally tall parents will have tall children, and short parents will produce short children.

Secondary disturbances of growth

Malnutrition is a well-known cause of growth retardation in many developing countries, and may also have been the cause

of the lower height in the Nordic countries in the past. Thus, Norwegian army recruits have increased their height by 9 cm in the last 75 years (Fig. 2-7). After periods of malnutrition, a child may have "catch-up" growth and be able to revert to its original growth channel. Only in cases of severe malnutrition may permanent stunting occur.

Systemic and metabolic disorders. Growth impairment (height as well as weight) is typical in children with chronic diseases of the gastrointestinal tract, kidneys, vascular system, etc. The diet may be adequate, but malabsorption (as in coeliac disease) may reduce the internal supply of nutrients.

Deprivation dwarfism (psychosocial growth retardation) may be caused by disturbances in the emotional contact between child, parents and environment (understimulation).

Endocrine disorders. A balanced hormone production is needed for optimal growth. Most important are the *growth hormone* from the pituitary gland, *sex hormones* from

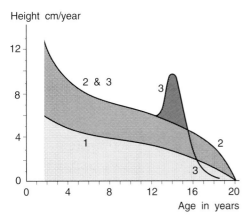

Height cm/year

Fig. 2-9. Influence of growth hormone and sex hormones on body growth. If both hormones are lacking, Curve 1 is followed. If only sex hormones are lacking, Curve 2 is followed. Curve 3 represents the normal growth curve with pubertal growth spurt, and early closure of the epiphyseal plates.

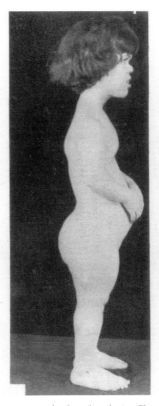

Fig. 2-10. A case of achondroplasia. Characteristic features are short extremities and a retruding maxilla. From(4).

testicles/ovaries and the *thyroid hormone.* The production of sex hormones and thyroid hormone are regulated by the pituitary gland, which again is regulated by factors produced in the hypothalamus (Fig. 2-8). The effect of growth hormone and sex hormones on growth is illustrated in Fig. 2-9. If both hormones are lacking, the child will follow Curve 1 ("basic growth"). If only sex hormones are lacking, the child will follow Curve 2, where the pubertal growth peak is lacking, but the growth period is extended. In normal growth (Curve 3), the pubertal peak is present, but the growth period is shortened. Lack of growth hormone results in pituitary dwarfism (nanosomia). The mean growth velocity may fall to about 3 cm/year resulting in a severe, but balanced, dwarfism.

The growth reduction is also present in the craniofacial complex, and dental development and eruption are retarded (Fig. 2-11). The condition may be treated with growth hormone injections. The effect of overproduction of growth hormone is gigantism, and may be caused by tumours of the pituitary gland.

Lack of sex hormones results in absence of a pubertal growth spurt, but, because of the extended growth period, final stature may be above normal (eunuchism). If the production of sex hormones starts too early (pubertas praecox), height will be above normal during childhood (Figs. 2-4, 2-12), but the final height will be below normal. The same pattern may also be observed in normal children, especially in girls. An early start of puberty may lead to excessive tallness (and some anxiety), but growth will proceed for a shorter time, and final height will be in accordance with constitution or a little less (Fig. 2-5).

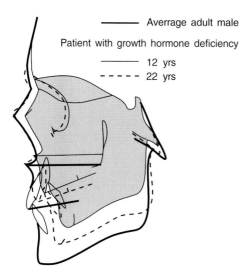

Fig. 2-11. Facial growth of a patient with growth hormone deficiency. Tracings at 12 and 22 years are compared with the normal adult mean.

The thyroid hormone regulates the general metabolism. In cases of hypothyroidism there will be a significant reduction in skeletal growth (cretinism). If the diagnosis is made early, replacement therapy may correct the aberrant metabolic behaviour.

Constitutional growth delay. Most children with growth impairment belong to this category in whom skeletal maturity is delayed, while all other physical parameters prove normal. These children will exhibit delayed growth and sexual maturation, but final height is normal.

CHILD HEALTH CARE

The aim of child health care offered by the Mother and Child Welfare Stations is to contribute to the best obtainable physical, mental and social health of every child in society. Of special importance are general and individual preventive programs, diagnosis of incipient and manifest diseases and handicaps, but certain therapeutic services

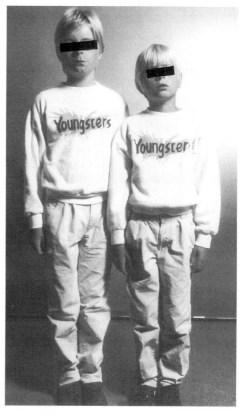

Fig. 2-12. Monozygotic twins at 8 years. The boy to the left has pubertas praecox. His height corresponds to 10.5 years, his skeletal maturation to 15.5 years. His brother has a normal growth pattern.

are also offered. The main working methods are *information to parents* by physicians, nurses, psychologists, dental personnel, etc., and also *regular health checks* prenatally as well as postnatally. The aim of the prenatal checks is early detection of conditions that could endanger the child during its fetal life or at parturition, e.g. maternal disorders, malnutrition, drug abuse, blood group incompatibilities between mother and fetus, but also inborn metabolic disorders, syndromes, etc., in the fetus itself. For early intrauterine diagnosis such modern methods as ultrasound scanning and transabdominal amniocentesis are available.

TABLE 2-2

Vaccination programs for children

Denmark	Pertussis at 5 & 9 weeks, and at 10 months Diphtheria-tetanus-polio (Salk) at 5, 6 & 10 months Polio (Sabin) at 2, 3 & 4 years Morbilli, Parotitis, Rubella at 15 months and 12 years Tuberculosis latest at 14-15 years
Finland	Polio (Salk) at 4, 5, 6, 18 & 24 months and at 6, 11, 16 & 18 years Diphtheria-tetanus-pertussis at 3, 4, 5 months and 2 years Tetanus at 12 years, 22 years, etc. Morbilli, parotitis, rubella at 15 months and 6 years Tuberculosis newborn, and at 11-13 years if tbc.neg.
Iceland	Diphtheria-pertussis-tetanus at 3, 4, 6 & 14 months Polio (Salk) at 6, 7 & 14 months and at 4, 9 & 14 years Morbilli, parotitis at 18 months Diphtheria-tetanus at 6 years Rubella at 12 years offered to girls at risk only
Norway	Diphtheria-tetanus-pertussis at 3, 5 & 10 months Diphtheria-tetanus at 11 years Polio (Salk) at 6, 7 & 16 months and at 7 & 14 years Morbilli, parotitis, rubella at 15 months and at 12 years Tuberculosis latest at 14-15 years
Sweden	Diphtheria-tetanus at 3, 4½ & 6 months and at 10 years Polio (Salk) at 9, 10 & 18 months and at 6 years Morbilli, Parotitis, Rubella at 18 months and at 12 years Pertussis to "risk groups" Tuberculosis to newborn at risk and to all at 13-14 years

From Nordisk lærebog i pædiatri, 1985.

During postnatal life, health controls are especially important to detect developmental disorders during the first year. Vaccination programs (Table 2-2), are also of great importance, as they have prevented or reduced the incidence of most of the diseases that formerly crippled or killed many children. Informing parents and later also children is an important task.

The effects of intensive health care for mother and child may be excellently demonstrated by the mortality statistics from Sweden 1915-1980 (Fig. 2-13). Deaths from infectious diseases are nearly eliminated. At present, most neonatal deaths are caused by malformation.

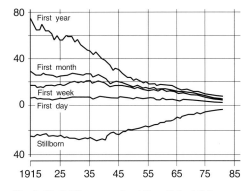

Fig. 2-13. Stillborn or dead Swedish children during the first years of life, from 1915 to 1981 (per 1,000 births). Adapted from Nordisk lærebog i pædiatri, 1985.

Background literature

Björk A. Kæbernes relation til det øvrige kranium. In: Lundström A, ed. *Nordisk lärobok i ortodonti*. Stockholm: Sveriges Tandläkarförbunds Förlagsförening, 1975.

Friis-Hansen B, ed. *Nordisk lærebog i pædiatri*, Chapters 1,2,4,7,9. København: Munksgaard, 1985.

Kaplan SA. *Clinical pediatric and adolescent endocrinology*. Philadelphia: Saunders, 1982.

Karlberg P, Taranger J, Engström I., et al. Physical growth from birth to 16 years and longitudinal outcome of the study during the same age period. *Acta Paediatr Scand*, Suppl. 258, 1976: 7-76.

Tanner JM. *Foetus into man*. Physical growth from conception to maturity. London: Open Books, 1975.

Zachmann M, Aynsley-Green A. Prader A. Interrelations of the effects of growth hormone and testosterone in hypopituitarism. In: Pecile A, Muller EE, eds. *Growth hormone and related peptides*. New York: American Elsevier, 1976.

Literature cited

1. Björk A. Timing of interceptive orthodontic measures based on stages of maturation. *Trans Eur Orthod Soc* 1972; **45**: 61-74.

2. Demirjian A. Dentition. In: Falkner F, Tanner JM, eds. *Human growth*. London: Bailliere Tindall, 1982.

3. Greulich WW, Pyle SI. *Radiographic atlas of skeletal development of the hand and wrist*. California: Stanford University Press, 1959.

4. Tachdjian, MO. *Pediatric orthopedics*, Vol 1. Philadelphia: Saunders, 1972.

5. Tanner JM, Whitehouse RH, Marshall WA, Healy MJR, Goldstein H. *Assessment of skeletal maturity and prediction of adult height* (TW2 method). London: Academic Press, 1975.

CHAPTER 3

MENTAL DEVELOPMENT

Theories of developmental psychology
Oral phase, infancy
Anal phase, early childhood
Oedipal phase, late childhood
Latency phase, early school-age
Genital phase, adolescence

When children and young people are given dental or other forms of care, it is important for the practitioner to try to see the world through a child's eyes. Knowledge of developmental psychology can help in understanding the reactions of children undergoing treatment, as well as in finding the best ways of dealing with both child and parents. In part, children's reactions are responses to the way they are approached by the practitioner, as well as to their experience of treatment. Frequently, these reactions are quite normal in terms of age. Developmental psychology deals not just with child development, but with the whole process of human development over a life span(1, 2).

When it comes to dental treatment, the most important and interesting areas of development are motoric, adaptive, verbal and social behaviors and personality. At a given age, a child may be at different stages for each of these areas, with motoric behavior, for example, fully advanced while personality and social behavior are relatively undeveloped (Fig. 3-1).

Motoric behavior includes both gross motor development, such as walking, and fine motor development such as finger movements and coordination. Knowledge of motor development is important when it comes to a child's ability both to sit still during treatment and to brush its teeth.

Adaptive behavior means adaptation to different situations requiring thinking, imagination and learning. Adaptation to the situation is the most important issue in dental treatment.

Verbal behavior includes all verbal messages from babble to sentence construction, vocabulary, and understanding different words. Knowledge of children's communication skills is important in all treatment.

Personality and social behavior are children's interaction with their total environment, especially parents, other grown-ups, children and, sometimes, the dental practitioner. Just how this development proceeds is dependent upon a number of factors including the interplay between heredity and environment (Fig. 3-2). The environmental factors which play the largest role in a child's early emotional development are, quite naturally, those existing in the im-

Developmental level

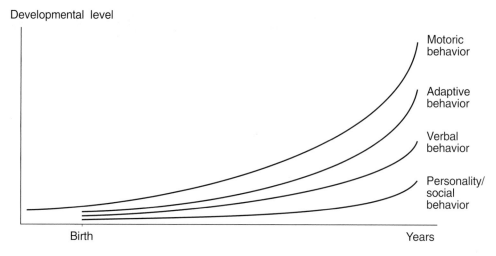

Fig. 3-1. Development of behavior in children.

mediate surroundings during the first years of life. The parents and the relationship with them have a completely dominant role during a child's early emotional development. Peers, relatives, other adults and teachers gradually become more important. Economy, housing and unemployment are all factors which can influence a child's development more indirectly.

THEORIES OF DEVELOPMENTAL PSYCHOLOGY

It can be said that development involves two concepts: maturity and learning. By maturity we mean those changes in the human which depend to greater degree upon innate abilities, i.e. heredity. While the concept of learning involves the ability to absorb from and interact with the environment. Through interaction with the environment the child learns different ways of relating to and coping with its surroundings, ways which may be termed characteristics and attributes of personality. In everyday life both maturity and learning

are involved in a constant interplay more or less indistinguishable from each other. However, the different schools of developmental psychology place different emphases on these attributes. The theory of maturity has its foremost advocate in Gesell(5), according to whom human development is predetermined and regulated by laws over which surroundings have little influence. The cognitive theories describe the processes of thinking, linguistic development, concept-formation and memory, while emphasizing that the driving force of development is to be found in the positive feelings which arise when a child, step by step, achieves new knowledge and experience. The foremost proponent of this theory, Piaget(7), viewed humans as having two innate tendencies important for coping successfully with life: the tendency to adapt to surroundings and the tendency to organize experience and knowledge. The psychoanalytical theories held by S Freud, A Freud, Mahler and Winnecott(4,3,6,10), emphasized the interplay of surroundings and society in the emotional development of the individual. The society within which a child grows up is accorded much greater significance by Erikson(1,2) than is usually the case in psychoanalytical theory. Skinner, who is a leading exponent of the theories of the psychology of learning, holds that it is of decisive importance for human development how well an individual is both guided and influenced by his surroundings(9). Here, development is seen simply as a series of behavioral changes. Irrespective of the extent to which heredity or environment are emphasized, the child's development is seen as a whole. This implies that one must take into consideration the child's innate qualities, its closest relationships (the family), together with all the associated socioeconomic and cultural circumstances. In the following, development will be described principally on a basis of the Erikson model(1,2).

Erikson, like Freud, holds that it is man's instinctive drives and their socialisation in interaction with his surroundings, family and society that are the motive forces in development. Erikson's theory is termed epigenetical, as a child's development follows a predetermined plan where different parts of the personality come into focus at different times during the developmental process. The emotional development of the personality goes through a series of eight consecutive phases, each involving development of fundamental personality traits. These have come to be called the eight ages, as they encompass the whole span of human development from birth to death. Erikson, like Freud, connects human personality development with physical development, assuming that certain bodily organs are differently "charged" with instinctive psychic energy at different ages. At each phase it becomes the task of both the child and its surroundings to create the specific patterns of behavior required for that phase. How well this succeeds is reflected in the continued development. The problem of achieving the behavioral pattern specific to each phase constitutes a crisis. The solution of that crisis in a positive

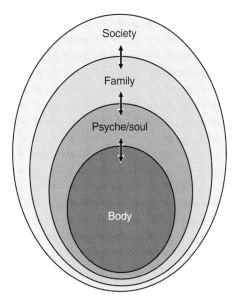

Fig. 3-2.

direction creates an invaluable basis for continued development, while a negative solution can imply problems for that continuation. The specific crisis should, within each phase, result in a fundamental, more or less balanced and favourable, adjustment of the being to self and surroundings. Thus, the being gradually develops both socially and in identity. It is generally held that no phase can be omitted without resulting in an unsuccessful solution of the crisis, with the child stuck, returning to an earlier phase, or eventually arriving at the next phase too quickly, accompanied by unsolved problems. The following describes the first five phases from birth to adulthood (Fig. 3-3).

ORAL PHASE, INFANCY: 0-1.5 YEARS

Basic trust *versus* basic mistrust

During infancy the mouth is the most important organ of the body and it becomes the organ of contact through which an in-

	Psychosexual stages	Psychosocial crises	Developmental characteristics **Significant relations**
I	Oral phase, infancy	Basic trust, *versus* basic mistrust	Attachment Sensomotoric intelligence Primitive causal connection Motor functions Continuity of existence **Parents**
II	Anal phase, early childhood	Autonomy *versus* shame and doubt	Language development Self-control Motor functions Play and imagination **Parents**
III	Oedipal phase, late childhood	Initiative *versus* guilt feelings	Creativity Self-awareness Moral development Problem solving/activity Gender identification Playing in groups **Parents/peers**
IV	Latency phase, early school-age	Industry *versus* inferiority	Practical/problem solving Learning skills Learning knowledge Working together Self-evaluation **Family of origin/school, peers, others**

Fig. 3-3. Psychosocial development according to the Erikson model(1,2).

fant obtains life-giving air and food, while at the same time being the organ with which it makes contact with its surroundings. The mouth, eyes, ears, nose and all sensation are important for the infant's interaction with its environment. During this early interaction the environment (the mother) is the donor while the child is the recipient. The child explores the body and surroundings via its mouth, skin and rhythm, while the parents convey a concept of the body and its surroundings, as well as feelings of basic security and trust.

At first, a child experiences no boundary between self and mother, on the contrary it feels fused with her, we call this symbiosis. Only after reaching 6-7 months old does a child begin to discover a boundary between self and environment, and the first person to develop form is usually its mother. A positive development during the first 6 months of life leads to the child learning to receive and retain that which it is given, while its mother feels herself a person who can give. Feelings of self-confidence and confidence towards the environment and existence are the beginning of the ability to make contact. Negative development can mean that a

Psychosexual stages	Psychosocial crises	Developmental characteristics **Significant relations**
V Genital phase, teens	Identity *versus* identity diffusion	Self image/identity Abilities/possibilities Formal operational thought Group activity/identity Gender activity/identity Gender role/relations with opposite sex Physical maturity **Family of origin/peer group**
VI Young adulthood	Intimacy *versus* isolation	Married life Relations to children Working relations Relation to values of life **Own family/colleagues/friends**
VII Adulthood	Generative *versus* self absorbation	Family structure/function Child rearing Working situation Involvement in society **Own family/colleagues/groups of interests**
VIII Maturity age	Integrity *versus* dispair	Reflection Winding up **Own family**

child shows resignation, becomes slack and indifferent; it will suck and sleep inadequately. Other patterns of negative development can be: children who reject; who refuse to suck/eat; who throw up; who ward off contact; who scream and are inconsolable. Consequences can be fundamental insecurity and distrust, including difficulties in developing the ability to make contact.

During later infancy (6-18 months) a child learns to chew and bite even though it may still prefer to suck. The ability to grip, with other motor functions and increased mental activity now develop, providing more of the qualifications necessary for interaction and activity. The child is now able to distinguish between itself and its surroundings and can retain what it receives in the form of feeling, contact and impressions.

Parents observe it can successfully manage longer periods without intensive contact, and its mother can distance herself for short periods which can gradually lengthen, the child begins to tolerate dissatisfaction and separation, while being trained in what Mahler(8) calls the individuation-separation phase. Positive interaction brings with it a deepened sense of security and trust, combined with the child's learning to receive and retain and to help itself towards the beginning of purpose of mind. Later in life, this appears as a capacity to form emotionally deep and lasting bonds. Negative interaction between the child and its surroundings can result in behavioral disturbances principally of two sorts: a child who clings and whines, refuses to accept what it is offered, or one which may become exaggeratedly demanding, urgently in need of feelings and attention, while constantly seizing and grabbing. The inner feeling is one of not getting enough and from this follows difficulty in entering and retaining lasting relationships later in life.

Children with disturbances from this phase, who experience feelings of mistrust, need very careful introduction to dental treatment, and it is advisable always to use the same confident, experienced practitioner. Such easy solutions as manipulation of the child's treatment resistance are not advisable.

The need to suck

Sucking is important for an infant's physical survival and its psychological development. Accordingly, as it grows, the need to suck diminishes both physically and psychologically, as it can eat more and more solid food, bite and chew. Through weaning from breastfeeding the child learns to leave the earlier phase and continues its process of maturation without feeling deserted or deprived of anything. The physiological need to suck ceases at 9-12 months old. The psychological need remains for a time, for example when the child is unhappy, tired or about to fall asleep, when it regresses then to an earlier level of development. A more prolonged need to suck may sometimes continue even beyond the age of 3 years, carrying with it problems of both bite and speech development. A "dummy" or "pacifier" may often function as a "social plug", hindering the seeking of contact with peers and adults. Grounds for this may be many. It can be learned behavior, but most believe that it derives from an early or still unsatisfied need to suck/a need for consolation for insufficient security. The dummy and sucking habits should be gradually replaced by other forms of contact, age-adequate activities, and stimulation.

ANAL PHASE, EARLY CHILDHOOD: 1.5-3 YEARS

Autonomy *versus* shame and doubt

This period derives its name from the Latin for rectal opening (anus) and by this time a child has normally achieved bladder and bowel control. The period could also be termed "the autonomy-period", i.e. when a child explores, experiences, and develops its physical functions, control over its own body and how to influence its surroundings. Parents convey whether a child should feel its body as good or bad, whether it is good or naughty, whether or not aggression and messiness are allowed, and whether or not the child's will is important.

The child has now developed a clearer self-image, a "me", that has begun to experience its own will, and this is why the period is often called "the defiant age". Stubborness, strong and contradictory feelings are typical of this age. The interplay between child and surroundings dictates how much it is able to do and to decide for itself. The pattern of behavior often shifts between "retaining", shown in frequently repeated activities, favorite toys, dishes, rituals and habits and; "letting go", demonstrated by constant change of activities, impatience and a tendency to throw away. Often the child will want different things at the same moment: an ambivalence that reflects difficulty in making up its mind.

A positive interaction between child and surroundings makes it possible eventually to find a balance in its patterns of behavior, activities, interests and feelings. The child gains confidence through knowing what it wants and the ability to be independent, to become someone who can/will something and be respected for that. Negative interaction can result in a compulsive repitition of the behavior pattern, constant exchange of one activity for another, and often suffering from feelings of ambivalence. Its fundamental attitude may be typified by shyness and doubt in its own ability, becoming submissive to external demands and wishes or, conversely, by expressing constant self-assertion and obstinacy.

Reaching treatment maturity

The end of the anal phase normally means a child has reached what is termed treatment-maturity, with the ability to sit still, and a patience span of approximately 10-20 minutes. It can now understand simple instructions and explanations according to the principle: tell, show and do. By now, it can do two things at once, such as sitting still and opening its mouth. It can also put a toothbrush into its mouth and pretend with it, but cannot yet perform correct tooth-brushing movements. It is important now to praise the child's abilities, at the same time not forgetting that physical contact and non-verbal communication are still very important.

OEDIPAL PHASE, LATE CHILDHOOD: 3-5 YEARS

Initiative *versus* guilt

While this phase of development derives its name from the Greek myth of King Oedipus it is usually called the early genital phase. At this time an interest in the genitals, sexuality and gender has become central. Children begin to ask questions about how they were concieved, and why girls and boys have a different appearance. They explore the significance of male and female, and experience in their families that it is

acceptable to be respectively boys or girls. Parents convey ideas of masculinity and femininity, of appraisal and appreciation of the child as person. It begins to understand that it cannot be a child forever, which may seem both painful and exciting. To ascertain its identity as boy or girl, the child will seek suitable people to imitate and identify with. Usually, the parent of the same gender becomes the object of identification. At the same time the child usually goes through a period of delight, falling in love with adults of the opposite gender, particularly the mother or father. The boy wants to be close to his mother, to convince her of his strength and his excellence, while the girl plays the coquette, displaying her excellence for her father. The parent of the same gender may be felt to be rival for the favour of the opposite parent. This induces conflict because the child also needs the rival as an object of identification, this is generally termed the Oedipus conflict. The positive solution is for the child to give up the conquest of the opposite gender parent and to identify instead with the same gender parent. Development of the superego or conscience gathers speed and is believed to result from this Oedipal conflict. In respectively striving for the favour of, and to identify with, each of the parents, the child assumes their values, morals and ways of life. Conscience may be a stern master and deviation may occasion guilt feelings. Curiosity inventiveness, a desire to explore and to play roles are typical of this age. Nevertheless, a child still needs defined boundaries and guidance. Too many prohibitions or warnings and, above all, burdening with guilt feelings, can turn curiosity and activity into passiveness. Positive interaction during this period provides a foundation for basic feelings of gender identity and initiative. Negative interaction can induce feelings of guilt, of not being good enough as a person, or as a man/ woman. Guilt feelings lead to lack of initiative and lack of creativity, and the child's gender identity may become uncertain.

A child should now be able to sit by itself and concentrate for up to half an hour. It is important to praise its appearance and gender. Correction should have a positive conotation, although it is still important to follow earlier principles, the child is now also able to use its imagination and to understand metaphor.

LATENCY PHASE, EARLY SCHOOL AGE: 5-12 YEARS

Industry *versus* inferiority

During the latency phase no bodily organ predominates and the child's inner life is believed to undergo no revolutionary changes, on the contrary, the main focus of this phase is the child in its social context. It is less egocentric and is increasingly interested in its role and a place in its social surroundings. School, peers, recreational activities and adults outside the home become increasingly important, with the child exploring the extra-familial world finding out what is to be learned, how to cope with peers and comparison with others. Parents and school mediate knowledge and exercise control, showing the child how it compares with others, and training the child to deal with adversity, while at the same time providing it with opportunities to succeed in what it tries to do. Frequently, the child is eager for knowledge, enjoys making conversation, begins conducting abstract discussions, enjoys collecting and categorizing, playing games and competing, and begins to borrow its own codes and rules from the adult world. While for many children this brings an increasing self-esteem, awareness and thirst for activity, for others, lacking knowledge and social competence, this period can produce feelings of inferiority.

Motoric skills are gradually maturing and the child is developing a more realistic view of society, and thus of dental treatment. This is the age when you can begin partnerships and make therapeutical contracts with a child. It wants explanations and has a growing ability for abstract thought; it often wants to be re-assured by hearing it is one of many children of the same age attending the clinic, and is capable of understanding generalizations.

GENITAL PHASE, ADOLESCENCE: 13 -19 YEARS

Identity *versus* identity diffusion

The genital phase and puberty are the onset of sexual maturity. Finite changes, both physical and psychological, occur in young people's lives. Childhood is left behind and the adult world approaches. During the teens, partially unsolved crises from earlier phases and the search for identity coupled with emanicipation from parents and home, frequently create enormous trials for both teenagers and parents.

The main function of this phase may be said to be the achievement of an inner identity (self-awareness, self-esteem) in interaction with the surroundings.

Such acquisitions from earlier phases as trust, autonomy, initiative and gender identity, for example, are "shaken up" and integrated with new experiences as part of a search for identity, the meaning of life and the future. Involved in this search, teenagers are frequently self-absorbed and uninterested in their surroundings, do not listen when spoken to, are dreamy and forgetful. Interest in personal appearance and clothes becomes important for both sexes. This interest is not solely focused on self, but embraces peers, parents, teachers, idols, ideologies, politics and religion. Just as teenagers oscillate between their inner and outer worlds, it is also typical for them to swing between the desire to be grown up and independent, with all the entailed privileges, and the desire to be little, dependent, and protected.

In face of their physical development and growing-up, young people experience fear, loneliness and emptiness. At the same time, there is a longing for freedom, to be taken seriously and to try out new values. Parents should show confidence in their children's ability to grow-up, and while still providing boundaries, must also be tolerant of their searching and aggressiveness. Young people often form groups with common interests and lifestyles. This provides the opportunity of measuring the group's ideals and interests against their own, and with the group as base they can test their parents' values and those of the adult world. For parents and teachers this self-assertion can be very trying.

During the teens emotional relationships develop from a platonic distant dreaming, through shorter, frequently changing, affairs to more adult and established pairing. Positive interaction will provide the opportunity to intergrate and modify the contributions from earlier phases with the developing teenage instincts, cognitive development and ideals, to form a stable inner identity. Negative interaction can result from negative reactions in this phase, but may also stem from inadequate solutions from earlier phases, or both. Consequences may be partial or total identity diffusion; a failure of the search for continuity in relationship with self and/or existence as a whole. Such "acting-out" behavior as asociality and substance abuse can be a manifestation that even the role of deviant may provide a means of filling identity void. Other young people loose themselves in brooding, isolating themselves in introverted inaccessibility that can, in extreme cases, lead to psychoses or deep depression.

Literature cited

1. Erikson EH. *Childhood and society*. New York: WW Norton, 1950.

2. Erikson EH. *Identity, youth & crisis*. London: Faber & Faber, 1959.

3. Freud A. *Normality and pathology in childhood*. London: Hogarth Press, 1966.

4. Freud S. *The ego and the id*. Standard Edition 19, London: Hogarth Press, 1966.

5. Gesell A, Amatruda CS. *Developmental diagnosis*. New York: Harper & Row, 1964.

6. Mahler MS. On the first three subphases of the separation-individuation process. *Int J Psychol Anal* 1972; **53**: 33.

7. Piaget J. *The psychology of intelligence*. London: Routledge & Kegan, 1950.

8. Segal H. *Introduction to the work of Melanie Klein*. London: Hogarth Press, 1966.

9. Skinner BF. *Science and human behavior*. New York: Macmillan, 1953.

10. Winnicott DW. *The child and the family*. London: Tavistock Publications, 1957.

CHAPTER 4

NORMAL DENTAL AND OCCLUSAL DEVELOPMENT

Tooth development
Tooth eruption
The chronology of tooth development and eruption
Occlusal development

TOOTH DEVELOPMENT

Morphogenesis

Tooth development starts from the dental lamina which is an epithelial thickening, appearing at the sites of the future dental arches. The positions of primary teeth are determined between the 6th and 8th week of embryonic development, as the dental lamina proliferates at specific locations, and buds into the underlying mesenchymal tissue. The epithelium induces condensation of the neural crest-derived mesenchymal cells, and these are thereby determined to an odontogenic lineage (Fig. 4-1A). During subsequent morphogenesis, the epithelium develops into a cap-like enamel organ (Fig. 4-1B), and the odontogenic mesenchyme is divided into two cell lineages. The dental papilla cells, which become surrounded by the epithelium, are the progenitors of odontoblasts and pulpal tissue, whereas the dental sac (follicle) cells which

surround the tooth germ, give rise to periodontal tissues. During the bell stage (Fig. 4-1C, D) the form of the tooth crown is determined, and the dentino-enamel junction is formed, as the *odontoblasts* and *ameloblasts* differentiate and start the secretion of dentin and enamel matrices, respectively.

The permanent teeth are initiated between the 20th week of prenatal and the 10th month of postnatal development and they arise from the dental lamina, lingual to the primary tooth germ (Fig. 4-1C, D). The growth of the jaws allows backward extension of the dental lamina distal to the primary molars, with subsequent initiation of the permanent first, second and third molars.

The number and shape of teeth are subject to strong genetic regulation. The epithelial dental lamina possesses all information that is needed for tooth formation. Via tissue interaction this information is shifted to the mesenchymal cells, which condense around the epithelial bud. The differentiation of odontoblasts is induced by the

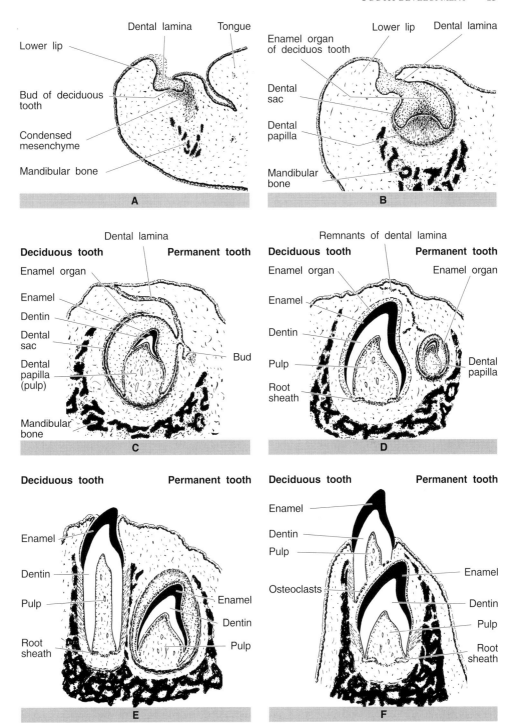

Fig. 4-1. Development and eruption of a lower primary incisor and its replacement by the permanent successor. Redrawn from(4).

enamel epithelium and the differentation of ameloblasts is controlled by the predentin matrix deposited by the odontoblasts. Disturbances in inductive interactions during the very early morphogenetic events may lead to numeric or morphological aberrations.

Deposition and structure of dentin and enamel

The organic matrix of dentin is deposited by the odontoblasts and starts at the sites of future cusps, thereafter, it spreads down the cuspal slopes. With advancing dentin deposition, the odontoblasts move towards the center of the dental papilla and eventually remain lining the dental pulp. The tubular character of dentin is established as the odontoblasts leave behind a cytoplasmatic process.

Ameloblasts differentiate from the enamel epithelium only after the first layer of predentin has been deposited. The dentinoenamel junction is established when the ameloblasts start the secretion of the organic matrix of enamel, the only hard tissue in the body that is formed by epithelial cells, thus differing in many aspects from other hard tissues. Enamel is composed of cylindrical rods (also called prisms), and each ameloblast is responsible for production of one enamel rod. Rodless enamel is, however, found at certain sites, e.g. at the outermost surface of primary teeth. The organic matrix of enamel consists mainly of two types of proteins, the amelogenins and enamelins. Inherited defects of enamel structure may involve mutations in the genes coding for enamel proteins (Chapter 15).

Enamel formation can be divided into three stages. During the formative stage the ameloblasts secrete the organic matrix of the enamel, about 30% of which mineralizes almost instantly. During the maturation stage, after the entire thickness of enamel

has been reached, the mineral crystals grow, and water and proteins are removed. The ameloblasts have an important function in the selective removal of components from the matrix. After enamel maturation, the enamel still remains porous and the ameloblasts form a protective layer on the enamel surface. The third stage of enamel formation is completed after eruption, when the addition of still more mineral results in reduction of the porosity.

Incremental lines are visible in histological sections of both dentin and enamel (Fig. 4-2). In enamel the lines are called the striae of Retzius, and they are prominent in most permanent teeth. In prenatal enamel they are rare. At the surface of enamel, the striae of Retzius are seen as *surface perikymata*, which run in horizontal planes across the crown (Fig. 4-2). The neonatal line is an enlarged stria of Retzius. As ameloblasts are particularly sensitive to environmental changes, disturbed enamel production may result from systemic disturbances, and is often seen as accentuated striae and perikymata (Chapter 15).

Root formation

Root formation starts when dentin and enamel deposition have reached the junction of the inner and outer enamel epithelia. By proliferation these epithelia form Hertwig's epithelial root sheath, which becomes located between the dental papilla and the dental follicle. The root sheath epithelium initiates the differentiation of odontoblasts, which subsequently deposit the dentin of the root. The apical end of the root sheath continues to proliferate and determines the shape and the length of the root.

The dental follicle gives rise to the cells and the fiber bundles of the periodontal ligament, and probably also to alveolar bone. In addition, those dental follicle cells, which come in contact with the root surface, differentiate into cementoblasts which se-

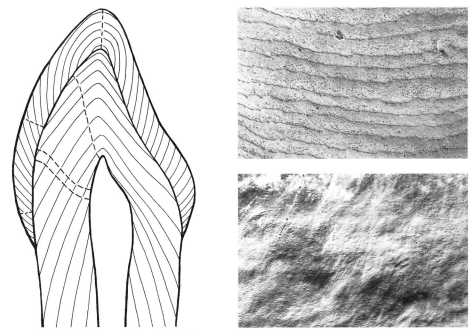

Fig. 4-2 *Left*. Schematic representation of incremental lines in dentin and enamel. The dotted lines represent the direction of dentin tubules and enamel rods. *Right top.* Scanning electron micrograph (SEM) of enamel of a premolar tooth illustrating perikymata lines. *Right bottom*. Similar SEM of enamel surface of a deciduous canine. Note absence of perikymata lines. From(8).

crete the organic matrix of cementum. Some recent evidence suggests that the first cementum layer, the "intermediate cementum", is an enamel-like material which is laid down by the epithelial root sheath cells. This material may have an important function in differentiation of cementoblasts from the dental follicle cells, as well as in anchoring cementum to root dentin. Cementum covers the root as a 50-200μ thick layer, and its main function is to attach the fibers of the periodontal ligament to the root.

Posteruptive maturation of teeth

Just after eruption the tooth will in several aspects be in an "immature condition" and maturation processes will proceed for several years:

– the enamel is fully formed at eruption, but its surface is still porous and inadequately mineralized. A "secondary" mineralization with ions from the oral milieu will penetrate into the hydroxyapatite lattice and make the enamel more "perfect" and resistant to caries.

– formation of dentin will proceed for the rest of life. At eruption the dentin is thin and the dentin tubuli are wide. Dentin formation will occur on pulpal walls, as well as on the walls of tubuli, making it thicker and less penetrable, thus, increasing the resistance of dentin to caries progress.

– at the time of eruption the cementum is still thin and the periodontal ligament consists of relatively few and unorganized fibres. After eruption the production of cementum continues and the

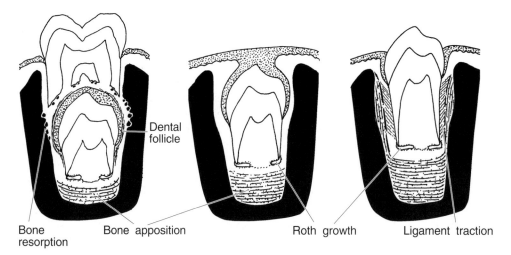

Bone resorption   Bone apposition   Roth growth   Ligament traction

Dental follicle

Fig. 4-3. Schematic presentation of histologic changes which accompany tooth eruption. The "eruptive force" has been suggested to be created either by localized bone remodelling (regulated by the dental follicle), by root growth, by periodontal ligament traction, or by vascular and tissue pressure.

fibres increase in amount, reorganize and link the tooth to the alveolar bone.

– at eruption the apical part of the root is incomplete. To obtain full root length and closure/narrowing of the apical foramen takes several years. The latter process is partly caused by formation of dentin, partly by formation of cementum.

All these posteruptive maturation processes are highly significant in cariology, periodontology and traumatology.

Anatomy of primary teeth

Primary teeth are, generally, smaller than the permanent teeth. The crowns are lower and more rounded. The cervical part of the crown is bulky with a marked cemento-enamel junction. The colour of the primary teeth is bluish-white. The pulp chambers and canals occupy a comparatively large portion of the primary teeth. The primary dentition is characterized by anatomical stability in number as well as in morphology.

For details of anatomical features see Appendix.

TOOTH ERUPTION

Eruption designates the movement of the developing tooth in axial direction from its original location in the jaw bone to its functional position in the oral cavity. Before the tooth breaks through the oral mucosa into the mouth, it has to escape its bony crypt by bone resorption occlusal to the crown, and bone deposition apical to the developing roots. Thereafter, the connective tissue between the reduced enamel epithelium covering the crown and the overlying oral epithelium is lost, and the two epithelia unite. The emergence of the tooth occurs without hemorrhage through the formed epithelial canal. The dentogingival junction is formed by the fused oral and dental epithelia (Fig. 4-3). The eruption of a tooth continues until it meets the teeth in the opposing jaw. It should be noted that the growth of the alveolar bone in the maxilla and mandible involves vertical and mesial drift of the teeth, also after they have reached their functional positions in the jaws.

The mechanism of tooth eruption

The exact mechanism of tooth eruption is still obscure. Tooth eruption is accompanied by multiple tissue changes, such as development of the root and periodontium, and resorption and apposition of the alveolar bone.

The following four causes have been most frequently suggested for tooth eruption:

– root growth

– vascular or tissue pressure

– bone remodelling

– periodontal ligament traction

Of these, the third and fourth possibilities have received most attention recently. Although lengthening of the roots accompanies eruption, root growth does not appear to be a major cause of eruption. Teeth without roots, and teeth with completed roots, may also erupt. Blood pressure and pressure from interstitial tissue fluids may contribute to the eruptive movement, but their significance for eruption is questionable.

Selective alveolar bone remodelling appears to play an important role, at least during the early stages of eruption. This coordinated bone remodelling, regulated by the dental follicle, appears to propel the tooth in an axial direction. According to this theory, no real "eruptive force" is needed, since tooth eruption would result from bone growth and be an example of how bone remodelling directs craniofacial growth.

There is, however, evidence that the cells and fibers in the periodontal ligament exert real pulling forces on erupting teeth. Both fibroblasts and the fibers in the ligament appear to be able to contract, and the directions of their arrangement during tooth development support a function in eruption.

In conclusion, it is likely that tooth eruption is a combination of several factors. It is conceivable that the selective bone resorption and apposition, brought about by the activity in the dental follicle, are important regulators of the early stages of tooth eruption. The traction by periodontal ligament cells and fibres, and possibly also vascular pressure, may be involved in the axial movement of the tooth after its emergence, and perhaps also in reactivated eruption later in life.

Shedding of primary teeth

Prior to eruption of permanent teeth, the roots of the primary teeth are resorbed, and their crowns shed. The pressure created by the erupting permanent tooth is generally believed to play an important role in primary tooth resorption. Dentinoclasts appear on the apical surface of the roots of primary teeth probably by a similar mechanism as when pressure stimulates the formation and activity of osteoclasts e.g. during orthodontic tooth movement. Also, when a permanent tooth is missing, the primary predecessor usually undergoes root resorption.

THE CHRONOLOGY OF DENTAL DEVELOPMENT AND ERUPTION

Data on the chronology of tooth development and eruption is usually given as mean values from series of observations, often from populations which in many aspects differ from ours. Therefore, it should be born in mind when deviations from

TABLE 4-1

Initiation of mineralization of primary teeth (mean ages)

Central incisors	14 weeks *in utero*
First molars	15½ weeks *in utero*
Lateral incisors	16 weeks *in utero*
Canines	17 weeks *in utero*
Second molars	18 weeks *in utero*

"norms" are judged, that deviations may arise because of such differences. Furthermore, the normal range *within* a given population may be large.

The pre-eruptive stages of the primary and permanent dentition

The mean ages for the onset of mineralization of the primary teeth are given in Table 4-1. The mineralization starts at the incisal edge/occlusal surface and progresses towards the apex. The formation of the primary dentition takes about 4 years (Fig.4-4). The crowns are mineralized about halfway at birth and become fully formed during the first year of life. Root formation is completed between the ages of 1.5 and 3 years.

Mineralization of the permanent teeth starts at birth with the cusps of the first molars (Fig. 4-5). The incisors and canines start their mineralization during the first year of life; the premolars and second molars between the 2nd and 3rd year of life; and the third molar between the 8th and 11th year of life. However, the normal range is wide. Thus, the second lower premolar may first appear on radiographs as late as 8-9 years of age. The crowns of the permanent teeth (except third molars) are generally completed between 5-7 years of age. Root development alone takes 6-7 years.

TABLE 4-2

Eruption of primary teeth. Mean age and standard deviation in months. Data from(7).

	Boys		Girls	
	$\overline{x}$	S.D.	$\overline{x}$	S.D.
Upper jaw				
1	10.01	1.67	10.47	1.82
2	11.20	2.25	11.55	2.34
3	19.30	3.04	19.18	2.86
4	16.08	2.45	15.93	1.91
5	28.89	4.12	29.35	3.55
Lower jaw				
1	7.88	1.86	8.20	2.25
2	13.23	2.84	13.11	3.20
3	19.92	3.33	19.47	3.03
4	16.39	2.25	16.12	2.08
5	27.14	3.92	27.07	2.94

Normally, the apex closes 3-4 years after eruption. The velocity of tooth formation is highest for the central incisors, lowest for canines and second molars. In general, the mandibular teeth develop earlier than the maxillary teeth. A marked sex-difference has been observed in tooth formation, girls being on average half a year ahead of boys.

The eruptive stage of the primary dentition

This stage spans, on average, from the 8th to the 30th month of life (Table 4-2). There is no distinct difference between the sexes, and the normal range is relatively small (SD = 1.5-4 months). The central incisors erupt first, followed by the lateral incisors, the first molars, the canines and the second

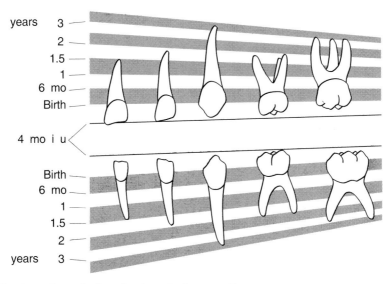

Fig. 4-4. The chronology of mineralization of primary teeth.

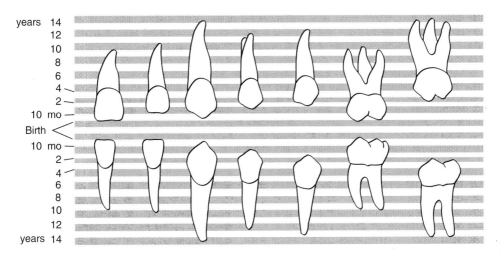

Fig. 4-5. The chronology of mineralization of permanent teeth.

molars. There appears to be little connection between the normal eruption time of primary teeth and factors such as skeletal maturity, body height or psychomotor maturity of the child. However, a genetic influence has been shown in reports on familial trends towards early and late eruption. Also severely retarded eruption or impaction has been reported as inherited traits (Chapter 15).

The functional stage of the primary dentition

From the time of eruption of the second primary molar at about 2.5 years of age to the shedding of the first lower incisors at about 6 years of age, the child's dentition may seem quiet, however, great activity is going on in the jaws:

TABLE 4-3

Eruption of permanent teeth. Mean age
and standard deviation in years. Data for
1, 2 and 6 from(7); for 3, 4, 5 and 7 from(5)

| | Boys | | Girls | |
	$\bar{x}$	S.D.	$\bar{x}$	S.D.
Upper jaw				
1	7.3	0.5	7.1	0.5
2	8.4	0.6	8.0	0.5
3	11.7	1.4	11.0	1.4
4	10.4	1.5	10.0	1.5
5	11.2	1.6	10.9	1.6
6	6.7	0.5	6.5	0.4
7	12.7	1.4	12.3	1.4
Lower jaw				
1	6.4	0.4	6.2	0.3
2	7.6	0.6	7.1	0.6
3	10.8	1.3	9.9	1.3
4	10.8	1.5	10.2	1.5
5	11.5	1.7	10.9	1.7
6	6.6	0.5	6.4	0.4
7	12.1	1.4	11.7	1.4

– root formation of primary teeth is completed

– root resorption of primary teeth is going
  on

– crown formation of most permanent
  teeth and also root formation of several
  permanent teeth are in progress.

The jaws are still small and to accomodate
the roots of the primary teeth and the developing crowns of the permanent teeth,
roots and crowns are densely packed (Fig.
4-6). The permanent incisors are situated
lingually to the roots of the primary incisors
with the labial surfaces of their crowns in
close approximation to the apices. Thus, the
forming permanent incisors are very vulnerable to trauma or apical infection of the
primary incisors. The permanent canines
are also developing lingually to the roots
of their primary predecessors, but above/
below their apices. The premolars are situated between the roots of the primary molars, thus vulnerable to bifurcal infections in
carious primary molars (Turner teeth). The
permanent molars are developing distally
to the second primary molars.

The relationship between the roots of the
primary dentition and the crowns of the
permanent dentition is not fixed during the
functional stage of the primary dentition.
Because of the vertical growth of the alveolar process, the primary teeth may move
away from the developing permanent teeth.
However, later on the eruptive movement
of the permanent teeth will again catch up
with the primary teeth.

The eruptive stage of the permanent dentition

This stage spans, on average, from the age
of 6 to 12 years (third molars excepted). The
eruption times are given in Table 4-3. Tooth
eruption begins upon the completion of
crown formation and/or the beginning of
rooth formation. The resorption and shedding of the preceding primary teeth are
integrated processes in the eruption of permanent teeth. The resorption and shedding
of the primary teeth take from 1.5 - 2 years
(incisors) to 2.5 - 6 years (canines and molars).

The average period between shedding of
a primary tooth and the emergence of its
permanent successor is between 0 days and
4-5 months. The toothless period is shortest
(0-6 days) after shedding of primary molars.
The toothless period in the mandible is, on
average, 2 weeks for the central incisor and

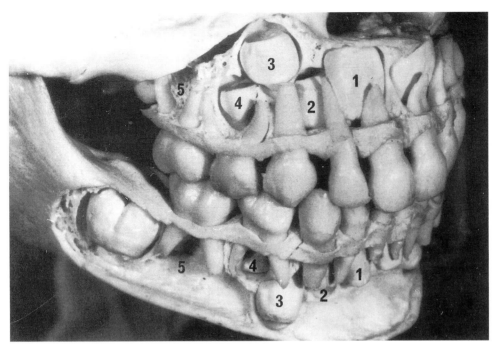

Fig. 4-6. Relations between the roots of primary teeth and the developing crowns of the permanent teeth during the functional stage of the primary dentition. The permanent crowns of the incisors [1,2] are positioned lingual to the roots of the primary incisors. The permanent canines [3] are positioned above/below the roots of their predecessors, and the premolars [4,5] are located between the roots of the primary molars. After(10).

6 weeks for the lateral incisor and canine. In the maxilla the corresponding periods are 6 weeks for the central incisor and over 4 months for the lateral incisor and the canine. In cases with crowding the length of the toothless period for the maxillary lateral incisor and the canine may exceed one year.

In general, the age at eruption of permanent teeth is more variable than that observed for the primary teeth. The variation is lowest for the first teeth to erupt (SD = about 0.5 year for incisors and first molars) and highest for the last teeth to erupt (SD = about 1.5 years for canines, premolars and second molars). There are some sex differences in the age at eruption of permanent teeth, girls being somewhat ahead of boys (Table 4-3). The sex difference is most pronounced for the canines, where the mean

difference is about 3/4 year. Racial differences in tooth eruption have also been documented. The teeth of the Caucasians erupt at a later age than the teeth of most other races. During this century there has been a tendency towards earlier eruption of permanent teeth in the developed countries ("secular trend"). This has mainly been attributed to the earlier onset of puberty, and indirectly to better child health and nutrition. In the individual child other general, as well as local, factors are also known to influence tooth eruption (Chapter 15).

The first tooth to erupt is the lower central incisor at an age of about 6.5 years. The last to erupt (third molars excepted) is the upper 2nd molar. The eruption is normally linked to the development of the second half of the root, but the eruption path of the

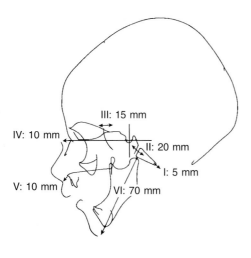

Fig. 4-7. Average incremental growth (mm) of the cranial base and the jaws from birth to adult age in males.
I: anterior margin of foramen magnum.
II: spheno-occipital synchondrosis. III: spheno-frontal suture. IV: glabella. V: maxillary sutural displacement. VI: mandibular growth.

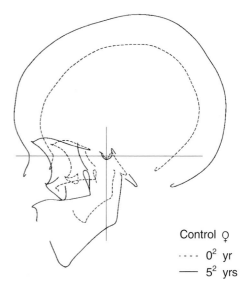

Control ♀
---- 0² yr
—— 5² yrs

Fig. 4-8. Facial growth in a normal girl from 2 months of age to 5 years and 2 months of age. Superimposition was made on the nasion-sella-line registered at sella. Note the magnitude of mandibular growth.

tooth is much longer than the increase in root length. Thus, the upper canine has to move from its initial position below the orbit and also has to catch up the vertical growth of the alveolar process. At the time of eruption 3/4 of the root is generally formed. Thereafter, 1.5-3 years are needed to complete rooth length, and even longer to close the root apices to the mature size.

Estimation of dental age

Observations on dental development may be helpful in evaluation of general growth disturbances, and also in children with unknown chronological age, e.g. adopted children from foreign countries. Other parameters used are body height, skeletal maturity, psychomotor skills, mental and social performance. The dental development is considered to be the most reliable. Dental age may be evaluated from the number of erupted teeth, but since several local factors may influence eruption (lack of space, early loss of primary teeth, aplasia etc.), it is recommended that dental age should be assessed from the pre-eruptive tooth formation as judged from orthopantomograms. Various stages of tooth development are given numerical values (scores). The sum of scores is compared to figures from a comparable population. Several such systems have been developed. The best internationally known method is that of Demirjian et al(3). This method has a high accuracy in the lower age groups, when dental age estimation is most needed. The method is presented in the Appendix, together with tables for transformation of scores into dental age, comprising data from a French-Canadian population.

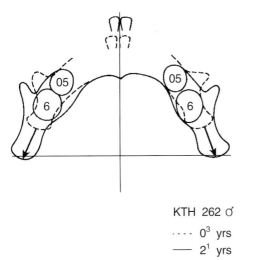

KTH 262 ♂

---- 0^3 yrs

—— 2^1 yrs

Fig. 4-9A. Sagittal and transverse growth of the mandible from 2 months to 22 months of age in a normal child. Tracings from axial cephalometric films have been superimposed on the anlage for the first permanent molars and registered according to the mid-sagittal plane. Note the backward and lateral growth of the ramus and the condyle to adapt to the sagittal and transverse growth of the cranial base.

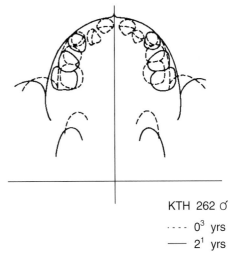

KTH 262 ♂

---- 0^3 yrs

—— 2^1 yrs

Fig. 4-9B. Sagittal and transverse growth of the maxilla in the child illustrated in Fig. 4-9A. Superimposition has been made on the anlage for the permanent incisors with registration according to the mid-sagittal plane. Note the markedly greater transverse growth posteriorly than anteriorly.

OCCLUSAL DEVELOPMENT

Dental occlusion, the interdigitation of maxillary and mandibular teeth is dependent upon developmental processes in three dimensions of the cranial base, the jaws and tooth eruption. The processes are under strong influence of genetic as well as functional factors. For detailed information considering growth of the face and the jaws, readers are referred to textbooks in orthodontics. In the following only the main elements of postnatal development of intermaxillary relations will be dealt with.

The main principles involved in the growth and development of the craniofacial skeleton are *displacement* and *surface remodelling* of bones. In the cranial base the dis-

placement type of growth in the sagittal plane occurs at the spheno-occipital and spheno-petrosal synchondroses and at the spheno-frontal suture. Apposition of bone at glabella and at the anterior border of foramen magnum serves to elongate the external cranial base. The average growth at the various growth sites is indicated in Fig. 4-7. Since the maxilla is attached to the anterior cranial base while the mandible is suspended under the middle cranial fossa, growth of the cranial base is of major importance for the intermaxillary relations and, thus, for the development of the occlusion. With growth in the synchondroses, the sphenoid bone, the frontal bone and the maxillary complex are displaced anteriorly in relation to the glenoid fossae. In addition, the frontal bone and the maxillary complex are displaced forward in relation to the sphenoid bone by growth in the spheno-frontal suture. Finally, the maxilla is displaced downward and forward in relation to the anterior cranial base by growth in the maxillary sutures. The sagittal relation between the jaws is maintained by marked growth of the mandible (Figs. 4-7, 4-8).

Sagittal growth of the anterior cranial fossa stops around 7 years of age, whereas the spheno-occipital synchondrosis continues growing until postpubertal age. In comparison, sutural growth of the maxilla continues until postpubertal age, and condylar growth continues until adult age.

The transverse growth of the cranial base is characterized by lateral displacement of the temporal bones and thereby the glenoid fossae. Only minimal transverse displacement type of growth occurs in the anterior cranial base postnatally. This difference in the transverse development of the anterior and middle cranial base is reflected in the transverse development of the jaws (Fig. 4-9).

For a detailed description of the rotation and remodelling of the jaws during growth readers are referred to the classic paper by Björk and Skieller(2).

Within the framework of this complex facial development the erupting teeth come into interdigitation. The individual variability in growth of the cranial base and the jaws is large and the coordination of development in the various components is not always perfect. This situation is partly controlled by the dento-alveolar compensatory mechanism which serves to coordinate the eruption and position of the teeth securing a normal relationship between the dental arches. The dento-alveolar compensatory mechanism is dependent on normal oral function and normal tooth eruption. Furthermore, the space conditions in the dental arches and the inclined-plane effect of opposing teeth during occlusion and mastication are significant factors. Thus, good interdigitation of the dental arches may serve to maintain normal occlusion in spite of aberrant jaw relationships. The dento-alveolar compensatory mechanism has been discussed in detail(1,2,9).

The dento-alveolar changes from birth to an established permanent dentition and their influence on occlusal development are discussed in the following sections.

Primary dentition

At birth the crowns of the primary teeth have been formed to a great extent, but root development has not yet started. Thus, the gum pads are low and the palatal vault is flat (Fig. 4-10). The gum pads are slightly lobulated indicating the position of the developing teeth. When the jaws are closed there is normally contact only in the posterior region of the gum pads, and the mandible is retruded in relation to the maxilla. During the first year of life, however, the sagittal jaw relationship improves, allowing the canines to erupt in a normal sagittal relation.

Occlusion in the posterior segments is first established around 16 months of age, when the first primary molars attain occlusal contact. The inclined planes of the cusps of the mandibular molar functions as a funnel for the palatal cusp of the upper molar to secure a proper occlusion. Once a good intercuspidation in all three planes is achieved, the jaws are normally closed to the same position each time. The established occlusion has a guiding role on the interrelation between the jaws and thereby for the proper positioning of later erupting teeth (canines and second molars). Further stabilization of the occlusion is created by the large mesiopalatal cusps of the upper second molars.

With the eruption of primary teeth, the alveolar processes develop, and there is a considerable increase in facial height (Fig. 4-11). The growth of the maxillary alveolar

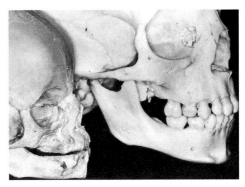

Fig. 4-11. The eruption of primary teeth is accompanied by the development of the alveolar processes with considerable increase in facial height.

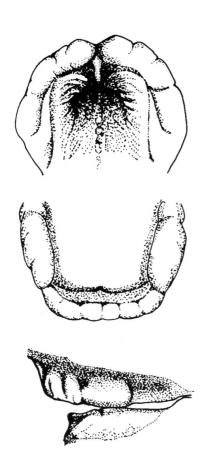

Fig. 4-10. The gum pads at birth. Adapted from(6).

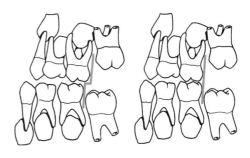

Fig. 4-12. When there is a mesial step in the terminal plane of the primary dentition, the permanent molars may erupt directly into normal occlusion (left). If the primary dental arches end in the same vertical plane, the permanent molars will erupt into a cusp-to-cusp relation.

process also results in an increase in palatal height. The primary teeth erupt almost perpendicular to the jaw bases. The interincisal angle is approaching 180°, and the occlusal plane is flat. During development, the dento-alveolar area generally moves anteriorly in relation to the basal structures of the jaws.

Spacing of teeth is common in the early primary dentition. Especially marked diastemata are often found between the lateral incisors and the canines in the maxilla and the canines and first molars in the mandible. These diastemata are referred to as "primate spaces".

The second primary molars erupt without proximal contact with the first primary molars. However, in most children the molars drift into proximal contact between the third and fourth year of life.

At two years the overjet is on average 4mm, with a range of 2-6 mm. With attrition of the teeth and growth of the mandible the overjet exhibits a steady decrease up to the

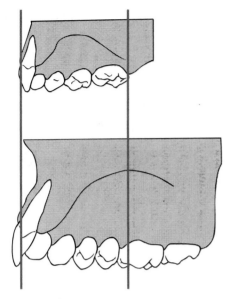

Fig. 4-13. The permanent upper incisors are more labially inclined than their primary predecessors. Consequently, the dental arch becomes wider and longer.

age of five years, where an edge-to-edge incisor relationship is common.

The primary incisors generally erupt into a rather deep overbite if there is no obstacle to hinder them. The individual variation is, however, large. On average, the overbite decreases up to the age of 5-6 years.

As to molar relations the primary dentition may, generally, be divided into two types:

– the primary dental arches end in a mesial step, i.e. the distal surface of the second molar in the mandible is mesial to the corresponding surface in the maxilla (Fig. 4-12 left)

– the dental arches end in the same vertical plan (Fig. 4-12 right)

Both situations are favourable for the later guidance of the first permanent molar into normal occlusion. It should, however, be noted that the occlusion undergoes dynamic changes with jaw growth, with dental attrition and mesial drift of the dental arches on the jaw bases. It would seem that at the time of eruption of the first permanent molar, a mesial step between the dental arches as shown in Fig. 4-12 at left is the most favourable.

Mixed dentition

By the time of eruption of the first permanent molar any initial spaces between the primary molars and canines have generally diminished or disappeared. The first molar erupts in contact with the second primary molar. If the primary dental arches end in a mesial step, the permanent molars may erupt directly into normal occlusion. If the primary dental arches end in the same vertical plane, the first permanent molars will erupt into a cusp-to-cusp relation. This is, however, normally later adjusted as a result of mesial drift of the lower molar in conjunction with the gain in space during eruption of the premolars.

Sufficient space for the permanent molars is created by the sagittal, vertical and transverse growth of the jaws. In the maxilla apposition of bone at the tubers occurs concomitantly with the development and eruption of the molars. In the mandible resorption at the anterior border of the ramus and especially the growth in width accomodate the developing molars. Dental development and tooth eruption are not always strictly coordinated in time with the growth of the jaws. Thus, it is not unusual for the upper molars to erupt into a marked buccal and the lower molars into a marked lingual inclination but the growth of the jaws may later bring the teeth into normal transverse position in the dental arches.

The permanent incisors are mesio-distally wider than their predecessors, with a mean difference of about 7 mm in the upper anterior segment and 5 mm in the lower.

Space is made available for the wider permanent incisors as follows:

– utilizing the natural diastemata in the anterior segments

– the protruded eruption path of the permanent incisors increases the perimeter of the anterior part of the arches (Fig. 4-13). In the sagittal plane the increase may be up to 5 mm. In the transverse plane the increase is less, about 3 mm measured between the canines. In the maxilla the transverse increase is noticeable at the time of eruption of the central incisors. In the mandible increase occurs at the time of eruption of the lateral incisors.

Thus, the space for the permanent incisors is normally sufficient, but there may be a slight temporary lack of space for the lower incisors ("physiological crowding"). The interincisal angle will on average be 135°, the overjet 3.5 mm and the overbite 2.5 mm, however, with large individual variations.

The emergence of the permanent incisors and first molars is followed by a pause in eruption. When the primary molars and canines are shed, there is a gain of space in the dental arches, since the space occupied by the primary canines and molars is greater than that required for the erupting permanent teeth. The mean surplus of space is about 1.5 mm in the maxilla and 2.5 mm in the mandible. The fact that this space ("leeway space") is greater in the mandible than in the maxilla facilitates a greater mesial movement of the lower permanent molar, which serves to normalize a cusp-to-cusp relationship of the permanent first molars. The large upper canines are best adjusted into the dental arch when they erupt concomitantly with the second premolars. The first premolars are then moving slightly distally in the arch.

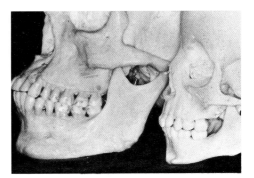

Fig. 4-14. The eruption of the permanent teeth is accompanied by considerable vertical growth of the alveolar processes.

Permanent dentition

Dynamic changes in the occlusion continue in the permanent dentition in conjunction with the growth of the jaws and alveolar processes. On average, the overjet decreases and the dental arches become shorter through mesial drift in the lateral segments. A slight "physiological" crowding will often develop in the mandibular incisor region in the post-pubertal period. This crowding is probably related to the late growth of the mandible, although it has repeatedly been suggested to be linked to the eruption of 3rd molars.

The mean overbite decreases slightly up to the age of 18 years. The alveolar processes increase in height till late adolescent age (Fig. 4-14), more posteriorly than anteriorly in relation to the anterior rotation of the mandible most often observed.

The transverse dimensions of the dental arches tend to remain relatively stable in the permanent dentition.

Even after growth has ceased dynamic changes in the occlusion may be observed compensating for occlusal and proximal wear.

ANATOMY OF THE PRIMARY DENTITION

The upper central incisor is shovel-shaped, like its successor. The palatal tuberculum is marked. The coronal pulp chamber is marked. There is one root canal, as in all primary incisors and canines.

The upper lateral incisor has an anatomy similar to a central-like permanent lateral incisor. The root and crown have a slender form.

The maxillary canine is a stout tooth with one root. The buccal aspect is dominated by a cusp with a marked ridge. The palatal tuberculum is pronounced. The root is long.

The mandibular canine has also a marked cusp, but the crown is thinner. The proximal surfaces are nearly parallel.

The upper first molar is a three-rooted tooth with three or four cusps. Two cusps are buccal. Lingually there is, in most cases, one large cusp. The buccal surface is characterized by a mesio-cervical tuberculum molare. The buccal and lingual surfaces have a marked occlusal convergence. The roots diverge from the crown but bend to form a claw-like configuration. The palatal and distobuccal roots may be partly merged.

The lower first molar has four cusps and two roots and appears narrow due to a marked convergence of the buccal and lingual surfaces. Two cusps are situated buccally and two lingually. The distal cusps are much smaller than the mesial ones. The buccal surface has a marked mesio-cervical tuberculum molare. The two roots, one mesial and one distal, are long, slender and curved.

The upper second molar has a rhomboid crown with four cusps. The occlusal relief is identical to that of the first permanent molar. The three roots are curved, with the greatest circumference exceeding that of the crown. The distobuccal and palatal roots may be partly united.

The lower second molar has five cups, three buccal and two lingual cusps. The long curved roots are similar to those of the first lower molar, but markedly compressed in the mesio-distal direction.

Upper jaw

Lower jaw

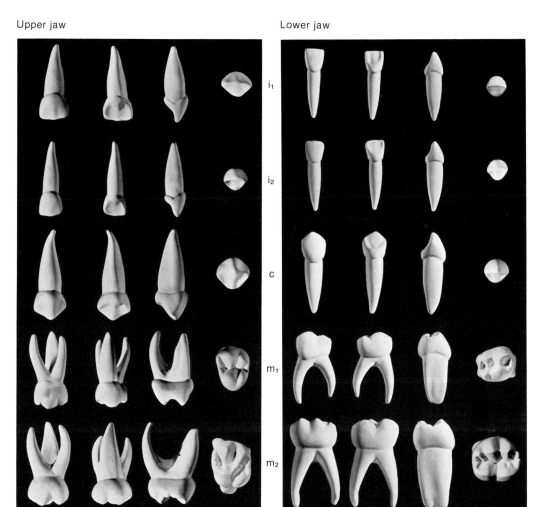

i_1

i_2

c

m_1

m_2

DENTAL AGE ESTIMATION

Tooth formation stages

Stage A Beginning mineralization of separate cusps.

Stage B Fusion of cusps.

Stage C Beginning of dentinal deposits is seen.

Stage D Crown formation completed down to the cemento-enamel junction.

Stage E The root length is less than the crown height.

Stage F The root length is equal to or greater than the crown height.

Stage G The walls of the root canal are parallel, and its apical end is still partially open.

Stage H The apical foramen is completed.

Using the Score System:

1. Pick out the stage for each tooth (1-7) in lower left quadrant.

2. Find the score for the appropriate tooth and sex in Table 4-A1 (e.g. tooth 46 at stage E in a boy gives the score 9.7).

3. The scores of all 7 teeth are added to give the **maturity score**.

4. The maturity score is converted to **dental age** in Table 4-A2. (e.g. score 45 in a boy is equivalent to 6.9 years).

TABLE 4-A1

Self-weighted scores for dental stages (7 teeth)

Boys

Tooth					Stage				
	0	A	B	C	D	E	F	G	H
37	0.0	2.1	3.5	5.9	10.1	12.5	13.2	13.6	15.4
36	-	-	-	0.0	8.0	9.6	12.3	17.0	19.3
35	0.0	1.7	3.1	5.4	9.7	12.0	12.8	13.2	14.4
34	-	-	0.0	3.4	7.0	11.0	12.3	12.7	13.5
33	-	-	-	0.0	3.5	7.9	10.0	11.0	11.9
32	-	-	-	0.0	3.2	5.2	7.8	11.7	13.7
31	-	-	-	-	0.0	1.9	4.1	8.2	11.8

Girls

Tooth					Stage				
	0	A	B	C	D	E	F	G	H
37	0.0	2.7	3.9	6.9	11.1	13.5	14.2	14.5	15.6
36	-	-	-	0.0	4.5	6.2	9.0	14.0	16.2
35	0.0	1.8	3.4	6.5	10.6	12.7	13.5	13.8	14.6
34	-	-	0.0	3.7	7.5	11.8	13.1	13.4	14.1
33	-	-	-	0.0	3.8	7.3	10.3	11.6	12.4
32	-	-	-	0.0	3.2	5.6	8.0	12.2	14.2
31	-	-	-	-	0.0	2.4	5.1	9.3	12.0

NB: Stage 0 is no calcification

TABLE **4-A2**

Conversion of maturity score to dental age (7 teeth)

Age	Score		Age	Score		Age	Score	
	Boys	Girls		Boys	Girls		Boys	Girls
3.0	12.4	13.7	5.0	25.4	28.9	7.0	46.7	51.0
3.1	12.9	14.4	5.1	26.2	29.7	7.1	48.3	52.9
3.2	13.5	15.1	5.2	27.0	30.5	7.2	50.0	55.5
3.3	14.0	15.8	5.3	27.8	31.3	7.3	52.0	57.8
3.4	14.5	16.6	5.4	28.6	32.1	7.4	54.3	61.0
3.5	15.0	17.3	5.5	29.5	33.0	7.5	56.8	65.0
3.6	15.6	18.0	5.6	30.3	34.0	7.6	59.6	68.0
3.7	16.2	18.8	5.7	31.1	35.0	7.7	62.5	71.8
3.8	17.0	19.5	5.8	31.8	36.0	7.8	66.0	75.0
3.9	17.6	20.3	5.9	32.6	37.0	7.9	69.0	77.0
4.0	18.2	21.0	6.0	33.6	38.0	8.0	71.6	78.8
4.1	18.9	21.8	6.1	34.7	39.1	8.1	73.5	80.2
4.2	19.7	22.5	6.2	35.8	40.2	8.2	75.1	81.2
4.3	20.4	23.2	6.3	36.9	41.3	8.3	76.4	82.2
4.4	21.0	24.0	6.4	38.0	42.5	8.4	77.7	83.1
4.5	21.7	24.8	6.5	39.2	43.9	8.5	79.0	84.0
4.6	22.4	25.6	6.6	40.6	45.2	8.6	80.2	84.8
4.7	23.1	26.4	6.7	42.0	46.7	8.7	81.2	85.3
4.8	23.8	27.2	6.8	43.6	48.0	8.8	82.0	86.1
4.9	24.6	28.0	6.9	45.1	49.5	8.9	82.8	86.7

Age	Score		Age	Score		Age	Score	
	Boys	Girls		Boys	Girls		Boys	Girls
9.0	83.6	87.2	11.0	92.0	94.5	13.0	95.6	97.3
9.1	84.3	87.8	11.1	92.2	94.7	13.1	95.7	97.4
9.2	85.0	88.3	11.2	92.5	94.9	13.2	95.8	97.5
9.3	85.6	88.8	11.3	92.7	95.1	13.3	95.9	97.6
9.4	86.2	89.3	11.4	92.9	95.3	13.4	96.0	97.7
9.5	86.7	89.8	11.5	93.1	95.4	13.5	96.1	97.8
9.6	87.2	90.2	11.6	93.3	95.6	13.6	96.2	98.0
9.7	87.7	90.7	11.7	93.5	95.8	13.7	96.3	98.1
9.8	88.2	91.1	11.8	93.7	96.0	13.8	96.4	98.2
9.9	88.6	91.4	11.9	93.9	96.2	13.9	96.5	98.3
10.0	89.0	91.8	12.0	94.0	96.3	14.0	96.6	98.3
10.1	89.3	92.1	12.1	94.2	96.4	14.1	96.7	98.4
10.2	89.7	92.3	12.2	94.4	96.5	14.2	96.8	98.5
10.3	90.0	92.6	12.3	94.5	96.6	14.3	96.9	98.6
10.4	90.3	92.9	12.4	94.6	96.7	14.4	97.0	98.7
10.5	90.6	93.2	12.5	94.8	96.8	14.5	97.1	98.8
10.6	91.0	93.5	12.6	95.0	96.9	14.6	97.2	98.9
10.7	91.3	93.7	12.7	95.1	97.0	14.7	97.3	99.0
10.8	91.6	94.0	12.8	95.2	97.1	14.8	97.4	99.1
10.9	91.8	94.2	12.9	95.4	97.2	14.9	97.5	99.1

Background literature

Björk A. Facial growth in man, studied with the aid of metallic implants. *Acta Odontol Scand* 1955; **13**: 9-34.

Björk A, Skieller V. Growth in width of the maxilla studied by the implant method. *Scand J Plast Reconstr Surg* 1974; **8**: 26-33.

Björk A, Skieller V. Normal and abnormal growth of the mandible. A synthesis of longitudinal cephalometric implant studies over a period of 25 years. *Eur J Orthod* 1983; **5**: 1-46.

Helm S, Seidler B. Timing of permanent tooth emergence in Danish children. *Community Dent Oral Epidemiol* 1974; **2**: 122-9.

Hägg U, Taranger J. Timing of tooth emergence. A prospective longitudinal study of Swedish urban children from birth to 18 years. *Swed Dent J* 1986; **10**: 195-206.

Mina M, Kollar EJ. The induction of odontogenesis in non-dental mesenchyme combined with early murine mandibular arch epithelium. *Archs Oral Biol* 1987; **32**: 123-7.

Mjör, IA, Fejerskov O. *Human oral embryology and histology*. Copenhagen: Munksgaard, 1986.

Nyström M, Peck L. The period between exfoliation of primary teeth and emergence of permanent successors. *Eur J Orthod* 1989; **11**: 47-51.

Slavkin HC, Bessem C, Fincham AG, Bringas P, Santos V, Snead ML, Zeichner-David M. Human and mouse cementum proteins immunologically related to enamel proteins. *Biochem Biophys Acta* 1989; **91**: 12-8.

Steward RE, Prescott GH. *Oral facial genetics*. St. Louis: Mosby, 1976.

Ten Cate AR. *Oral histology, development, structure and function*. St.Louis: Mosby 1989.

Thilander B, Rönning O. *Introduction to orthodontics*. Stockholm: Tandläkarförlaget, 1985.

Literature cited

1. Björk A. Sutural growth of the upper face studied by the implant method. *Acta Odontol Scand* 1966; **24**: 109-27.

2. Björk A, Skieller V. Facial development and tooth eruption. An implant study at the age of puberty. *Am J Orthod* 1972; **62**: 339-83.

3. Demirjian A, Goldstein H, Tanner JM. A new system of dental age assessment. *Hum Biol* 1973; **45**: 211-27.

4. Ham AW, Cormack DH. *Histology*. Philadelphia: Lippincott, 1987.

5. Hurme VO. Ranges of normalcy in the eruption of permanent teeth. *J Dent Child* 1949; **16**: 11-5.

6. Leighton BC. The early development of normal occlusion. *Trans Eur Orthod Soc* 1975; 67-77.

7. Lysell L, Magnusson B, Thilander B. Time and order of eruption of the primary teeth. *Odontol Revy* 1962; **13**: 217-34.

8. Risnes S. Circumferential continuity of perikymata in human dental enamel investigated by scanning electron microscopy. *Scand J Dent Res* 1985; **93**: 185-91

9. Solow B. The dentoalveolar compensatory mechanism: background and clinical implications. *Br J Orthod* 1980; **7**: 145-61.

10. Van der Linden FPGM, Duterloo HS. *Development of the human dentition - an atlas*. Hagerstown, Maryland: Harper & Row Publishers, 1976

CHAPTER 5

THE CHILD AS A DENTAL PATIENT

THE CHALLENGE OF TREATING CHILDREN

To have a confident and relaxed patient in the dental chair is one of the most important prerequisites for successful treatment. However, many people feel upset or even frightened and anxious when visiting the dentist, often associating the scene with unpleasant dental experiences in childhood(4). The dentist treating children, therefore, may lay the foundations for their future attitudes towards dental treatment, whether it be confidence and trust or fear and anxiety.

Childhood involves learning. Training in tolerance and coping with stress are part of growing up. In a sense, the dentist can be regarded as a teacher of the child patient by building up good habits.

Treating children is a never-ending challenge to the dentist, since each child and each situation is unique. A skilful and experienced child psychiatrist once said when asked how to handle children: "In a given situation you act in a certain way, sometimes it turns out right, sometimes wrong, but the more knowledge and experience you get, the more often it probably is right". This chapter attempts to provide an introduction to that knowledge.

CHILDREN'S BEHAVIOUR

General experiences

The behaviour of children at the dentist depends on a number of factors, which also interact with one another. The various factors and their interplay are schematically illustrated in Fig. 5-1.

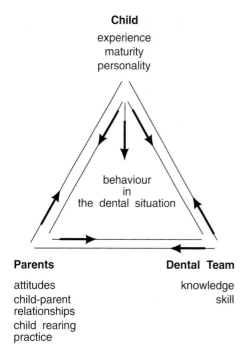

Child

experience
maturity
personality

behaviour
in
the dental situation

Parents   **Dental Team**

attitudes   knowledge
child-parent   skill
relationships
child rearing
practice

Fig. 5-1. Schematic illustration of factors influencing the child's behaviour at the dentist. The arrows represent the psychological interactions that take place between child, parent(s) and dental team.

Generally, the child's experience with people it has met and those who surround it in daily life is of great importance. This is basically a matter of trust and goes back to the first year of life. Homburger Erikson(3) refers to this as basic trust, which is founded very early, and he emphasizes its importance for the child's harmonious development. To feel safe, to trust people and have confidence in them serves as the basis for being able to cope, Fig. 5-2. This trust can also be applied to the dental situation.

Early experience of medical and/or dental treatment

Painful experiences from medical or dental treatment may be a serious obstacle to the

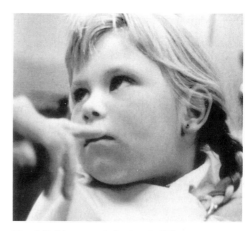

Fig. 5-2. "Are you to be trusted?"

future cooperation of the child. Therefore, treatment should be made as painless as possible. Optimal pain control is the key word for good professionalism, and the value of learning to master good injection techniques cannot be emphasized enough. It should be kept in mind that the level of pain tolerance varies as much in children as adults. Small children may not be able to distinguish between unpleasantness and pain. Methods to achieve good pain control are given in Chapter 7.

Maturity of the child

Small children, usually under the age of four, cannot distinguish between imagined and real danger. They often react primitively, scared by unexpected and sudden movements (Fig. 5-3), bright light and sharp and pointed objects, all of which may be easily encountered in the dental setting. Every child therefore should be treated according to its level of maturity, Fig. 5-4. Small children are also afraid of being left alone, and need the security of a grown-up and, particularly, of people they know and trust. To have a parent or some close relative accompany the child is therefore recommended.

As the child acquires experience, the ability to master new things and situations also increases. Instinctive reaction will be replaced successively by knowledge and cognitive skills. Besides increased ability to evaluate and master fear, the mentally maturing child also gains the power to concentrate on a fixed purpose, to endure and to motivate itself according to the demands of the environment. Rud & Kisling(6) showed that the child, when reaching a mental development stage corresponding to three years of age, is able to cooperate in the dental situation. A small child needs more time and more attention to accept dental treatment than an older child!

Some age-related characteristics relevant to the dental situation

Although the behaviour of the child is more closely related to its mental development than to its chronological age, some typical age-related characteristics can be pointed out. For reasons mentioned previously, the cooperation of the child under the age of three is limited and unpredictable. Dental treatment should, therefore, be kept to a minimum.

The **3-year-old** is still often shy with strangers, but the socialization process has started, and the child wants to imitate and to comply within reasonable limits. The child's perception of time and patience are limited and must be considered in treatment planning.

The **4-year-old** has acquired a certain degree of self-confidence and independence and can be without a parent in the dental office. The child is now generally a sociable person who wants to imitate grown-ups and is talkative and willing to help. Curiosity and lots of imagination are other characteristics which can be used to facilitate the handling of the child.

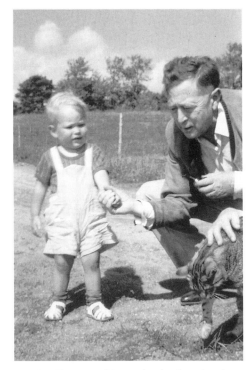

Fig. 5-3. To meet a big cat for the first time in your life is frightening when you are only 2 years old.

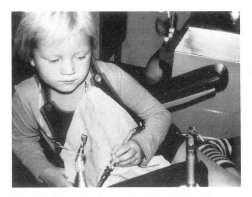

Fig. 5-4. Introduction to the dental situation.

The **5-year-old** is in the most harmonious pre-school period and is usually a very adaptive dental patient. The child is very sensitive to praise and flattery. Fine motor movements are now developing, although and views, and this is a suitable time for the child to begin to take responsibility for his/her own oral hygiene procedures.

The **teenager.** It is well known that teenagers easily come into conflict with the adult world, which may also affect the relationship with the dentist. Keeping in mind that this period is often characterized by insecurity and sensitivity to criticism and reproaches, the teenager should otherwise be regarded as an adult in the dental situation.

Personality

Each child has its own personality, although some characteristics and traits may be less stable, and rather represent a development stage. To obtain information about the child, its temperament, habits and behaviour in general, may be very useful.

The sturdy, robust and the delicate, vulnerable child – The robust child seems indefatigable, is venturesome and keen on new discoveries. Not easily thrown off balance and often having a certain self-esteem, such children are usually easy to deal with, Fig. 5-5.

The opposite is the cautious, delicate child who gives up easily and seems pessimistic about its own capabilities to cope with stress and new situations. At the extreme, such children seem vulnerable and "thin-skinned". They are often generally anxious, and may react to stress by feeling ill, having stomachaches or even by vomiting. Their pain tolerance is often low. Special attention and patience are needed for these children. One has to proceed very slowly with introductory measures, repeat the various steps many times but also to work efficiently, since these children tire easily. It should be kept in mind that a child may appear delicate for some time due to general illness or fatigue, without constantly being that way.

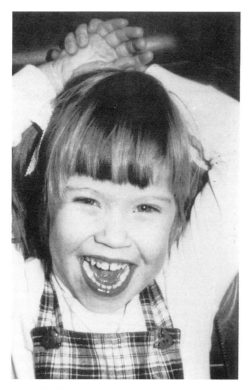

Fig. 5-5. I love my dentist.

the child is still not capable of learning how to use an optimal toothbrushing technique.

The **6-year-old** is in a less harmonious period, is often apprehensive and may have spells of bad humour. This is in the transition period to logical thinking; the child starts to argue in a logical way and may be hard to persuade.

The **7 and 8-year-olds** are generally sensible and reasonable. Fine motor movements are now well developed. Logical thinking develops rapidly. The egocentricity so typical of the preschool child vanishes, the child can function in a group, understands the significance of rules and can take responsibility to some extent. Children of this age are often categoric and rigid; things are either good or bad.

The **period from 9 years of age to prepuberty and puberty** is harmonious and active. The child is receptive to adult ideas

The stable and the easily affected child – The emotionally stable child behaves calmly and placidly. The opposite type seems emotionally more undisciplined, is impulsive and may burst into theatrical laughter or tears. These children may have a lively imagination and may also be domineering. When meeting stress, they may loose control and fall into hysterical crying fits, during which they are almost impossible to communicate with. They need calmness and reassurance, but also a firm and determined approach.

The expressive, easily contacted and the reserved, withdrawn child – While some children are open, warm and natural in their contact with other people, others are more difficult to reach. Sometimes one may get the impression that they are detached and prefer to remain secluded. Such children are sometimes called schizothyme because of their uncommunicativeness and introverted temperament. Time, patience and lots of kindness are necessary to reach them.

The characteristics mentioned, although within the normal range, are extremes, and most children's personalities fall somewhere in between. Furthermore, their behaviour is generally governed more by their experiences in interpersonal relationships and by the way they are approached in the specific dental situation than by personality traits. However, occasionally one does encounter children with whom the psychologic approach has to be considered carefully(9).

"Children begin by loving their parents; as they grow older, they judge them; sometimes they forgive them."

Oscar Wilde

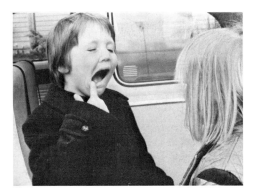

Fig. 5-6. It is sometimes tempting to impress, exaggerate and spread fear among playmates.

PARENTS

Every home has its own rules, often unspoken, unique patterns of communication, attitudes and traditions that are continuously imposed on children, who learn by observing and imitating the people around them. It is, therefore, not surprising that family attitudes, especially those of the mother, have been found to have great influence on child behaviour(7). Accordingly, dental anxiety in an inexperienced child is often closely related to that of the mother. Venham et al(8) found that a mother with self-esteem, confidence and responsiveness, who was actively intervening at home to promote the independence and sociability of her child, facilitated its ability to cope at the dentist. However, the mother who lacked self-confidence, was permissive and easily annoyed, insecure and doubtful about limit-setting, and therefore avoided restrictions, more often had children with cooperation problems.

When a child reaches school age, teachers may also serve as models. Negative modelling may occur through playmates who enjoy making trouble, Fig. 5-6.

A comfort to the imperfect parent: if you were perfect, your child would get no experience in dealing with the not too perfect members of the genus homo sapiens.

Anonymous

CHILD - PARENT RELATIONSHIPS AND CHILD REARING

The behaviour of a child at the dentist reflects the relationship between child and parents. A good relationship is characterized by a balance between the respective needs of child and parents. The basic needs of a child, which are also elements in rearing children, can be summarized:

– affection

– approval

– authority

To receive *affection* and love is fundamental for a child's harmonious emotional development. Most children are loved by their parents. Rarely, a child is rejected because of its mother's emotional disturbances. If there is no substitute for such a mother, this may result in lifelong emotional disturbance. Rejected children also present problems for the dentist. They are often introverted, suspicious and sometimes aggressive. These children need much attention and kindness even if they are disobedient and resentful. To penetrate their protective walls may take a great deal of patience.

To get *approval*, to be accepted as one is, and to have a feeling of adequacy are necessary for the child to develop self-confidence and self-esteem. These needs for encouragement and support are usually met, as the majority of parents are proud of their children. Some parents, however, constantly make too great demands and, thus, promote the development of a frustrated child who feels inadequate and inferior. Extremely demanding parents may constantly nag and criticize the child as they cannot accept it as it is. These children may also present management problems for the dentist and, like rejected children, they require kindness and patience.

To use *authority* is perhaps the most difficult part of rearing a child. It includes limit-setting, rules, discipline and consistency. The aim is to develop the child's independence and tolerance to frustrations and to teach it to cope with fear and stress. Authority also means serving as a model. To set a good example, and to do this consistently, is certainly not an easy task.

PARENT MANAGEMENT

Generally, a good dentist-parent relationship develops without any particular effort. Sometimes, however, the parents need advice and instruction on how to best contribute to good treatment for the child, for instance to avoid a negative approach when preparing it for a dental visit. Some parents, in their eagerness to give the child all the best in life, become too concerned, too protective and, therefore, unwilling to make demands. These parents may be widely read in child psychology. However, too much information, often fragmented and confusing, may lead to uncertainty about what is best for the child. Parents may choose to let it make its own decisions instead of taking the responsibility of setting limits. These children are often uncooperative with the dentist, as they are not used to demands. Parent counselling about proper and specific demands made of children is necessary. If presented with understanding and confidence by the dentist, the parents are often grateful. A few parents are, however, openly hostile and refuse to accept any kind of demand on their children.

Counselling them may be difficult, requiring much diplomacy and tact. A parent's own dental anxiety often lies behind such hostility and suspiciousness. If possible, the other parent, or another relative should accompany the child to the dentist.

A frequently discussed question is whether or not a parent should be present during treatment of their child. A parent who does not hinder the establishment of good contact between child and dentist and who does not interfere with the treatment may just as well be present. If, however, the parent cannot control their anxiety in front of the child or otherwise interferes, or if the child takes undue advantage of the parent's presence, the parent should not be there. Note, however, that a request or an appeal to the parent not to be present during treatment of the child should be based on confidence and trust.

To summarize, the "difficult" parent is often:

– dentally anxious;

– unsure of how to handle the child at the dentist, and grateful for help and advice;

– guilty about the uncooperative behaviour of the child and being partly responsible for the child's dental condition;

– underestimating themself as a parent;

– underestimating the resources of the child to cope with frustrations and stress.

What the parent needs is:

– honest information about the child's dental needs;

– positive reassurance;

– to be able to accept that their child is an independent person with its own resources for coping with stress.

THE DENTAL TEAM

Children are extremely sensitive to body language and unspoken communication. An atmosphere in the dental office characterized by calmness, confidence and professionalism usually creates cooperative children and satisfied parents. Good professionalism is characterized by:

– self-knowledge and confidence, a realistic knowledge of both your skills and limitations; courage to admit failures and, if necessary, refer a child you cannot manage to another dentist;

– the ability to work efficiently, with optimal pain control, to balance the demands on the child against the treatment needs, and to find acceptable modifications of treatment if necessary;

– understanding and respecting children and ability to imagine how they experience the dental situation;

– parent counselling with respect and understanding, honesty and empathy;

– using the different skills of the members of the dental team, the dental assistant, the dental hygienist and the dentist, each may be better at some tasks than others.

There is no shortcut to achieving this, knowledge is the basis, and to obtain the skills requires training.

Psychological interactions

The complex interactions, both verbal and non-verbal, that take place in the dental setting between the child, the parent and the members of the dental team are difficult to perceive, unmeasurable and sometimes not possible to control. However, they are of the utmost importance in creating the atmosphere, Fig. 5-1.

FEAR AND ANXIETY

Fear of being hurt is necessary to protect a child from danger. At the same time, fear presents the greatest management problem for the dentist. Fear and anxiety can make children more difficult to treat and lower the pain threshold, resulting in a vicious circle.

The words fear and anxiety are often used together and without distinction. Strictly speaking, however, there is a difference between them, Fig. 5-7. Fear is concrete. That is, it has a real background, and you can express in words what you are afraid of. Anxiety, sometimes expressed as fear of the unknown, is diffuse and is not related, as fear is, to any specific threat. The proportions of reality are lost, as well as the ability to rationalize the threat.

Very young children have limited experience of the world and its dangers, and their fear is sometimes called primitive, based on instinct rather than realistic understanding of danger. Homburger Erikson(3) says that fear and anxiety during childhood are so close that they cannot be separated. The power to rationalize the threat behind fear and anxiety increases as the child grows older.

Low level fear and anxiety may help a child, enabling it to make the cognitive and emotional transition to the actual treatment. In other words, the child should be given time to cope. Conversely, it has been shown that a child who is exposed to unfamiliar treatment without warning, is more often subject to a higher and more permanent level of fear and anxiety.

When fear and anxiety are manifest over a long period and result in behaviour changes, they have become a phobia. Phobic reactions often remit spontaneously during childhood, but may be triggered again in response to specific emotional crises in adulthood. Infantile phobias (fear of thunder, darkness, snakes, etc.) are considered

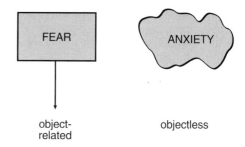

Fig. 5-7. Illustration of the difference between fear and anxiety. Fear is concrete, anxiety diffuse.

normal and necessary parts of emotional development, but such phobic reactions can be associated with unfamiliar situations. Thus, some children exhibit phobic reactions at their first dental appointment, even though they have had no previous negative dental experience.

Factors determining how the child will react to fear and anxiety

1. *The degree of fear*, depending how the child perceives the situation is related to the child's own experience and to the environment, whether the child is surrounded by secure, confident people or not.

2. *Ability to cope* with fear is related to the child's maturity and personality.

3. *Motivation to cope* with fear is related to the demands from surroundings, child-rearing practices, and those imposed by the dental visit.

Expressions of fear and anxiety

Children usually reveal their emotions more openly than adults, although there are exceptions, and expressions of fear and anxiety are several. Depending on the child's maturity, personality, experience of earlier frightening situations, and the demands from the parents and/or the dentist it might react by:

– flight

– aggressiveness

– crying

– evasiveness

– apathy and withdrawal

– regression

– vomiting or stomachaches

– trying to suppress and hide the fear.

A child who cries usually gets more sympathy than the one who is aggressive, fighting and abusive. The fear behind these different expressions may, however, be the same. It is also important to realize that a child may be very well behaved due to parental discipline despite being frightened. This is usually revealed by frightened eyes and a tense expression.

Alleviating fear and anxiety

The most effective methods of alleviating fear and anxiety in children are to instill receptive attitudes through positive modelling, reduce uncertainty by giving helpful information, give emotional support through positive non-verbal communication and eliminate pain through effective analgesia. It should be noted, however, that offering more information than needed may be just as anxiety-provoking as offering too little.

Since the reduction and elimination of fear and anxiety is part of a learning process, a step-by-step approach, reinforced by repetition appears to give the best and most lasting results (see Child management).

UNCOOPERATIVE CHILDREN

Main reasons

Fear and anxiety are the main components of uncooperative behaviour in children. The reasons are related to the child, the parents and the dental team, and they can be summarized as:

– insufficient maturity;

– illness, fatigue;

– developmental crises;

– general anxiety;

– low pain tolerance;

– bad experience from previous treatment;

– negative parental attitudes;

– basic deprivation from unfavourable social conditions;

– overindulgence, faulty upbringing;

– extensive dental treatment needs;

– inadequate management by the dental team.

These reasons are *not* ranked according to significance, their relative importance is difficult to establish as they are interrelated and partly dependent on each other. Complexity is apparent from the discrepancy between parents' and dentists' views of cause: parents mainly blamed the dentist, dentists most often blamed the parent (Table 5-1).

How common is it?

A study of acceptance of dental treatment among Swedish children(2) showed that the prevalence of dental fear was 3% in 4-16 year-olds; 8% sometimes reacted in such a

TABLE **5-1**

Main reason for uncooperative behaviour of preschool children, as seen by the dentist and by the parent, in per cent of children. From (5).

Main reason for uncooperative behaviour of the child	Dentist	Parent
Previous dental treatment	6	54
Urgent need of dental care	3	1
Previous illness and/or physical traumatic injuries	3	10
Attitudes in the family/child-rearing	44	7
Socioeconomic factors	2	1
Personality of the child, such as general anxiousness, stubborness	21	15
Immaturity of the child	15	1
Don't know	6	11
Total (n = 186)	100	100

way that treatment could not be carried out without physical restraint or excessive delay; more than 50% of 3-year-olds resisted in some way. Cooperation improved with increasing age, the rate of improvement being most pronounced among the youngest. It was also shown that the level of cooperation decreased with each new appointment in preschool children who had extensive treatment needs.

Strategies

With the uncooperative child, the first step is to find the reason(s). If it is very young, observe it and ask the parent about the child's behaviour in other stress situations and in general. Try to gain the confidence of parent and child. Assess the treatment needs and the demands you are going to be making, then plan your approach and describe it.

CHILD MANAGEMENT

Various techniques are used to eliminate or reduce dental fear and anxiety. Besides re-

ducing fear, they also aim at teaching the child coping strategies and motivation. They can be used both for introducing the dental situation and for reconditioning the dentally fearful child.

Most of the techniques are based on learning theory, that children are perceptive and both learn and relearn easily. *Modelling* involves the child watching a cooperative child of the same age either directly in the dental chair or on film, after which the child is supposed to imitate the good behaviour. The tell-show-do technique is probably the most commonly used(1). Reinforcement for modifying behaviour means that positive behaviour is rewarded while negative behaviour is disapproved of. *Behaviour shaping* is a combination of tell-show-do and positive reinforcement (encouragement). It includes the following:

– tell-show-do

– encouragement

– observing the reactions

– rating the acceptance

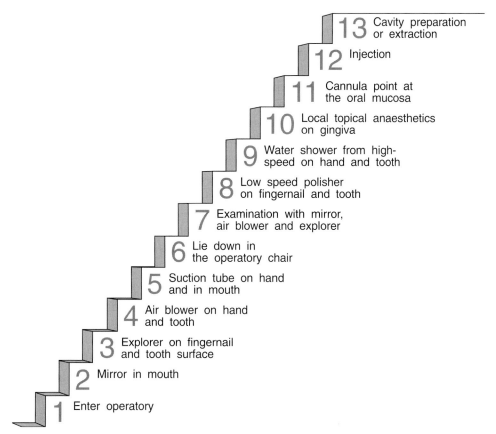

Fig. 5-8. Introductory steps to the dental situation. The steps escalate from the least to the most stress-provoking.

– if positive, introduce a new step

– if negative, further training on the present step

– repetition of these stages according to a hierarchy of treatment steps from the easiest to the most difficult to accept, Fig. 5-8.

Guidelines for behaviour shaping

General instructions

The aims are to build up confidence and to attain positive acceptance of dental treatment. The technique is based on the tell-show-do-method, using positive encouragement, initially small demands which gradually increase, and by training. Inform about your procedures. Try to establish a good relationship by developing two-way communication. Tell about and show your facilities. Show understanding for the child's feelings and situation. Observe and be sensitive to all signals from the child, especially the non-verbal. Equipment is best presented logically, step by step from the least to the most anxiety-provoking, Fig. 5-8. As each step is positively accepted, the child is praised for the desired response and behaviour. How detailed and how fast the

TABLE 5-2

Rating of acceptance. Categories of behaviour at different levels of acceptance and their influence on treatment. From(2).

Rating	Categories of behaviour	Level of acceptance	Influence on treatment
1	Active physical resistance, protests, screaming. No cooperation	No or negative	Treatment cannot be carried out without physical control or undue delay. Raised hands interfering with treatment.
2	Signs of resistance such as strained muscles. Reserved attitude. No answers, following directions with poor cooperation.	Reluctant	Raised hands but no interference with treatment, which can be carried out without undue delay.
3	Relaxed, calm eyes, talking and showing interest in the procedures. Good cooperation.	Positive	Treatment can be carried out immediately (after proper information).

steps should be processed is adapted to the individual. Carefully observe the child's reactions and behaviour, and let this guide you, helping you to control the situation and decide the limits for the particular child. Effort should be made to ensure that each visit ends with positive acceptance. The gradually increasing demands may be repeated at each visit to maintain the skills of the child.

Rating of acceptance – The child's behaviour is observed and rated according to the categories of behaviour, Table 5-2.

Further training – If the child reacts in a negative way to a particular step, further training is given and the achieved behaviour is rated. When a new step is introduced, it is according to tell-show-do with a successive approach. For instance, test the explorer or the polishing instrument at first on your own fingernail, then on the child's fingernail and finally on a tooth surface.

Ask for the child's experience. Communicate with eye and facial expressions. Encouragement is always given when progress is achieved.

Next visit
The next visit starts with further training. Efforts are made to achive positive acceptance at a higher level of the stimulus hierarchy.

Repeat tell-show-do and help the child to try. If not successful, the child can be forced to try (there must be a guarantee of no harm and no pain and the parent must be informed and approve).

If the child cannot be brought to accept treatment after reasonable efforts, the situation should be re-evaluated:

– check the treatment plan again to see if it can be modified or postponed.

– talk to the parents realistically, they may have ideas about how to solve the problem.

– perhaps the timing is wrong and the child has other problems at home or school.

– try somebody else accompanying the child, a change may have a positive effect.

– should the child be sent to another dentist?

– does the child suffer from severe emotional disturbance or for other reasons is unable to cope with stress in the dental situation?

In addition to psychological techniques, there are other methods of increasing cooperation and reducing fear, such as premedication, use of nitrous oxide sedation and general anesthesia. These methods are discussed in Chapter 7.

Literature cited

1. Addelston HK. Child patient training. *Fort Rev Chicago Dent Soc* 1959; **38**: 358-66.

2. Holst A. Crossner C-G. Direct ratings of acceptance of dental treatment in Swedish children. *Community Dent Oral Epidemiol* 1987; **15**: 258-63.

3. Homburger Erikson E. *Childhood and society*. (Norton 1987) Swedish ed. *Barnet och samhället*. Stockholm: Natur och kultur, 1977.

4. Kleinknecht RA, Klepak RK, Alexander LD. Origins and characteristics of fear of dentistry. *J Am Dent Assoc* 1973; **86**: 842-8.

5. Mejàre I, Ljungkvist B, Quensel E. Preschool children with uncooperative behaviour in the dental situation. Some characteristics and background factors. *Acta Odontol Scand* 1989; **47**: 337-45.

6. Rud B, Kisling E. The influence of mental development on children's acceptance of dental treatment. *Scand J Dent Res* 1973; **81**: 343-52.

7. Shoben ED, Borland L. An empirical study of the etiology of dental fears. *J Clin Psychol* 1954; **10**: 171-4.

8. Venham LL, Murray P, Gaulin-Kremer E. Child-rearing variables affecting the preschool child's response to dental stress. *J Dent Res* 1979; **58**: 2042-5.

9. Venham LL, Murray P, Gaulin-Kremer E. Personality factors affecting the preschool child's response to dental stress. *J Dent Res* 1979; **58**: 2046-51.

CHAPTER 6

CLINICAL AND RADIOGRAPHIC EXAMINATION

Case history
Clinical examination
Radiographic examination
Recording of findings
Epicritic evaluation

A thorough examination and diagnosis of the child dental patient is important for several reasons.

First of all, delivery of any type of medical or dental service can only be successful when based on a comprehensive diagnosis based on a thorough examination of the patient.

Secondly, since child dental services in Scandinavia cover the entire child population, the dentist is, in many cases, the medical practitioner, who sees the child most frequently.

For this reason dentists should be able to make initial diagnosis of some of the major medical conditions occurring in childhood. Examples of such conditions are: growth disturbances, infections, child abuse and neglect.

Finally, young children's first contact is an important determinant of their future behavior towards dentistry.

During the first visit, children and parents form their opinions about the attitudes of the dentist and his team towards the treatment of children. Thus, it is important that the examination of the child is performed in a friendly and relaxed atmosphere. Dental personnel should be fully aware of this and meet the parents with a warm and supportive attitude. It is important for them to focus on child and parents as people and not primarily as patients. This also gives the dentist a good opportunity to form an impression of the general background of children and parents, their attitudes to dentistry, and their expectations.

This chapter gives a general description of the case history, clinical and radiographic examination of children, leading to diagnoses for individual patients. Details of examination of teeth, periodontal tissues and occlusion will be given in other chapters.

The examination should cover the following:

Case history
    personal data (name, age, etc.)
    present complaint(s)
    family history
    general medical history
    dental history

Clinical examination
    general appearance
    face
    oral mucosa
    periodontal tissues
    teeth
    occlusion

Radiographic examination

In a few cases, laboratory tests such as biopsies, bacteriological tests, etc. are required to establish a final diagnosis. Description of these techniques, are found in relevant textbooks.

CASE HISTORY

The case history should give the personal data of child and parents (name, age, etc.) and a description of the present complaint(s) of the child. At this point it may be advantageous if the dentist gets a quick look at the child's mouth and teeth. In practice, the case history should take the form of a relaxed conversation rather than an enquiry. Standardized forms can be used to obtain the case history, but their use should always be followed by an interview.

The complete case history consists of a family history, a medical history and a dental history. Important information collected under each of these headings is shown in Table 6-1.

The family history

The purpose of this is to provide relevant

TABLE 6-1

A list of important information, which should be obtained during recording of the case history.

Family history
    occupation of parents
    social status
    number of siblings
    attendance in dayinstitutions

Medical history
    mother's health during pregnancy
    birth weight
    birth complications
    child's health during first year of life
    childhood diseases and previous medical treatment
    medication including adverse reaction to drugs
    traumatic injuries
    disorders of the circulatory, respiratory, digestive or nervous systems
    sleeping disturbances

Dental history
    past dental care, including the child's reaction
    oral habits
    oral hygiene habits
    food habit patterns (diet history)
    fluoride therapy

information about the social background of the child and, most important, its family.

Such factors as the number of children, the housing conditions, the parents' occupations, the child's attendance at dayinstitutions and schools, are important in selecting a realistic plan for preventive and restorative dental services.

This history should also include the occurrence of any familial genetic diseases, oral or general.

It should be emphasized that the information required for an adequate family history is considered confidential by many parents. Thus, the dentist should be very tactful in attempting to obtain it.

General medical history

Known disease or symptoms of unknown disease should be identified. The general medical history brings the oral and dental problems into a broader perspective of total patient care.

Congenital or aquired diseases or functional disturbances may, directly or indirectly, cause or predispose to oral problems (e.g. craniofacial syndromes, juvenile rheumatoid arthritis, diabetes, hematologic diseases) or they may affect the delivery of care and treatment of oral disease to the individual child.

The history includes information about pregnancy, delivery, neonatal period and early childhood.

    Pregnancy
        duration
        maternal health
        medication
        other
    Delivery
        complications
        breech presentation
        other
    Neonatal period
        birth length
        birth weight
        icterus
        respiratory problems
        feeding problems
        deformations
        neonatal teeth
        other
    Child's health during first year of life
        somatic development
        psychomotor development
        traumatic injuries
        diseases

Previous history should specially review hospitalizations, illnesses, traumatic injuries and previous and current medical treatment. Information about infectious diseases (e.g. childhood diseases; otitis media), immunizations, allergies (including adverse reaction to drugs), and sleeping disturbances should be obtained.

Finally, current and past problems as well as any current signs and symptoms of disease in the head, respiratory, cardiovascular, gastrointestinal, neuromuscular and skeletal systems should be included in the general medical history. When necessary this information should be supplemented with information from hospital records and the family physician.

Dental history

The child's past experience with dental services should be reviewed. The kind of dental treatment received, including pain-control measures and acceptance of earlier dental treatment, give the dentist important background for evaluation of the child's past behavior in the dental situation and may reveal treatment procedures which have been especially trying.

Factors of importance for future dental health should be identified as part of the dental history, including day-to-day oral hygiene, dietary and sucking habits.

Dental history also aims at identifying etiological explanations for such unusual conditions as rampant caries, atypical attrition, gingival recession, etc., noted during the initial, brief inspection.

CLINICAL EXAMINATION

General appearance

As mentioned, the dentist is, in many cases, the medical person who sees the child most

TABLE 6-2

Examination of the head and neck of children suspected of congenital or acquired craniofacial anomalies.

Structure	Diagnostic procedure
Cranium	inspect for shape deviations and asymmetry.
	measure head circumference.
Ears	test gross hearing.
	inspect ears for size, shape and position; pits and tags.
Eyes	test gross vision.
	evaluate gross eye movements; strabismus; hyper- or hypotelorism; exophthalmos; iris coloboma; ptosis; conjunctivitis.
Nose	evaluate olfactory capability.
	evaluate patency of nasal airway.
	evaluate gross deviations of nasal septum.
Face	inspect skin for inflammation, scarring, eruptions, ulceration.
	observe gross facial movements.
	inspect for asymmetry of facial bones or soft tissues.
	observe for function and range of mobility of the jaw.
Neck	evaluate musculature (torticollis) and range of motion.
	palpate for lymphnodes.

frequently. Thus, the dentist has the opportunity to identify medical and functional problems which may have gone unnoticed and can contribute to an improved health service by making appropriate referrals.

Assessment of general appearance should start before the child is seated in the dental chair. If the dentist personally fetches the child from the waiting room and walks with it, this gives an excellent opportunity to form a first impression of the child's stature, proportions, posture, head, mouth, breathing and gait. This assessment may indicate growth disturbances, central nervous system disorders, neuromuscular disorders or orthopedic problems worthy of further examination.

Examination of the skin for colour, pigmented lesions, bullae, scarring, dryness and scaling, may indicate the presence of systemic disease. The hands should be examined with emphasis on webbing, or syndactyly of fingers (indicative of a syndrome) and evidence of habits. The quality and the shape of the nails should be assessed. In ectodermal disorders the nails may be missing or be of poor quality. In chronic respiratory diseases or congenital heart disease, the fingernails may be markedly convex and the fingers clubbed.

The colour, amount and quality of the hair should be evaluated. In certain types of ectodermal dysplasia and various metabolic diseases the hair is missing or sparse and thin.

Examination of the head and neck

If the family history, the patient's past history or the gross clinical examination give rise to suspicion of congenital or acquired craniofacial anomalies, a systematic examination of the head and neck should be carried out. This should include assessment of each anatomic structure for integrity, function, development and pathology. Also minor anomalies should be assessed since such anomalies are present in many multiple congenital anomalous syndromes and since it has been shown that in newborns with three or more minor anomalies, 90% have a major anomaly. Even with early care and evaluation many anomalies and developmental problems are not identified until early childhood and the dentist should thus be aware of variations from the normal that may signify other problems.

Table 6-2 suggests a sequence and certain elements of a clinical examination to diagnose pathology in the head and neck region.

Intraoral examination

Usually intraoral examination is the child's first contact with dental instruments. For this reason the dentist should use simple intraoral examination procedures to accustom the child to manipulations with mirrors, probes and other instruments in the oral cavity. A "tell-show-do" technique should be employed to its full extent. During and after the intraoral examination the dentist should take the opportunity to show parents what has been found.Most parents welcome explanations and discussions on their children's dental conditions.

The oral cavity should be examined in a systematic way in order to avoid omission of important conditions.

The equipment needed for routine intraoral examination can be limited to a few instruments. The examination can almost always be performed with the child in the dental chair. Though in some cases it may be an advantage to perform the examination with the child seated in the parent's lap.

Examination of oral mucosa

The oral mucosa should be examined after being wiped clean, starting with the inside of the lips and continuing to the mucosa on the inside of the cheeks, including the upper and lower alveolar sulci. The palate is inspected using a mirror. The mucosa of the tongue and the floor of the mouth are examined after careful retraction of the tongue.

During examination of the oral mucosa, which may include palpation, any ulcerations, changes in color of surface, swellings or fistulae are noted. When examining the alveolar processes special attention should be given to any minor swellings or any retraction of the gingival margin, which could be a sign of an interradicular pathological process.

The presence and attachment of frenulae should be examined with special emphasis on the possible complicating effects of high insertion of such frenulae on the periodontal tissues.

Examination of periodontal tissues

Periodontal tissues are examined for inflammatory changes. The gingival margin is gently checked with a blunt periodontal probe for areas with bleeding.

A complete periodontal examination of all teeth for loss of attachment is hardly feasible on a routine basis. There is little reason to recommend periodontal probing in the primary dentition unless general medical conditions motivate this. In the permanent dentition, loss of attachment may be seen during the teens. Thus, if juvenile periodontitis is not suspected from radiographs, it seems reasonable to postpone systematic periodontal probing until that age.

Deposits on the teeth can be either hard or soft. Calculus is, however, an unusual finding before the teens, although some cases of calculus in the primary dentition can be found on surfaces close to the orifices of the salivary gland ducts. The amount of deposits as well as the color should be noted.

Examination of teeth

Variations in number, morphology, color and surface structure should be observed under good light and after careful isolation and drying. Cleaning of the teeth may have to be done to detect minor changes in the enamel surface. This is especially important in the case of very mild hypomineralization as in the earlier stages of dental fluorosis.

In the case of traumatically injured teeth, the color and transluscency of the injured tooth or teeth should be evaluated carefully using both reflected and transmitted light. Slight color changes are often found as one of the first signs of early intrapulpal damage after trauma. Variation in the angulation of the light beam is often necessary to reveal minor changes in translucency.

Initial carious lesions can only be detected after meticulous cleaning and drying of the teeth. Such lesions should be examined for surface roughness or actual loss of surface continuity. However, in the case of initial lesions great care should be taken not to expose the subsurface lesions with the probe. Examination of lesions with distinct cavitation should include such signs as the color, size and depth of the lesion. All previous restorations should be examined for overhang, marginal breakdown and recurrent decay.

Examination of occlusion

Finally, the patient is examined for malocclusion including any deviations in dental development, occlusion of the two arches and space conditions.

RADIOGRAPHIC EXAMINATION

Indications for pedodontic radiography

The use of radiographs should be based on selection of individuals with clinical signs and symptoms likely to benefit from a radiographic examination. Some major categories or oral problems that are frequent indicators for radiography are:

caries
pulpal pathology
traumatic injuries
problems of eruption
anomalies of development
orthodontic evaluation
history of pain
evidence of swelling
unexplained tooth mobility
unexplained bleeding
deep periodontal pocketing
fistula formation
unexplained sensitivity of teeth
evaluation of sinus condition
unusual spacing or migration of teeth
lack of response to conventional dental
    treatment
unusual tooth morphology, calcification
    or color
evaluation of growth abnormalities
altered occlusal relationship
aid in diagnosis of systemic disease
familial history of dental anomalies
postoperative evaluation

Film size

In principle, the largest film size that fits or is accepted by the child, should be used to maximize the information from each exposure. The space is limited and it is recom-

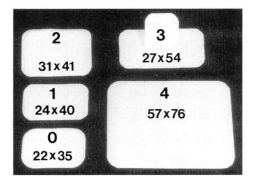

Fig. 6-1. The most common film sizes for intra-oral use in children. The numbers are according to the ISO standard.

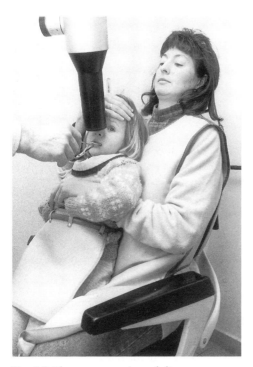

Fig. 6-2. The accompanying adult may sometimes have to restrain young children, when the radiograph is very important.

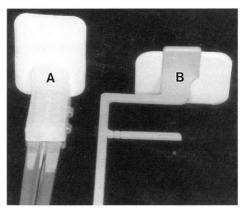

Fig. 6-3. Two different film holders with an x-ray beam guide, one for periapical radiographs (A) and the other is designed for bitewing radiographs (B).

mended to keep a selection of different film sizes in the office. Intraoral films are available in different sizes classified from 0 to 6 according to the ISO standard. The most commonly used film sizes for intraoral ra-diography in children are shown in Fig. 6-1. It is recommended to have at least 3 film sizes available; a small film for periapical use and bite-wings in small children (e.g. Size 1), an adult bitewing film (Size 2) which can also be used as an occlusal film in small children and an occlusal (Size 4) for use in older children.

Small children do not always behave as instructed and this gives rise to modified radiographic techniques in children. Some children can overcome their fear by having the radiographic procedure demonstrated. However, with the very young sometimes radiographs have to be taken of unwilling children. In such cases it is necessary for the accompanying adult to assist as shown in Fig. 6-2. The child is seated on the adult's lap, the child's forehead is held with one hand while the other grasps both the child's wrists. The child's movements are thus under satisfactory control.

Periapical radiographs

The radiographic technique for children is, in general, the same as for adults, i.e. the *parallelling* or the *bisecting-angle technique*. The parallelling technique usually gives a

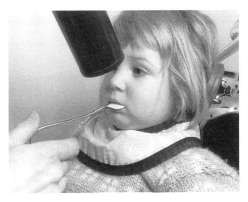

Fig. 6-4. A needle holder is useful for correct placement of the film and for keeping it in correct position in very young patients. Dental personnel should wear a lead apron in such cases.

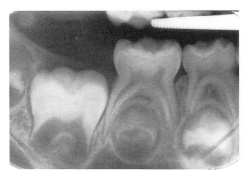

Fig. 6-5. A needle holder has been used as film holder to keep the film in correct position. Note the oblique lines at the lower corners, caused by sharp bends of the film-corners. Such bends help the child to tolerate the film placement.

more accurate and precise radiographic reproduction of the tooth dimensions than the bisecting-angle technique. The parallelling technique often requires a film holder to obtain parallellity between tooth and film. A film-holding device may also have an x-ray beam guide. Examples of film holders are shown in Fig. 6-3. Though the use of film-holders is recommended with children; it may not be tolerated by some and the bisecting-angle or a modified technique has to be used. A needle holder is useful to keep the film in the correct position during exposure (Fig. 6-4). Dental personnel should avoid the primary x-ray beam while using the needle holder. Fig. 6-5 illustrates a periapical radiograph in a 4-year-old child taken using a needle holder for correct placement of the film.

In the bisecting angle technique the vertical angulation should be perpendicular to an imaginary bisecting plane which divides the angle between film and tooth in half. This technique is useful, for example, in children of less than 3 years for the frontal region of the upper jaw. Trauma to the teeth occurs frequently at this age. To x-ray the actual teeth in such cases the biggest possible film (e.g. film No. 2) should be placed in the occlusal plane. The child is asked to bite on the film and the cone is adjusted according to the bisecting-angle technique (Fig. 6-4).

Three-dimensional localization is necessary for information about the relative position of structures, for example, in cases with dental injuries, or the presence of supernumerary teeth. Two projections which are at 90° to each other might facilitate a three-dimensional localization in the lower jaw. In the upper jaw, however, the superimposition of other structures could make this method unsuitable. Another possibility is to take two radiographs with slightly different horizontal or vertical angulation. This technique will provide three-dimensional localization according to geometric rules. If the relative movement is in the opposite direction to the movement of the x-ray beam, the object is located buccally to the reference object and vice versa when the object shows the same movement as the x-ray beam.

Injuries to the teeth

Since frontal teeth are usually the most often affected, the bisecting angle projection will give a satisfactory reproduction of the wounded area if the vertical angulation is varied. The x-ray beam has to follow nearly

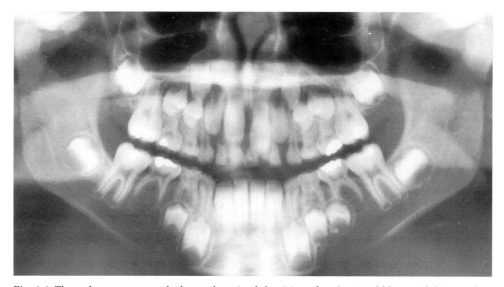

Fig. 6-6. The orthopantomograph shows the mixed dentition of an 8-year-old boy with late tooth formation and eruption. In most individuals the mineralization of the second premolar starts before 2.5 years of age and the crown is complete about 7 years; it is likely that this patient will have hypodontia of 45. Information about the position of the buds is also obtained from an orthopantomograph, e.g. notice the mesial position of 35 in this case.

the same line as the fracture in the bucco-lingual direction to visualize a horizontal fracture in the root. Often the fracture will be radiographically recognized as a circle because the x-ray beam shows some deviation from the fracture line. In younger patients the permanent tooth buds in the frontal region of the upper jaw will be projected over the apex of the underlying primary teeth when a periapical radiograph is taken. Another exposure, with the film placed in the occlusal plane will give a satisfactory projection of the apex.

In cases where comparison with previous radiographs is important, as in the control of traumatic injuries, it is important to standardize the radiographic technique. A film holder with a beam guide is then strongly recommended.

Bitewing projection

The diagnosis of approximal caries is most efficiently performed using the bite-wing projection. This technique is also important for diagnosis of osteitis in the bi- or trifurcation of primary molars.

If radiographic information about large areas within the oral region is needed, several methods are available. Both intra-oral and extra-oral films might be used. Intra-oral full mouth surveys consist of 10 to 20 radiographs. Extra-oral radiographs require intensifying screens and the reproduction of details will be poorer than intra-oral radiographs.

Extra-oral panoramic radiographs

This technique gives a useful view of anatomic structures in focus. Some structures in front of and behind the object will be blurred. Panoramic radiography should be used, on specific clinical indications, to clarify root formation, developmental disturbances and eruption problems, for example.

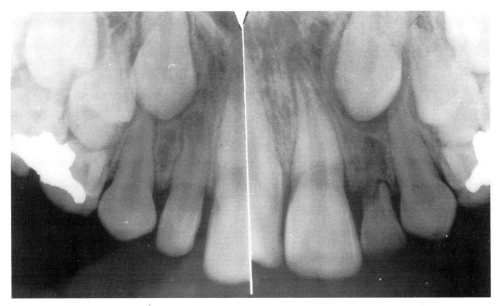

Fig. 6-7. Intraoral radiographs of a 9-year-old girl with hypodontia of the upper left lateral [22]. The other lateral [12] has a small clinical crown and a short root. Intraoral radiographs provide excellent reproduction of details compared with extraoral film-screen combinations.

It is not recommended for screening purposes in children. The panoramic technique requires an exposure time of several seconds and some patients have difficulties in being quiet during the exposure. As a general rule, any radiograph should be avoided if it is likely to be worthless due to patient movements during exposure or incorrect film placement.

Interpretation and diagnostic considerations

All information on the radiograph should be utilized by careful and systematic interpretation. The basis of judgement of pathology is knowledge and experience of normal anatomy and its variants.

A perfect diagnostic test should always be positive in the presence of disease and negative in its absence. Unfortunately, tests are biased, which causes two types of error: overregistration (false positives) and underregistration (false negatives). There are thus four alternatives: true positive, true negative, false positive and false negative.

The statistical probability that a positive diagnosis is correct will be positively correlated with the prevalence of the disease. As an example, with declining caries incidence the relative number of overdiagnoses is likely to increase.

Crown – Caries should be diagnosed according to a quantitative assessment index according to the depth of the radiolucency in enamel and dentine. Several indices have been proposed. Traditionally, only the approximal surfaces have been examined radiographically. However, caries in the occlusal surfaces may also be revealed radiographically.

Severe changes in mineral contents of enamel, or defects related to tooth shape, may be disclosed even before the tooth erupts.

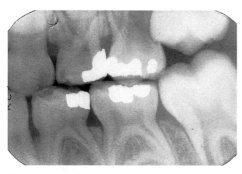

Fig. 6-8. All information on a radiograph should be utilized. In addition to information about absence/presence of caries and restorations, this radiograph provides important details of the ectopic eruption of 26 and pathologic root resorption of 65.

Missing teeth – Delayed tooth eruption or any suspicion of hypodontia (e.g. due to family history) should be followed up by a radiographical examination of the jaw(s). Extra-oral panoramic radiographs give a reproduction of the jaws which offers an excellent opportunity to identify and count teeth and buds (Fig. 6-6). In addition, the developmental stages and tooth morphology might be compared in and between individuals. It is important to notice that great variation exists in the onset of tooth-mineralization and eruption. The reader is referred to tables with eruption times. Such tables should include both mean values and the ranges. In general, crown completion occurs approximately 3 years prior to eruption, but a missing bud diagnosed radiographically at a certain time is not conclusive until it is verified some years after its normal mineralization starts.

Developmental failures may involve any tooth in the dental arch, but the observed frequency is highest for the second lower permanent premolar (Fig. 6-6) and the upper permanent lateral (Fig. 6-7).

Congenital absence of teeth often follows a hereditary pattern. Hypodontia in the primary dentition is very often connected with hypodontia in the permanent dentition.

Root – Physiologic root-resorption of the primary teeth may start from 4 years old. Pathologic root resorption may occur due to trauma or pulpal pathology or as sequelae of orthodontic tooth movement. Ectopic eruption of permanent upper canines for example, may cause root-resorption of the lateral incisor, or eruption of the first permanent molar may cause resorption of the second primary molar (Fig. 6-8). General disturbances in root morphology are seen in odontodysplasia and the affected teeth show a ghost-like appearance in radiographs due to severe disturbance of dentin formation.

After traumatic injuries it is important to examine radiographically the extent of the pulp cavity and the stage of root formation. Information about root fracture and displacement of the root are provided by the radiograph. The relationship between a displaced primary incisor and the underlying permanent tooth bud should be examined.

Pulp – Changes which are possible to monitor radiographically are those affecting the pulp walls as internal resorption or secondary dentin formation (obliteration). Mineral deposits within the soft pulp tissue may also be seen. Pulpal changes are often sequelae of traumatic injuries to the tooth or deep caries.

Generalized pulpal changes may occur in dentinogenesis imperfecta, where the pulp chambers sometimes are completely obliterated due to dentin formation after eruption.

Marginal bone – It is important to diagnose juvenile periodontitis with loss of attachment at an early stage. Information about bone height from the bite-wing radiograph should be utilized. Among older school children (>12 years) defects may be revealed adjacent to the first permanent molar.

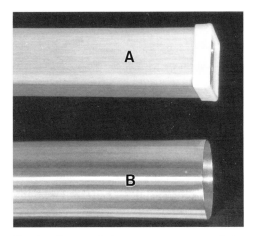

Fig. 6-9. Open-ended cones are recommended. A square (A) and a round opening (B) are shown. A square cone reduces the radiation.

Radiation protection in oral radiology

The low-level ionizing radiation used in dental radiology, has potentially adverse biological effects. Rapidly growing tissue is the most sensitive to radiation. Although the risk is very low, children are more susceptible to late effects of radiation than adults. It is impossible to quantify the risk exactly and the main risk to the children is cancer induction.

Radiation to children should be kept low through appropriate use of radiographs. The expected impact on the child's treatment from a radiograph should be considered to exceed the costs in terms of radiation.

Minimizing radiation exposure for every film is an important task for the dentist:

Use of thyroid shields and leaded aprons to decrease the dose to the patient including scattered radiation to the gonads. Use the fastest available film with acceptable diagnostic characteristics, which is, at the moment, a film in speed group E

(e.g. Kodak Ektaspeed). The use of Ektaspeed compared with conventional Ultraspeed allows more than 40% reduction of exposure.

Long and open-ended cones reduce the risk of scatter radiation to the patient and operator. The cone may be round or rectangular. A rectangular cone which has the same shape as the film, reduces the absorbed dose 2-5 fold (Fig. 6-9).

Use of a film holder reduces the probabilities of the need for a second exposure. It keeps the film flat, provides a guide for the x-ray beam and gives better exposure geometry.

Oral radiographs of asymptomatic children

Since the 1920s the bitewing (BW) technique has been used extensively in dental radiographic examination. The introduction of radiography represented a great advantage to dentistry because it could reveal dental decay at an early stage and thereby proper treatment could be instigated before further decay took place. The BW-technique has been used in screening procedures for dental disease on recall visits. Quality in dentistry has traditionally been associated with regular recall visits once or twice a year including radiography.

The use of radiography for screening of asymptomatic individuals may have a favorable risk-benefit ratio, e.g. mammography of postmenopausal women. In dentistry radiography has been used for several decades in screening during a period of increasing caries incidence. The declining incidence of caries and slow progression rate in enamel and a change in attitude toward the use of the ionizing radiation are all factors indicating the need for rethinking of radiographic practice. Attention should also be paid to the built-in errors in radio-

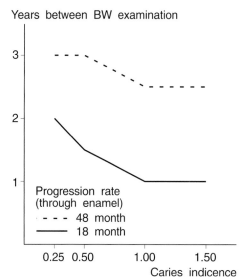

Fig. 6-10. The frequency of bitewing radiographs. The model is based on estimates of progression rates and incidence of caries. Five percent probability that a lesion will reach the inner half of dentin before detection, is accepted.

graphic examination, especially errors which lead to overtreatment, as a major concern is to avoid unnecessary fillings.

It is still reasonable to screen for caries using radiographs on asymptomatic individuals. However, some considerations should be based on the following "key questions" before radiography:

Is it impossible to obtain the information needed by a careful, clinical examination?

Does the anticipated radiographic information result in improved care for the patient?

The frequency of bitewings should have a scientific basis. The value of periodic bitewing radiographs depends on the incidence of caries and caries progression. When selecting a schedule for bitewing radiographs, an acceptable risk for deep dentinal lesions developing in the interval between two radiographic examinations should be considered, and at which stage of caries a restoration should be placed.

A theoretical model for selecting the appropriate intervals between bitewing examinations, can be outlined. In Fig. 6-10 the curves give alternative strategies according to the progression rate through the enamel. The model is based on data from more than 700 individuals from 10 to 22 years of age from Sweden and U.S.A., less than half received some fluoride prophylaxis. From the curves based (Fig. 6-10) on the actual data it can be read that a 3-year interval is acceptable if the likelihood that a new carious lesion will develop is low (low incidence) and if new or existing lesions are likely to progress slowly.

Screening for disturbances in tooth eruption

General screenings for developmental anomalies, are not indicated. The eruption of the upper permanent canines, for example, should be considered by clinical means, and radiographic examination performed only on individual indications. The radiographic examination should be based on clinical findings about eruptional disturbances and not chronological age. If the canines cannot be palpated at the age of 11 or an asymmetric eruption takes place, radiography is indicated.

Recording of findings

An accurate recording is just as important as a careful examination.

Two types of recording are performed:

1. recording of findings made during examination of the child, and

2. recording of treatment performed during subsequent visits.

Recording of findings made during the examination forms the basis for formulation of a treatment plan for the individual child. A number of different forms have been designed for this purpose. It is important that a uniform chart is designed for each dental service system, enabling transfer of information from one clinic to another.

Irrespective of records, all pertinent findings collected during the examination should be recorded. Radiographs should be mounted and marked with patient identification data and the date of exposure. Mounting frames with pockets protecting the radiographs from both sides and making mounting and remounting possible without damage to the films are preferable. For extra-oral exposures it may be helpful on later occasions if exposure data are recorded.

A complete record of all treatment procedures performed should be made at every visit. The information should be recorded in such a way as to permit later evaluation of earlier treatment.

The continuous and careful recording of all findings and of all relevant treatment and procedures forms important information for the dentist who is going to treat the patient in future. As an example, the reaction of the child patient to the administration of local anesthesia or nitrous-oxide/ oxygen analgesia should preferably be recorded at each visit.

Lack of cooperation and the reactions of the child and the parents to dental procedures should also be recorded, preferably in objective terms, to serve as a comparison for future visits. Records of treatment are also important in the re-evaluation of past treatment and in the evaluation of the response of the patient and the parents to past preventive and restorative procedures.

Epicritic evaluation

A systematic approach to pedodontics includes regular follow-up to evaluate the effect of previously delivered preventive and therapeutic services to the individual patient. On such occasions, the initial diagnoses may have to be modified. Such essential factors as the reactions of both child and parents to dietary advice and oral hygiene instruction can change from one visit to another. Such changes should obviously tend to result in modification of the treatment plan.

A good relationship between child, parents and the dental team, and a systematic recording of all relevant information is an important prerequisite for such epicritic evaluation.

CHAPTER 7

SEDATION AND ANESTHESIA

Need for management of pain and anxiety
Definitions
Methods for pain and anxiety control
Local analgesia/local anesthesia
General analgesia
Conscious sedation
General anesthesia

NEED FOR MANAGEMENT OF PAIN AND ANXIETY

Dental care is for most people associated with pain and anxiety. Painful procedures have proved to be one of the most important factors behind fear and anxiety in connection with dental treatment. The response of the individual child to pain and distress is complex and influenced by a number of psychological factors. Children at the age of 1.5-2 years have been pointed out in some studies as being extremely sensitive to pain. Preschool children and young schoolchildren up to the age of 11-12 years can usually not distinguish between pain and discomfort and pain and touch. When children develop the ability to think abstractly at about 12 years, their reaction to pain is more like that of an adult. Most children at this age will also be able to take full responsibility for whether local analgesia should be used or not. Before that age, the dentist has the responsibility. Parental attitudes to painful procedures also have an influence.

Painful procedures cause fear and anxiety, equally fear and anxiety enhance the sensation of pain. A trustful and informative atmosphere in the dental office, a cautious use of the child's suggestibility and the use of adequate technique of pharmacological pain and anxiety control will greatly reduce the discomfort of dental treatment.

The rules and regulations governing dental practice in different countries contain important differences as to the rights of the dentist to utilize various methods of pain control. There are also many variations in the right to prescribe medication. The trade names and range of pharmacological prescriptions are usually specific for each country. This chapter will therefore deal with basic principles.

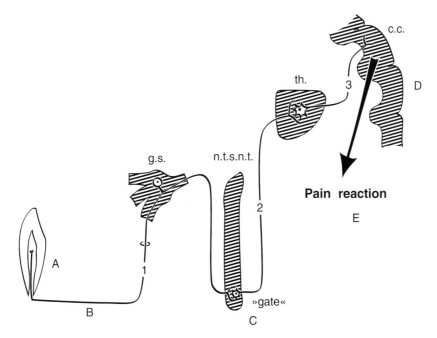

Fig. 7-1. The classic pain tract from a tooth in the trigeminal nerve. 1: First neuron. 2: Second neuron. 3: Third neuron. g.s.: ganglion semilunare. n.t.s.n.t.: nucleus tractus spinalis nervi trigemini. th.: thalamus. c.c.: cortex cerebri - gyrus postcentralis. The letters indicate, where the different pain-controlling mechanisms work: A: Peripheral acting analgesics and glucocorticosteroids. B: Local analgesics. C: Central acting analgesics, acupuncture, *descending* central control from higher centers. D: Central acting analgesics, nitrous oxide, general anesthesia, sedation, neuroleptics, hypnosis.

DEFINITIONS

Pain is defined as an unpleasant sensation, arising from noxious (harmful) stimuli and mediated in the nervous system. Most pain will arise in the periphery, being inflammatory in origin, but painful impulses can also arise along the peripheral nerves (neurogenic pain), or even in the central nervous system itself (central pain or psychogenic pain). In Fig. 7-1 the classic pain tract from a tooth is shown and in Fig. 7-2 a model of synapsis in pain transmission.

Pain may be acute or chronic. Nature's intention, undoubtely, with acute pain, is to supply the living organism with a mechanism of warning of impending threats to the living tissues. Chronic pain, is pain bothering the patient over a long period of time (months, years). In children's dentistry it is usually acute pain that has to be dealt with.

Anxiety seems to be generated by an internal threat, a feeling that all is not well, in contrast to *fear*, which has an external object, or what the patient sees as a real danger. Fear is therefore, easier to control than anxiety. Understanding and information are undoubtedly the best way to deal with anxiety and fear.

Both pain and anxiety produce stress, whereby such stress hormones as the catecholamines (adrenaline and noradrenaline) and the glucocorticoids (cortisol and cortisone) are released. The catecholamines generated from the adrenal medulla, make the patient feel uncomfortable (tachycardia, palpitations, nausea, and sweating in hands

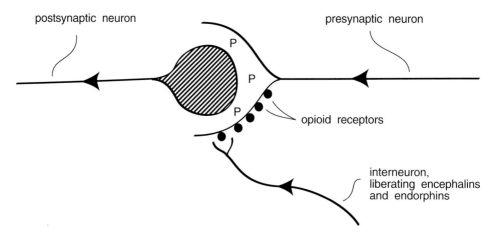

Fig. 7-2. Model of synapses in pain transmission. Substance P, a neurotransmitter, is released when a nociceptive impulse reaches the synapses. The release of substance P can be inhibited by an activation of the presynaptic opioid receptors, i.e. encephalins, endorphins, nitrous oxide, placebo, and hypnosis, or central acting analgesics.

and armpits), while the glucocorticosteroids normally will leave the patient uncaring, although they, of course, play an important physiologic role. In the healthy, this stress response will be without long-lasting consequences.

Analgesia literally means "without pain", while *anesthesia* means "without feeling". The term local analgesia is therefore more correct than local anesthesia, as not all sensations, only pain, are removed by this procedure.

Local analgesia is defined as a reversible, temporary cessation of painful impulses from a particular region of the body.

General analgesia is a state of reduced pain perception in a conscious patient.

Sedation describes a depressed level of consciousness which may vary from light to deep. At light levels of sedation, *conscious sedation*, the patient retains the ability to independently maintain an airway and respond appropriately to verbal commands.

The protective reflexes are normal or minimally altered and the patient may have amnesia. In *deep sedation* some depression of the protective reflexes occurs and although more difficult, it is still possible to arouse the patient.

General anesthesia describes a controlled state of unconsciousness accompanied by partial or complete loss of protective reflexes including the inability to independently maintain an airway or respond purposefully to verbal commands.

METHODS OF PAIN AND ANXIETY CONTROL

The term control relates to both the prevention and treatment of pain or anxiety. If the pain (or the anxiety) is allowed to start, the pain tract can be remembered by the brain ("pain tract printing"), and can be difficult to "erase". In all cases, prevention is therefore better than treatment. If pain is ex-

TABLE 7-1

Methods for pain and anxiety control.

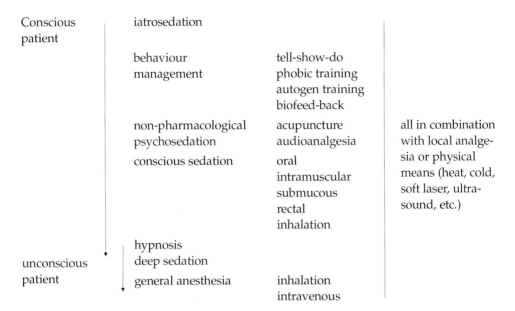

Conscious patient	iatrosedation		
	behaviour management	tell-show-do phobic training autogen training biofeed-back	
	non-pharmacological psychosedation	acupuncture audioanalgesia	all in combination with local analgesia or physical means (heat, cold, soft laser, ultrasound, etc.)
	conscious sedation	oral intramuscular submucous rectal inhalation	
unconscious patient	hypnosis deep sedation general anesthesia	inhalation intravenous	

pected during operative dentistry, local analgesia is given before starting. If pain is expected after a surgical procedure, it is wise to administer an analgesic *before* the operation in order to lessen or hinder the pain before it starts. It may also be necessary to combine conscious sedation or general anesthesia, which work at the end of the pain tract, with local analgesia, which works at the beginning of the pain tract to prevent "pain tract printing".

Table 7-1 summarizes the different approaches to pain and anxiety control, because much anxiety is actually based on the fear of impending pain.

LOCAL ANALGESIA/ LOCAL ANESTHESIA

Local analgesia (see definitions, p. 94), the most important means of pain control in dental practice, is here described in greater detail.

Local analgesia (LA) works by stabilizing the cell surface membrane of the nerve cell against sodium-ion influx. This means that sufficient concentration of the analgesic agent in and around the nerve cell will hinder its depolarizing and thus initiate an impulse. Interestingly enough, many drugs affecting the CNS (antidepressives, neuroleptics, antiepileptics, and antihistamines) have a structure similar to LA, and apparently their effect on the CNS cells can be looked upon as a similar "surface membrane stabilization".

The LA-efficiency is increased and prolonged, and the LA-toxicity is decreased by the addition of vasoconstrictors. In this respect, adrenalin appears to be the most effective and safe vasoconstrictor.

Indications and contraindications

LA can be used in any situation connected with pain or discomfort. It can also be used diagnostically to confirm or rule out suspi-

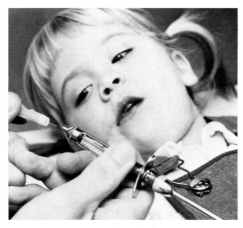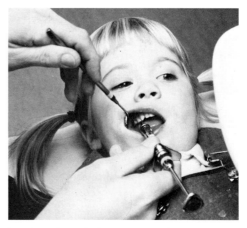

Fig. 7-3. Instruments should always be openly displayed. In the right-hand picture the procedure of local analgesia is demonstrated by a sham operation observed by the girl in a hand-mirror.

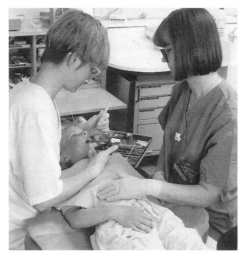

Fig. 7-4. During injection, the assistant should be in a position to grasp the child's arms should they be thrust upwards.

cions of pain cause. In certain cases, it can be used to treat forms of referred pain from muscles or joints, especially such long-acting LA as bupivacain (Marcain®) which erases the pain tract print. If LA is infiltrated profusely into an area of surgical intervention, the postoperative pain and edema will be less, as LA stabilizes *all* cell membranes, and thus reduces the inflammatory response mediated by the prostaglandins.

LA should be used routinely when conscious sedation or general anesthesia is used, in order to block the pain tract peripherally, i.e. where the pain arises during dental treatment.

A child's unwillingness or inability to cooperate remains as one of the few *contraindications* to local analgesia. LA is also contraindicated in case of genuine allergy to the agents, though this is actually very rare. It is also not advisable to inject patients with bleeding and coagulation disorders due to the risk of uncontrollable hematomas. LA with adrenalin is *not* contraindicated for patients being treated with tricyclic antidepressants, if injected slowly, and aspiration is performed before injection. LA with adrenalin is *not* contraindicated for patients with hypertension or cardiac arrhytmia, if the same precautions are taken. In these patients, it is actually the amount of endogenously produced adrenalin, due to stress and pain, that is the problem!

Preparation of the patient

When an LA-injection is administered for the first time, the dentist should take time to explain to the child what is going to happen and what will be felt during and after injection. This information must be adjusted to the age of the child. It is important to tell the child the truth, in non-dramatic language that will "soften" the emotional words. Never say a painful or uncomfortable procedure is not going to hurt or be felt. The child should be allowed to see the equipment (Fig. 7-3). Demonstrations of syringes and needles *should not be overdramatized*. The dental assistant can be of great help to the patient (Fig. 7-4). Finally, it is important to emphasize to children the avoidance of self-inflicted bite-wounds in anesthetized tissues.

Methods of administration

Local analgesia can be applied in the following ways:

– topical (ointments, sprays, mouth washes)
– infiltration
– blocks
– PDLA-injection
– jet injection.

Topical application

The most important indication for this is undoubtedly the preparation of the mucosa (and the patient!) for injection and can be achieved by application of flavoured 50 mg/ml lidocain ointment to the mucosa for 2 minutes (Figs. 7-5, 7-7).

Benzocaine or lidocain in smaller concentrations can also be part of ointments used for "teething" in small children.

Topical application of flavoured 5 mg/ml lidocain solution for mouthwashes before impression taking or x-ray can help children with pronounced gag reflexes.

Infiltration

Infiltration means the application of local analgesic solution around the nerve endings

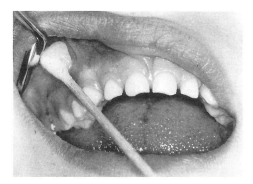
Fig. 7-5. Topical application of local analgesia – ointment in a cotton roll or an applicator.

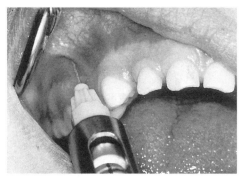
Fig. 7-6. Infiltration of local analgesia in primary dentition.

(Fig. 7-6). If the adjoining bone plate is sufficient thin, the solution can penetrate and diffuse into the bone affecting the nerves to the pulp and periodontal ligament of an individual tooth. Infiltration analgesia of teeth can be used with greater degree of success in deciduous than in permanent dentition.

Use only sharp needles, a thin one (30 G) will not necessarily be felt less than a standard one (27 G). Inject slowly after aspiration, self-aspirating syringes are preferable (Fig. 7-7). Use solutions at room temperature, never directly from the refrigerator. A good trick is to apply finger pressure to the area, where you are going to inject, it will distract the patient's attention. If you have to inject in the incisive canal, first place your LA on

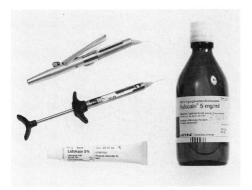

Fig. 7-7. Syringe for PDLA, self-aspirating syringe, ointment for topical application and mouthwash solution.

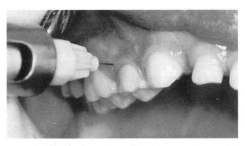

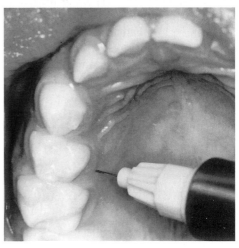

the labial aspect, and then in several phases make transpapillary injections from the buccal aspect. The same approach can be used whenever the palatal mucosa is to be injected (Fig. 7-8). Be careful with injection just opposite the apices of the upper central incisors, it can be very painful for the patient. Place an infiltration around the infraorbital foramen, and then wait a minute or so. Infiltration can, in principle, be made anywhere in the oral cavity, including the palate.

Fig. 7-8. Transpapillary injection starting from the buccal and continuing into the palatal mucosa.

Blocks

By far the most used block is the mandibular foramen block (Figs. 7-9, 10). The patient should open maximally, and the needle be introduced just lateral to the pterygomandibular fold at its deepest point (the pterygoid notch). In order to secure a good block, the needle should be introduced into the tissues without any resistance. If resistance is felt, the needle is slightly withdrawn and redirected. The most common obstacle is the strong medial tendon from the temporal muscle along the temporal crest.

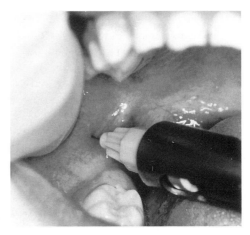

Fig. 7-9. Mandibular block analgesia in a preschool child.

PDLA-injection

PDLA means periodontal ligament analgesia, and has been relatively recently introduced in dentistry. A thin needle (30 G) is introduced into the periodontal ligament until bony contact. Then a small amount of solution, usually about 0.2 ml, is injected with a special forcing syringe, as the resistance against the injection (plunger pressure) is rather high (Fig. 7-7). It is important to inject *slowly* (Fig. 7-11). Every root is injected approximally, i.e. two injections per root. Injections on the facial aspect should be avoided due to the thin layer of alveolar bone.

Indications for PDLA are:

– supplementation of conventional analgesia (e.g. hypersensitive hypomineralized teeth)
– intrapulpal injection during painful pulpextirpation
– extraction of deciduous teeth and permanent premolars
– hemostasis from a bleeding papilla or sulcus, before filling therapy or impression
– diagnostic aid in localizing a painful tooth.

Contraindications for PDLA are:

– acute periodontal infection
– deep periodontal pockets.

Hypomineralization of enamel in the permanent successors, after PDLA, of primary teeth has been reported from experiments in animals, but has not been confirmed by clinical observations in humans.

Jet injection

The principle in jet injection devices is high pressure infiltration across the mucous membrane in a limited area. It works well in such firmly attached mucosa as the palate, but seems to be insufficient on such loosely

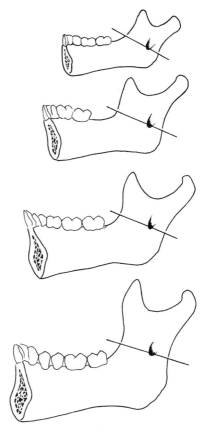

Fig. 7-10. The position of the mandibular foramen changes during growth. However, the foramen is always situated on the line where the ramus is narrowest, two-thirds of the way back from the anterior concavity.

bound mucosa as the facial aspect of the alveolobuccal sulcus. The indications for jet injection are, as such, rather restricted to pre-anesthetizing the palatal mucosa before conventional needle injections.

Side effects and complications

In general, very few side effects and complications actually arise following local analgesia in dentistry. The most common problem is without doubt that the efficacy of the procedure is less than desired, making both patient and dentist unhappy!

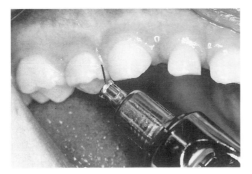

Fig. 7-11. Periodontal ligament analgesia, mesial root first upper right primary molar

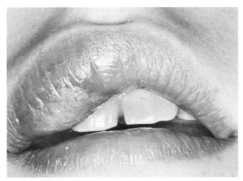

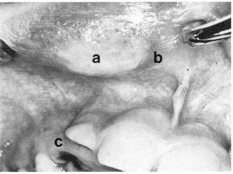

Fig. 7-12. Bite wounds often cause considerable swelling. The greyish-white central area (a) is surrounded by a reddish border (b). Extraction alveolus (c).

The most common systemic side effect is *syncope* or *fainting* which is loss of consciousness due to a decreased blood supply to the brain. It may be caused by three factors: 1) vasovagal collapse from fear and anxiety, sudden pain, or high temperatures; 2) toxic reaction due to intravascular injection of the solution or injection of too much solution at one time; and 3) hyperventilation due to anxiety, as the CO_2-concentration in blood decreases, the brain arteries constrict. If the patient faints, he or she should be placed in a recumbent position with elevated legs. The airway should be secured by bending the head back or forcing the mandible forward.

Also the *recommended maximum dosage* per sitting should be adhered to. For *adults*, they are:

– local analgesic
  without vasoconstrictor: **200 mg**
– local analgesic
  with vasoconstrictor: **500 mg**
– adrenalin or noradrenalin (i.v.): **100 µg**
– felypressin: **none**

For some commercial products this means that the maximum adult dosage would be:

– 3% Citanest with Octapressin: 16.7 ml
– 2% Xylocain with adrenaline: 25 ml
– 3% Carbocain Dental: 6.7 ml

The recommended child dosage can easily be calculated from the listed formula, when the adult dosage is known:

$$\text{Child dose} = \text{adult dose} \times \frac{\text{age in years}}{\text{age in years} + 12}$$

This formula can also be used in conjunction with calculation of maximum dosages of other drugs.

As mentioned previously, genuine *allergic reaction* to local analgesic solutions is very rare and consists of skin eruptions, sometimes bronchial constrictions, and fall of blood pressure. In case of proven allergy (skin test), one of the other products can be tested.

Most complications and side effects are of local origin, the most common being self-in-

TABLE **7-2**

The American Society of Anesthesiologists' Physical Status Classification.

Classification	Description
Class I	A healthy patient **Example**: inguinal hernia in an otherwise healthy patient
Class II	A patient with mild systemic disease **Examples**: chronic bronchitis; moderate obesity; diet controlled diabetes mellitus; old myocardial infarction; mild hypertension
Class III	A patient with severe systemic disease that is not in incapacitating **Examples**: coronary artery disease with angina; insulin-dependent diabetes mellitus; morbid obesity; moderate to severe pulmonary insufficiency
Class IV	A patient with incapacitating systemic disease that is a constant threat to life **Examples**: organic heart disease with marked cardiac insufficiency, persisting angina, intractable arrhythmia; advanced pulmonary, renal, hepatic, or endocrine insufficiency
Class V	A moribund patient not expected to survive for 24hours with or without operation **Example**: ruptured abdominal aneurysm with profound shock
Emergency(E)	The suffix E is used to denote the presumed poorer physical status of any patient in one of these categories who is operated on as an emergency (e.g. 2E).

flicted bite of anesthetized tissue (Fig. 7-12), which is best treated with chlorhexidine gel 10 mg/ml. Hematomas sometimes arise during injection. The patient should be told of their nature and that the swelling and discolorations will disappear.

In summary, local analgesia is a very useful and safe way of controlling pain and discomfort in pedodontic practice. Its success, however, partly depends upon the person administering the procedure.

GENERAL ANALGESIA

The most commonly used and recommendable analgesic for children is paracetamol. This is given prophylactically in children undergoing surgical procedures to avoid postoperative pain, or to manage acute pain due to inflammatory processes.

It is good practice to administer an analgesic if pain is expected, *before* the pain appears, instead of waiting for the pain to cause discomfort and distress to the patient.

Dosages of paracetamol are:

– children under 1 year : 60 mg
– 1-6 years : 60-120 mg
– 6-12 years : 50-300 mg

The first dosage is given perorally immediately, before the local analgesia is injected, and followed by the same dosage every 4-6 hours for the following two days. In children under the age of 12 combination with codein should be avoided. For larger children such antirheumatics as naproxen or ibuprophen can be recommended in the following doses:

Naproxen: 10-15 mg/kg/24h, divided into two daily doses.

Ibuprophen: 20-40 mg/kg/24h, divided into three daily doses.

It should be mentioned that acetylsalicylic acid (aspirin) is contraindicated for postoperative pain due to its anticoagulant effect. Acetylsalicylic acid is *always* contraindicated for children of less than 2 years because of risk of toxic reaction.

CONSCIOUS SEDATION

Consious sedation can be achieved by oral, intramuscular, submucous, or rectal administration, or inhalation of a drug. Oral administration of tranquillizing and anxiety-suppressing drugs has long been the commonest method of achieving conscious sedation. The *benzodiazepines* are today the drugs of first choice. Benzodiazepines are also available as rectal preparations. Barbiturates, propanidiol derivates, chloral hydrates, and antihistamines are preparations recommended for conscious sedation, but for such different reasons as difficulty in estimating the correct dose, marked side effects, narrow therapeutic latitude, are no longer in regular use in Scandinavia. The main indication for the use of conscious sedation is anxiety.

Contraindications can be assessed as: when patients are grouped according to anesthetic risk (Table 7-2), the dentist may take the responsibility for assessing patients in Classes I and II while sedation of patients in Classes III and IV should be decided in consultation with a phycisian. For further details see below.

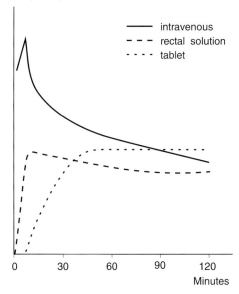

Diazepam, plasma conc.

— intravenous
--- rectal solution
.... tablet

Fig. 7-13. Plasma concentrations of diazepam after single intravenous, oral and rectal administration.

Oral and rectal administration of benzodiazepines

The benzodiazepine group of drugs contains several chemical variations: oxazepam, diazepam, lorazepam, nitrazepam, flunitrazepam, and midazolam. Some authors claim there are more similarities than differences in clinical effect. The maximum plasma concentration is obtained after 0.5-2h depending on the preparation used (Fig. 7-13).

Benzodiazepines are contraindicated for drug abusers and in outpatient practice for children under the age of one year. The presence of myasthenia gravis or porphyria is an absolute contraindication. Hyperactivity may occur in very small children (paradoxical excitation). In oral administration of sedatives, a fractionated dose produces a better effect than a single dose. Addiction occuring after administration for such a single event as dental treatment, has not been demonstrated. The preparation should be supplied by the clinic, with instructions as to the dose and the times at which it should be taken. The patient should be accompanied to the clinic, and children should not be left unsupervised on the day of sedation. Driving, even of a bicycle, is not permitted within 12 hours.

Benzodiazepines *by mouth* may be indicated to avoid 'treatment stress', alleviate mild anxiety before dental treatment, and facilitate sleep on the night before the treatment. They may also be indicated prior to dental treatment of medical poor risk patients, particularly those with cardiovascular disease, given either in fractionate or single doses. The doses recommended for diazepam are:

Children aged below 8 years:
  0.5-0.8 mg/kg body weight

Older children and young adults:
  0.2-0.5 mg/kg body weight

The recommended dose for sleep disturbances on the night before dental treatment is 2-5 mg, depending on body weight.

Results from clinical studies suggest that all administration of benzodiazepines increases the patient's ability to cooperate during the treatment, that dental surgeons sometimes overestimate the potential of the drug to suppress anxiety, but may also use doses that are too low. Experience has shown that it is often difficult to orally sedate children who have reached the "defiant" stage of development.

Rectal administration of diazepam is widely used for conscious sedation in preschool children in Scandinavia (Fig. 7-14), particularly in children under the age of three. Fast absorption through the rectal mucosa results in a maximum plasma concentration after 10-15 minutes (Fig. 7-13).

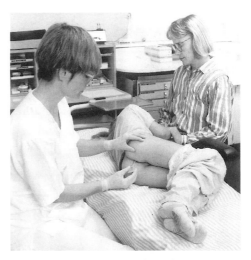

Fig. 7-14. Administration of rectal sedation by the dentist in an anxious preschool child before dental treatment.

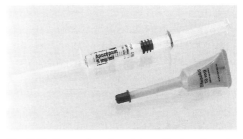

Fig. 7-15. Examples of rectal applicators for administration of diazepam.

The recommended dose in preschool children is 0.8-1 mg/kg body weight and in older children 0.5 mg/kg body weight.

Inhalation sedation: nitrous oxide/oxygen sedation

For inhalation sedation, nitrous oxide/oxygen is the method most commenly used and its high success rate and safety are well documented.

Nitrous oxide/oxygen sedation is defined as a state of sedation with a varying

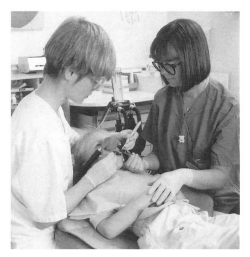

Fig. 7-16. Nitrous oxide/oxygen sedation.

degree of analgesia induced by inhalation of a mixture of nitrous oxide and oxygen while retaining an adequate laryngeal reflex. Sedation with nitrous oxide/oxygen is started by giving the patient 100% oxygen for 2-3 minutes; the nasal mask is adjusted to prevent leakage and the gas flow regulated (Fig. 7-16). Nitrous oxide is then administered in increasing amounts until a sufficient deep sedation has been achieved. On conclusion of the dental treatment, 100% oxygen is given for 5 minutes. Although the patient is able to leave the chair after the first 5 minutes, he or she is not ready to leave the clinic for about another 20 minutes.

Nitrous oxide is a poor anesthetic, but susceptible patients may loose consciousness with a 50% mixture of nitrous oxide. Nitrous oxide is always administered with oxygen to safeguard the patient's supply of oxygen. The peak alveolar concentration is attained within a few minutes of inhalation. The gas is quickly eliminated after termination of administration.

Nitrous oxide has little to no effect on respiration, blood circulation, and metabolism.

Chronic exposure to low doses of nitrous oxide has been reported as constituting a health hazard, as shown by the increased frequency of spontaneous abortion, liver and kidney disease, and neurological conditions in dental staff.

Nitrous oxide does not bind to body fluid or tissue. It was long believed that nitrous oxide was not metabolised, but we now know that it is metabolised by bacteria in the intestine where free radicals are formed and that it interferes with the metabolism of vitamin B_{12}. These discoveries are probably without importance for the patient, but they may explain the side effects occurring in dental staff who are chronically exposed to low concentrations of excess gas owing to inadequate scavenging or leakage.

Side effects of nitrous oxide, as described by patients are excitation (oversedation), nausea, vomiting, dysphoria, sweating, restlessness, anxiety, panic, headache, nightmares, tinnitus, urinary incontinence.

In a study carried out in Sweden in 1982, of 823 patients given N_2O/O_2 sedation during dental treatment, 8.3% exhibited side effects, 0.1% of which were due to oversedation.

The administration of nitrous oxide/ oxygen sedation requires special equipment (Fig. 7-17). The machine must always supply not less than *20% oxygen* (Sweden 40%) in the gas mixture. The gas flow must be continuous and the apparatus equipped with a *fail-safe device*, i.e. if the oxygen pressure falls, the supply of nitrous oxide automatically stops. If the gas supply is broken off the patient must be able to breathe air via an *"emergency air-valve"*. Re-breathing or addition of air is not permitted and the tubes must have *low breathing resistance*. Excess gas and exhaled gas must be effectively eliminated by scavenging.

Indications are:

- fear - anxiety;
- resistance to treatment;
- medically compromised patients;
- muscle tone disturbances;
- muscle relaxation;
- pronounced gag reflexes;
- treatment stress;
- the nature of the dental treatment (e.g. if analgesia in several quadrants is required).

It is a general rule that patients belonging to anesthesia risk Classes III and IV (Table 7-2) must be treated in collaboration with a responsible doctor or anesthetist. For patients in anesthesia risk Classes I and II the following contraindications apply:

- partial obstruction of the respiratory airways;
- psychosis;
- pregnancy;
- other:
    recent otological operation
    sinusitis
    porphyria
    family history of malignant hyperthermia.

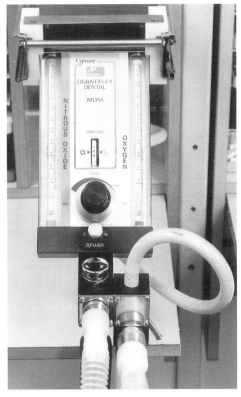

Fig. 7-17. Machine for nitrous oxide/oxygen sedation.

GENERAL ANESTHESIA

Some patients lack the physical or mental ability to cooperate during treatment or do not tolerate local anesthesia. Dental treatment under general anesthesia may then be the only solution. Moreover, some surgical procedures are so long and tiring that no other form of treatment can be considered.

The prevalence of serious complications in association with dental treatment under general anesthesia is very low when performed in a hospital clinic. Indication for dental treatment under general anesthesia, however, must be restricted because anesthesia itself exerts great physical and mental stress on the organism compared with the alternative methods. Treatment under general anesthesia is an expensive, but necessary, method of treating some children. It should be the last recourse when all efforts to treat a child in the conventional manner have failed.

Indications for dental treatment under general anesthesia:

- treatment of severely mentally and/or physically handicapped children who lack the ability to cooperate during treatment;

- severe management problems in patients with a genuine psychiatric disorder;
- complicated surgical procedures in young children;
- accumulated treatment needs in
  disabled children,
  children living in remote areas,
  children under the age of three or
  children with severe dental fear;
- intolerance of local anesthesia.

In Scandinavia dental treatment under general anesthesia requires the assistance of an anesthetist who selects the method of anesthesia according to the child's condition and the nature of the treatment to be performed.

Every possible effort should be made to return the child to routine therapy in future. After dental treatment under general anesthesia, adequate prophylactic dental care should start as soon as possible.

Background literature

Allen GD (ed). *Dental anesthesia and analgesia* (local and general). Baltimore: Williams & Wilkins, 1984.

Hallonsten A-L. Nitrous oxide-oxygen sedation in dentistry. Academic thesis. *Swed Dent J* 1982; suppl 14.

Coplans MP, Green RA (eds). *Anesthesia and sedation in dentistry*. Amsterdam: Elsevier, 1983.

Dionne RA, Laskin DM (eds). *Anesthesia and sedation in the dental office*. Amsterdam: Elsevier, 1986.

Lundgren S (ed). The use of sedation in outpatients. *Acta Anaesthesiol Scand* 1988; **32**: suppl 88.

Malamed SF. *Sedation – a guide to patient management*. St. Louis: CV Mosby, 1985.

Wall P, Melzack R (eds). *Textbook of pain*. Edinburgh: Churchill Livingstone, 1984.

CHAPTER 8

DENTAL CARIES: ETIOLOGY, CLINICAL CHARACTERISTICS AND EPIDEMIOLOGY

Caries etiology
Clinical characteristics
Epidemiology

Dental caries is a progressive demineralization and disintegration of the calcified dental tissues that occurs underneath a layer of bacteria on the tooth surfaces. It is thought to be caused by acids formed by plaque bacteria through metabolism of dietary sugars. An international multidisciplinary research effort in recent decades has done much to clarify the main etiological issues of dental caries.

The most dramatic increase in dental decay is thought to have occurred during the last part of the 19th and the beginning of the 20th centuries. This coincided with an increase in sucrose consumption associated with the industrialization and urbanization then taking place in Europe.

CARIES ETIOLOGY

The role of sucrose

The role of sucrose in dental caries is supported by extensive data collected in Europe during the two world wars where a sharp reduction in sucrose consumption was followed by a marked caries reduction.

The correlation between sugar consumption and dental caries has changed during the last two decades due to the introduction of fluoride as a preventive agent.

Fluoride increases the resistance of the teeth (Chapter 9) and is not directly involved in the caries challenge as such, except possibly by reducing acid formation by bacteria to a small degree. Sucrose consumption, thus, still provides the cariogenic challenge even if the correlation with caries is reduced.

A large number of other epidemiologic studies clearly confirm the correlation between sucrose consumption and dental decay. The people of the isolated island of Tristan da Cunha in the Atlantic had a very low caries rate. With the introduction of sucrose, the prevalence of caries increased from 5% to 30% DMF teeth. In Japan it was observed that caries increases when sucrose consumption exceeds 10 kg per individual per year. Data from Norway and Britain support these studies. Norwegian children consuming about 21 kg of sucrose per year during World War II established a good state of dental health compared with pre-war conditions, when the consumption was much higher. A close correlation exists between sugar available for confectionary production and the caries rate.

Data from Australia provide additional evidence: institutionalized children who consumed virtually no sucrose between meals had, at 11 years, an average of one tooth with caries, whereas the non-institutionalized population exhibited between six and seven decayed teeth.

Patients suffering from hereditary fructose intolerance are unable to consume fructose or sucrose. The caries experience in this group is known to be extremely low.

The often cited Vipeholm study was performed in a Swedish mental hospital in the late 1940s and early 1950s. This study showed that the frequency of toffee consumption and sugar clearance are the most important factors in the etiology of dental caries.

Another Scandinavian study showed that experimental caries could be induced within 23 days when a test panel rinsed nine times a day with sucrose. More recent experiments in Britain of similar design have confirmed this finding.

A Finnish clinical study where sucrose was substituted with the non-fermentable sugar alcohol xylitol in a group of students during a 2-year period resulted in development of very few cavities.

A large amount of data accumulated from animal experiments supports the view that sucrose is essential in the etiology of caries. Rats, hamsters and monkeys experience high caries incidence when sucrose is included in their diet. Other fermentable low molecular weight sugars such as glucose and fructose also induce caries in animals, but not to the same degree as sucrose.

Sucrose appears to be able to cause formation of a particularly adhesive dental plaque of high acidogenicity. If such a plaque is available, other fermentable mono- or disaccharides become good substrates for acid production. However, only sucrose appears to be able to induce large amounts of highly cariogenic plaque on smooth surfaces.

A few unprocessed products like honey and figs are known to cause dental caries to a certain degree. These products most likely only represent a marginal problem. Starch has a very low caries potential. Starch and starchy food were previously, but erroneously, suspected of being a major dietary factor in the development of dental decay. Combinations of starch and sucrose, however, have a high cariogenic potential.

The role of bacteria

The significance of the infective agent in the caries process, the bacterium, was unequivocally established by Orland and co-workers in the 1950s. Modern microbiological techniques, including studies of germfree animals, clearly demonstrated that caries-susceptible animals developed no cavities on high sucrose diets, until cariogenic microorganisms were introduced. In subsequent experiments the relative cariogenic potential of different oral bacteria was evaluated in monoinfected or gnotobiotic animals.

Such studies showed that *Streptococcus mutans* was by far the most cariogenic bacterium in animal systems. *S. mutans* produces an extracellular glucan, a glucose polymer, in the presence of sucrose, allowing *S. mutans* to establish on tooth surfaces and form an adhesive and highly cariogenic plaque. *S. mutans* is acidogenic and aciduric and this is presumably another important aspect of its high cariogenic potential.

Whereas the unique property of *S. mutans* as an infective agent in dental caries in animals is indisputable, no general agreement has been reached concerning its role in

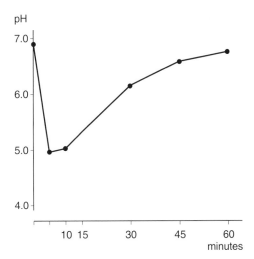

pH

Fig. 8-1. Changes in plaque pH following a 1 min rinse with 10 ml sucrose (15% w/v). The plaque was accumulated during a 3-day period with frequent sucrose rinses.

human caries. Although this bacterium in most individuals can be isolated from cavities there are also many reports of failure to isolate *S. mutans*. Microorganisms such as *Actinomyces viscosus* and *Lactobacillus casei* are capable of fermenting sugars and are often associated with human dental caries.

Recent studies where African populations have been shown to harbour high numbers of *S. mutans* and exhibit low caries rate indicate that *S. mutans*, as such, is not pathogenic. However, it becomes pathogenic when sucrose is added to the diet.

The pathogenesis of dental caries includes the establishment of the caries conducive bacterium on the tooth surface and formation of an acidogenic plaque.

The next phase in the process which leads to cavity formation in the teeth includes repeated cycles of lactic acid generation in the plaque, which cause dissolution of the mineralized dental tissues (Fig. 8-1). White spots appear on the tooth enamel underneath the plaque. This process will usually take several months, but can also occur in

matter of weeks under extreme challenges. The early changes are mainly caused by a selective dissolution of the more soluble crystal components in the surface enamel. Deeper layers of enamel which become exposed at later stages have a lower resistance and the demineralization proceeds more rapidly in this region, undermining the surface enamel. At one stage the surface breaks, bacteria enter the newly formed cavity in large numbers and the speed of the process increases. Later, a visible cavity is formed from which the demineralization of the internal regions of the tooth spreads.

The role of host-specific defense mechanisms

The major factors in the mechanism of dental caries are fairly well understood and have been outlined above. However, there is no doubt that there is wide individual variation in the response to caries challenge. It is well known that fluoride in drinking water confers an increased resistance. This aspect of caries prevention will be discussed in Chapter 9.

Many local resistance factors such as the level of IgA in serum and in saliva against salivary microorganisms have been investigated, but no clear correlation between such factors and caries resistance has been observed.

Salivary antibacterial systems like lysozyme, lactoperoxidase and thiocyanate have been compared in different groups of patients. No correlations to clinical caries have been observed. *S. mutans* is present in both caries-resistant and caries-susceptible individuals as discussed above.

The migration of workers in Europe in recent decades has shown that people from traditionally low-caries areas in southern Europe rapidly acquire a high rate of caries when they move to the industrialized countries in northern Europe.

These observations indicate that hereditary factors are of less importance in resistance to dental decay than was previously thought: sucrose consumption and use of fluorides are the dominating factors.

Caries activity tests

There is a need for a simple laboratory test by which the individual's caries activity can be determined. A large number of such laboratory tests have been devised based on:

– the ability of salivary samples to ferment sugar
– measurements of the buffer capacity of saliva
– plaque pH telemetry
– counts of Lactobacilli in saliva and, more recently,
– or the number of S. mutans in saliva.

However, it is generally accepted that simple scientific methods for prediction of the individual rate of caries incidence are not available at present. A careful clinical examination, recording the traditional signs of initial or manifest caries lesions may still be the best way of judging individual caries activity.

CLINICAL CHARACTERISTICS

The clinical picture of the caries lesion in children and adolescents differs in a number of aspects from that in adults. First of all, the lesion is often observed in its early stages. Secondly, the morphological characteristics of the primary dentition and the young and erupting permanent dentition modify the clinical symptoms of the disease.

The diagnosis of the lesion is performed using direct vision and different diagnostic aids (probes, dental floss and radiographs). Prior to the inspection of the enamel sur-

face, removal of plaque covering the surface is often required. This is important not only on free smooth surfaces, where the gingival part of the surface is often covered by a layer of plaque, but also on the occlusal surface of erupting permanent teeth, which are often covered by a gingival flap resulting in heavy plaque accumulation.

Diagnostic aids should be considered as such, i.e. as an aid to the visual examination of the enamel surface. Probing should only be performed with a very slight pressure due to the danger of damaging the enamel surface and radiographs should be used only after clinical examination and on individual indications.

Predilection sites

The most commonly observed locations (the predilection sites) in both the primary and the permanent dentition are pits and fissures, proximal surfaces and the gingival parts of free smooth surfaces. In the primary dentition less pronounced fissure systems are found than in the permanent molars. This is especially true in the first primary molars, where only a few isolated pits may be found.

The high frequency of spacing in the molar areas in the primary dentition of young preschool children reduces the number of proximal lesions. With increasing age proximal contacts are established, which may give rise to an increase of proximal lesions in primary molars.

The relatively high prevalence of caries of the upper primary central incisors is partly due to the fact that the incisal papilla at this age is situated close to the mesiolingual aspects of those teeth. This structure gives rise to increased accumulation of plaque, which in turn may lead to inflammation of the papilla followed by even greater retention of plaque.

In the primary dentition a particularly rampant type of caries may develop as early as in the first year of life (Fig. 8-2). In this type of caries large smooth-surface lesions on the labial and palatal surfaces of the incisors are seen. Since this type of caries is often caused by extensive and prolonged bottlefeeding, it has been named "baby bottle caries", "nursing bottle syndrome", "bottle mouth" and "nursing mouth". A similar clinical picture may be seen following the use of sucrose-sweetened medicine, dummies dipped in sugar, at will breastfeeding and other similar practices. The frequency of this special type of caries is decreasing in many parts of Scandinavia, but is high in many developing countries.

In the permanent dentition, attention should be given to pits on the palatal surface of the upper incisors. The upper lateral incisor usually has a well-recognized pit, but these may also be found on the upper central incisors.

On the free smooth surfaces, lesions are located in close proximity to the gingival margin. As the permanent tooth erupts, arrested lesions may be found on some parts of a surface at the same time as new lesions develop on other parts.

The buccal surface of the lower permanent molars and the palatal surface of the upper permanent molars often present a pit. This site is particularly in risk of caries during that period of the eruption, where the gingival margin is located close to the pit.

In the posterior areas of the permanent dentition the upper molars erupt with a buccal inclination and the lower molars with a lingual inclination. During the period before these teeth have reached an upright position, the upper buccal and lower lingual surfaces frequently show initial carious lesions.

The pit and fissure lesion – The initial pit and fissure lesion presents itself as a discoloration of the fissure system. Such discolorations may be either dark or white.

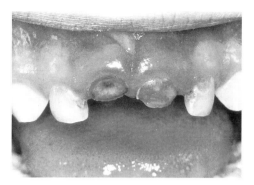

Fig. 8-2. Rampant dental caries in a 2.5-year-old boy due to extensive bottlefeeding.

The manifest pit and fissure lesion causes undermining of the enamel, as the lesion spreads at the amelodentinal junction. At this stage gross loss of substance may not yet have developed, and probing should only be performed with great care using only slight pressure. On inspection, such lesions usually manifest undermining of the enamel as a greyish discoloration extending laterally from the entrance of the fissure. In later stages, the enamel breaks down and the lesion is easily detected on visual inspection.

The proximal lesion – Lesions on proximal surfaces cannot be detected clinically during the initial stages. At later stages the buccal and palatal aspects of the lesion can, however, often be inspected after removal of plaque and gentle retraction of the interdental papilla. Especially in the primary dentition, such lesions may extend buccally and palatally as an initial decalcification from the lesion located under the contact area.

In more advanced stages, proximal lesions will result in undermining of the enamel. This in turn will result in a dark or greyish shadow, which can be observed from the occlusal aspect extending centrally from the proximal surface. In the primary dentition this sign may not be apparent until the lesion is very advanced, due to the broad contact areas found between primary molars.

The smooth surface lesion – On free smooth surfaces the carious lesion can be detected from the earliest stages. The initial decalcification results in an increased porosity of the enamel which is observed clinically as a loss of translucency. In the initial stages the lesion shows a loss of lustre and a slight roughness of the surface on probing. This latter sign is clearly demonstrated when a probe is run gently from the sound enamel onto the lesion. No clinical loss of surface continuity can be demonstrated and great care should be taken not to destroy the thin surface layer covering the subsurface lesion.

More advanced free smooth surface lesions show loss of substance which can be detected clinically as true cavities. In the early stages of this process, loss of substance may be limited to one or two areas within the original lesion. As the process progresses the entire lesion will show loss of surface-continuity, eventually exposing the carious dentin.

The acute and the chronic lesion

For the clinician an important part of the diagnosis is to evaluate the acuteness of the caries found.

No exact method of measurement of acuteness can be recommended at present, but a number of signs can be used for estimation.

The acute initial smooth surface lesion can be distinguished from the arrested initial lesions by the surface texture. As mentioned previously, acute initial lesions show a typical surface roughness. In contrast, if such lesions become arrested a hard transparent surface layer will cover the under-

lying subsurface lesion. This picture is typically found on free smooth surfaces, where initial lesions have developed in relation to the gingival margin. With the continuous eruption of the tooth, such lesions may become arrested, leaving a white spot covered by hard, smooth and shining enamel.

The acuteness of a lesion with loss of surface continuity and exposure of dentin can be evaluated from a number of different signs. Large lesions extending into less caries-prone areas of a given surface are usually considered to be acute lesions. These often show discoloration of the enamel margins typical of the undermining of the enamel by the carious lesion in the dentin. White opaque enamel circumscribing the actual cavity is thus a sign of high acuity.

Once the enamel is broken down, the lesion in the dentin can be observed. Acute dentinal lesions show only slight yellowish discoloration and the dentin is very soft and feels moist on probing. In contrast, less acute lesions show a darker discoloration with a harder dentin.

EPIDEMIOLOGY

In most of the Nordic countries, dental health of children and adolescents is recorded regularly, and data reported to central and/or local authorities using various recording levels and indices. These systems, mainly created for planning purposes, make data on, for instance, dental caries easily accessible.

Denmark was the first Nordic country to institute a National Recording System in 1972. In this system, caries data of all children are reported to the authorities annually. In Sweden, where the separate counties are responsible for the organization of dental care, the recording systems vary, but in general, dental caries in 4-, 12-, 15-, and 19-year-olds is reported.

In Finland, dental caries data are reported for all age groups annually in the same way as in Denmark. In Norway and Iceland, there are no official recording systems, but caries prevalence data are available through epidemiological studies performed in various age groups.

Caries indices

The index most commonly used to describe dental caries is the DMF-index, based on a count of units that are either decayed, missing due to caries, or filled. The unit of measurement can be the tooth or the surface (DMFT or DMFS). In the DMFS-index, the problem of missing teeth is handled differently by different investigators.

For primary teeth, the designations d, m and f are used. Instead of m, the letter e is sometimes used, originally denoting "indicated for extraction", but often simply used instead of an "m". The dmf-index is valid up to the age of 5, when exfoliation of primary teeth starts. Between 5 and 9 years of age the dmf-index is, therefore, confined to primary canines and molars. After the start of the eruption of the permanent teeth, it is common to describe dental health only by the DMF-index.

The DMF-index is a purely quantitative index and gives no information about extent and progression of disease. It is also cumulative, which means that a DMFS-score of 12 in a 15-year-old may indicate 12 open cavities needing treatment, as well as complete freedom from caries or fillings, but 4 first permanent molars extracted at an early age. The various components of the index are therefore often analyzed separately.

Even though the DMF-index has disadvantages, it is commonly used in epidemiologic studies. Indices to measure caries progression have also been constructed, especially for use in longitudinal studies and in clinical trials.

In Scandinavia, caries prevalence is still high, with 80% or more of children and young people affected when they reach their late teens. The number of teeth or surfaces that are damaged have been, however, much reduced during the last two decades, and the DMF/dmf-scores generally lowered in all age groups.

Dental caries of the primary dentition

About 50-70% of preschool children in the Nordic countries are still affected by dental caries. The teeth most commonly attacked are the molars and the upper anterior teeth, while canines and lower anterior teeth seldom show any sign of dental caries. The surfaces most commonly affected are the occlusal surfaces, specially those of the second molars, while proximal molar surfaces usually do not become carious until proximal contacts are established at the age of 5 or 6.

The most common surfaces for caries to start used to be the occlusal surfaces, or the surfaces of the upper anteriors. Today, however, bitewing radiographs in a 4- or 5-year-old child with no occlusal decay may reveal caries on the proximal surfaces.

Dental caries of the permanent dentition

In the permanent dentition, the occlusal surfaces of the molars are still the most affected.

In 1987, only 20% of Swedish 13-year-olds had any proximal surface filled or with cavitation into the dentine. Caries in permanent incisors or canines is becoming increasingly rare, and mainly found in those children in each age group who have the highest DMF-score.

Changes in dental caries prevalence

As has been mentioned, the prevalence of dental caries in the Nordic countries, as well as in most countries in Western Europe and North America, has declined during the last 10-15 years. Fig. 8-3 shows the mean dmf score in groups of 4-year-old children examined between 1967 and 1987, with the same caries criteria and examination methods employed in all studies. The shape of the curve may be representative for many age groups, with the most pronounced disease reduction during the 1970s.

Fig. 8-4 shows a similar development on the permanent dentition over a 14-year period based on data from the Danish national recording system.

The average DMF/dmf-scores in virtually all age groups have decreased by 40-70%. The reduction is largely due to an almost complete elimination of the M/m score and a reduction of the F/f score, the latter partly caused by a change in treat-

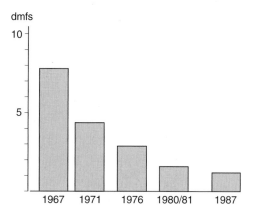

Fig. 8-3. Mean dmfs of 4-year-old children in Umeå, Sweden examined over a 20-year period.

ment philosophy. The D/d component can be high if initial lesions are included, but in general only teeth or surfaces with actual cavitation are included in the DMF-score.

Obviously, the etiology of this decline is multifactorial. In the Nordic countries the reason for this decline has been attributed to the effect of a combination of a widespread use of fluorides, not least of fluoride tooth-

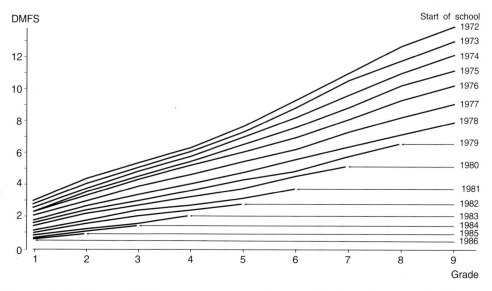

Fig. 8-4. Decline in mean DMFS over a 14-year period based on Danish national data. Each line represents a group of children according to the year of start of school.

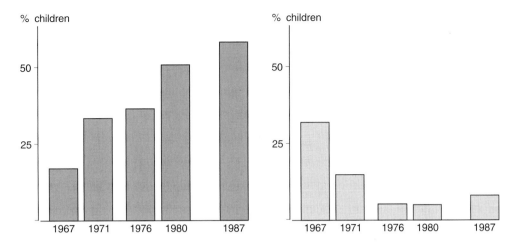

Fig. 8-5. Proportion of 4-year-old children who are caries free (left) or have a dmfs >10 (right) over a 20-year period.

paste, and an organized dental care for all children and adolescents.

There is, however, still a wide variation in caries prevalence between countries, as well as between various regions in the respective countries, due to differences in resources allocated to dentistry and to differences in the extent of the dental health programs.

With a decrease in prevalence, follows a more skewed distribution of the disease. This means, that a given fraction of all DMF/dmf teeth can be found in a smaller and smaller fraction of the children. An example of this is shown in Fig. 8-5, where the children also included in Fig. 8-3 are divided into "caries free" and "with > 10 dmfs". The group of caries-free children is continuously increasing, but the number of children with a high dmfs has not decreased to the same extent during the later part of this period in this population.

Fig. 8-6 shows a similar development over a 9-year period in 12-year-old Danish children.

The group that has the highest number of DMF/dmf teeth or surfaces, the most caries-active group, has thus reduced in size in recent decades, but is still a group of major

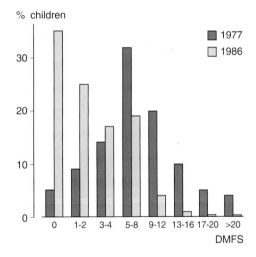

Fig. 8-6. Distribution of 12-year-old (5th graders) Danish children according to DMFS over a 9-year period.

concern. To identify these children at an early age, analyze the reasons for their poor dental health and institute adequate, individualized, preventive programs is of vital importance if the dental health of Nordic children is to be further improved.

Background literature

Thylstrup A, Fejerskov O, (eds). *Textbook of cariology*. Copenhagen: Munksgaard, 1986.

CHAPTER 9

DENTAL CARIES: PREVENTION

Fluorides
Oral hygiene
Diet
Preventive dental care

Caries prevention has attracted a great deal of interest during the last century, obviously due to the difficulties and costs associated with treatment of dental caries. The principles on which caries prevention was originally based were mechanical hygiene (toothbrushing) and change in diet (reduced sucrose consumption). Although both principles are sound from a scientific point of view even today, the results were mainly disappointing; only a small segment of the better educated part of the population was able to obtain significant caries prevention by these methods. Exceptions were periods when sugar rationing was enforced during the two world wars. These periods showed unequivocally that sucrose consumption was *the major factor* in the etiology of dental caries. The introduction of fluoride prophylaxis in the form of water fluoridation in the late 1940s and the extensive use of topical fluoride, starting 20 years later, has given us methods which are markedly more effective. The caries rate in the Western world has dropped to manageable levels during the last two decades. All data available point to the significance of the widespread use of fluoride-containing toothpaste as the major factor explaining recent successful caries prevention.

However, it is now realised that fluoride can not give one hundred per cent protection against caries. Caries has also appeared in regions of the world which traditionally did not suffer from it (Africa, some parts of Asia and South America), most likely due to urbanization and increased sucrose consumption. Caries prevention by fluoride is not easily applicable in areas where the population has no tradition in the use of toothpastes and the conditions do not allow water fluoridation.

The present chapter contains a brief, practically oriented account of caries prevention and stresses the importance of use of fluoride, of mechanical oral hygiene and the significance of diet and dietary counselling.

FLUORIDES

As mentioned above, the introduction of fluorides in caries prevention has been associated with remarkable success. It was first experienced in the United States in connection with water fluoridation programs introduced during the 1950s and the 1960s. Caries incidence was shown to be reduced in both children and adults upon the introduction of water fluoridation. It was assumed that the major mechanism of action of fluoride was systemic, with improvement of the chemical and physical properties of enamel, causing a reduced dissolution rate at low pH. However, the marked reduction in caries incidence in the Western world during the last two decades cannot be explained in terms of a systemic effect only, because the effect on the adult population with all their teeth erupted is as marked as in children. The conclusion concerning *the local* mechanisms involved was that the effect was as great, and in many authors' opinion, greater, than the systemic effect. The exact mechanism of the cariostatic effect of fluoride is thus not completely understood even now. The observed effects of fluoride on caries that could not be explained by established concepts, forced scientists to reconsider their positions and provide new ideas more consistant with the observed facts. This has been a slow and painful process and is not yet complete.

Systemic application of fluoride

The systemic route for application of fluoride was originally thought to be the most important. The observation that fluoride in the drinking water was associated with mottled enamel made this a natural conclusion at the time. The finding that even in populations which received only 1 ppm of fluoride in drinking water, about 10% exhibited symptoms of mild dental fluorosis gave further support to this concept. It should also be realized that chemical analysis of fluoride in water and in enamel was much more difficult to perform then, and this also caused slow progress in research. Clinical findings during the last two de-

cades indicate that the original emphasis on systemic fluoride, as the dominating mechanism of caries prevention, was not justified. It appears that fluoride present in plaque fluid during a caries attack may be more important. It is however generally accepted that systemic fluoride application provides some protection for the teeth against dental caries. It is well known that deciduous and permanent teeth exposed to fluoride during formation, erupt covered with a thin surface layer of fluoridated apatite of lower solubility than normal enamel. This layer of permanently bound surface fluoride clearly provides increased resistance against caries. It should also be realized that most of the data available on the level of fluoride in surface enamel are too low, because they are obtained by surface etching of successive layers of the enamel. The observed concentration of fluoride in the outer layer of the enamel is, thus, an *average* of the fluoride in a three-dimensional layer of enamel. With a steep gradient from the surface, decreasing in the deeper layers, such an average would give misleading results. There is reason to believe that the outer layer of enamel in newly erupted teeth contains a higher concentration of fluoride than previously thought, probably near to that of fluorapatite. However, it has been shown that the fluoride-rich surface layer of enamel which is a result of systemic fluoride application, is lost by wear. It is thus plausible that this aspect of systemic fluoride application provides only temporary caries prevention.

Another mechanism for systemic fluoride caries prevention has been suggested by Dutch researchers. It has been known for a long time that tooth enamel contains Mg, Na, CO_3, F and several other ions. One view is that the apatite lattice seems to be a "friendly host" for a large part of the periodic table and that tooth enamel is a single phase apatite. Another more recent view is that tooth enamel consists of three phases:

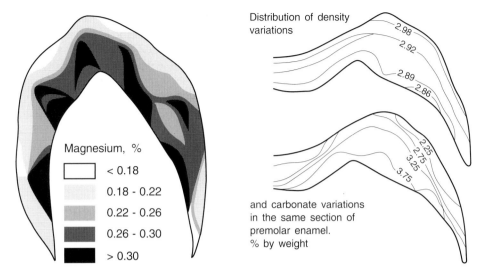

Fig. 9-1. The figure shows distribution of carbonate and magnesium in sections of teeth. Carbonate and magnesium are associated with enamel components that are more solute than hydroxyapatite and the areas which contain much carbonate or magnesium are thus susceptible to caries. Some authors assume that teeth exposed to fluoride before eruption contain less carbonate and magnesium.

magnesium whitlockite

$(Ca_9 Mg (HPO_4) (PO_4)_6)$,

a sodium- and carbonate-containing phase

$(Ca_{8,5} Na_{1,5} (PO_4)_{4,5} (CO_3)_{1,5})$,

and a slightly carbonated hydroxyapatite

$Ca_{10} (PO_4)_6 (OH, CO_3Cl, F)_2$.

Magnesium whitlockite, sodium- and carbonate-containing apatite are more soluble than slightly carbonated hydroxyapatite. This model can, to some extent, explain why Na, CO_3 and Mg are lost preferentially during early caries and partial dissolution of enamel.

Several studies have shown that the rate of acid dissolution of teeth containing pre-eruptively acquired fluoride is lower than in other teeth. It has also been shown that there is an inverse relationship between fluoride and carbonate content as a determinant of tooth susceptibility to caries. Research has come to the conclusion that the pre-eruptive effect on caries by fluoride is due to the presence of fluoride ions in the enamel during enamel mineralization, a condition which catalyzes the formation of slightly carbonated hydroxyapatite over that of magnesium whitlockite and Na- and CO_3-containing apatite; the former being less soluble than the latter, as discussed above.

The soluble components of enamel are located along the gingival margin and in the fissures. An improvement of the quality of enamel in these regions may be of particular significance because these locations are predilection sites for caries (Fig. 9-1). The concept that systemic fluoride directly alters the morphology of teeth giving shallow fissures and well-rounded cusps, has not been scientifically proven.

Two mechanisms are thus available to explain the pre-eruptive effect of F; one which emphasises the importance of fluorapatite or fluoridated hydroxyapatite in the surface, and one stressing the catalytic effect of fluoride on the enamel organ inducing formation of a "better" enamel containing smaller amounts of the more soluble enamel components. A combination of both mechanisms also appears conceivable.

Practical aspects of systemic application of fluoride

The easiest and cheapest method of systemic application is to use water fluoridation. Although a large number of studies have shown the caries preventive benefit of such administration, fluoridation has not gained a strong foothold outside USA.

A number of different factors are responsible for the limited acceptance of fluoridation of drinking water. In the past, different side-effects of fluoridation have been claimed, ranging from mongolism, cancer, and urinary problems to less defined allergic symptoms. However, none of these associations have been substantiated by research.

In rural areas large parts of the population are served by water plants with very limited technical equipment or by water from private wells. Thus, implementation of water fluoridation in such areas must be considered an unrealistic approach.

Administration of fluoride tablets may serve as an alternative to fluoridation of drinking water.

Fluoride tablets are not, however, used as frequently as could be expected. This is mainly due to the difficulty of ensuring that parental interest is maintained over a long time. In those studies where excellent co-operation has been obtained, ingestion of fluoride tablets has almost always resulted in a statistically significant reduction of dental caries.

For the administration of fluoride tablets a dosage schedule has to be followed. The dosage recommended varies with age. The recommended dosage should be adjusted to the fluoride content of the drinking water, thus making fluoride analysis necessary.

Epidemiological studies using refined criteria for classification of enamel changes have indicated an increase in the prevalence of slight enamel opacities in children consuming fluoride tablets.

When fluoride tablets are recommended, use should start at the age of 6 months and continue during the period of tooth development which means up to the age of about 12 years. In order to have a simultaneous local effect sucking or chewing of the fluoride tablets should be recommended.

Topical application of fluoride

As discussed above recent observations in many countries indicate that the effect of topically applied fluoride is of more importance than pre-eruptively applied fluoride. In particular, the widespread use of fluoride-containing toothpaste is thought to represent a major factor in the prevention of dental caries. The old concept that the mechanism by which topically applied fluoride prevents caries was by the exchange of surface OH groups with fluoride. The F content of tooth enamel is such that only about 2% of the OH groups can be replaced by fluoride in bulk enamel, and 10% in surface enamel. This is clearly not sufficient to explain the clinical effect of topically applied fluoride. The present view of the mechanism is that presence of fluoride in plaque fluid during a caries challenge causes this fluid to be supersaturated with respect to fluorapatite, and subsequently causes precipitation of this phase on the surface of the enamel as a substitute for the more soluble hydroxyapatite lost during the challenge. The stronger the challenge (the lower the pH) the more fluoride is incorporated in the precipitated phase. When pH drops so low that plaque fluid remains undersaturated with respect to fluorapatite, tooth enamel dissolves slowly, even in the presence of high concentrations of fluoride. This latter point has recently been demonstrated by induction of caries lesions in

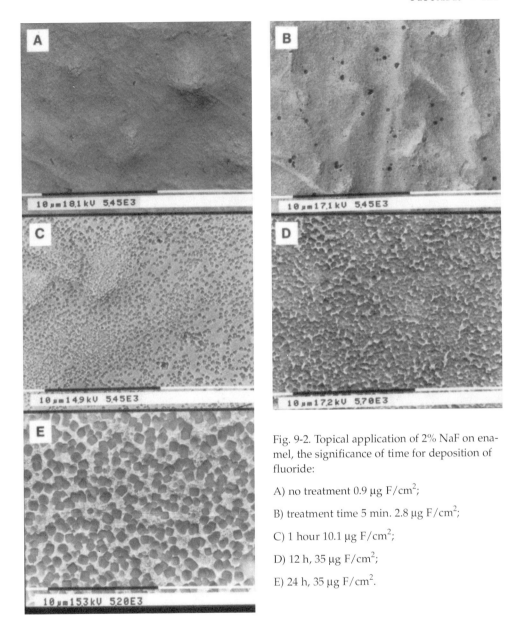

Fig. 9-2. Topical application of 2% NaF on enamel, the significance of time for deposition of fluoride:

A) no treatment 0.9 µg F/cm^2;

B) treatment time 5 min. 2.8 µg F/cm^2;

C) 1 hour 10.1 µg F/cm^2;

D) 12 h, 35 µg F/cm^2;

E) 24 h, 35 µg F/cm^2.

shark enamel (34,000 ppm of F) in the human mouth under adverse conditions (i.e. under thick layers of plaque).

If the oral hygiene is less than satisfactory, low pH may develop in plaque, and fluoride will have a reduced effect. The formation and dissolution of calcium fluoride on teeth during and after a topical application of fluoride is probably the key to understanding the cariostatic mechanism of fluoride. CaF_2 was previously thought to be rapidly lost from the tooth surfaces due to the low concentration of fluoride in saliva. However, recent experiments performed

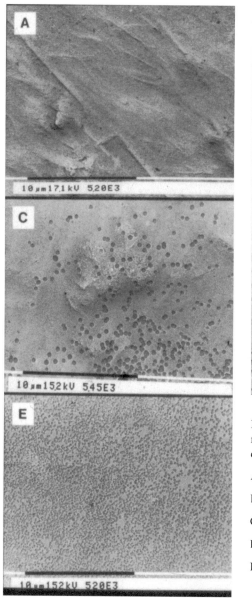

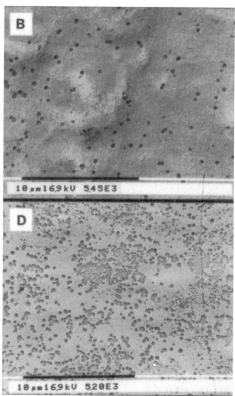

Fig. 9-3. Topical application of fluoride on enamel, the significance of concentration of fluoride for deposition of fluoride (over 1h).

A) no treatment 1.0 µg F/cm^2;

B) 0.25% NaF 2.5 µg F/cm^2;

C) 0.5% NaF 5.5 µg F/cm^2;

D) 1.0% NaF 5.8 µg F/cm^2;

E) 2.0% NaF 10.1 µg F/cm^2.

both *in vitro* and *in vivo* have shown that calcium fluoride persists in the mouth for weeks and months after a topical application of fluoride. This is due to surface absorption of phosphate ions (HPO_4^{2-}) to the calcium fluoride crystals. A dissolution-limiting phase is formed which renders CaF_2 insoluble at neutral pH in the oral cavity. When the pH is lowered during a caries challenge, the solubility limiting phase on the surface of the calcium fluoride is lost and the crystal dissolves and provides fluoride (and calcium ions) during the caries attack, thus decreasing the dissolution rate of enamel. CaF_2 crystals on enamel thus probably constitute a pH-controlled

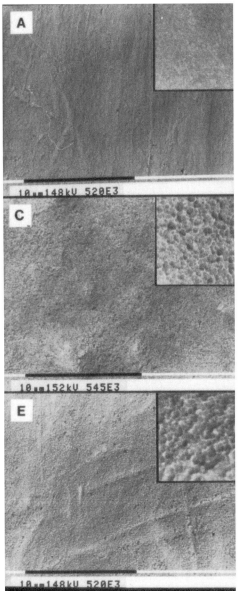

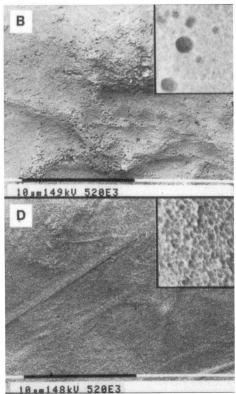

Fig. 9-4. Topical application of fluoride on enamel, the significance of pH for the deposition of fluoride (one 5-min application of 2% NaF).

A) no treatment 0.9 µg F/cm^2;

B) treatment with solution with pH 7, 2.7 µg F/cm^2;

C) treatment with pH 5.5, 12.1 µg F/cm^2;

D) treatment with pH 4.5, 33.2 µg F/cm^2;

E) treatment with pH 3.5, 30.4 µg F/cm^2.

reservoir of fluoride on the enamel which provides fluoride ions when they are needed, for extended periods of time. Calcium fluoride can presumably also form in plaque due to high concentrations of calcium in plaque fluid. CaF$_2$ in plaque may serve a similar function to CaF$_2$ on enamel. There are also new data indicating that calcium fluoride, or rather calcium fluoride-like material formed on enamel or in plaque during topical application of fluoride contains phosphate, and thus represents mixed crystals, which seem to exhibit different dissolution properties dependant on the conditions under which they are formed (i.e. fluoride concentration, pH and time of exposure). This is a field of considerable interest where more research is needed.

Conditions which favour CaF_2 formation on enamel are increased concentration of fluoride, increased length of exposure and lowered pH (Figs. 9-2, 9-3, 9-4).

Fluoride may also function by catalyzing the transformation of dicalcium phosphate dihydrate (CaHPO$_4$ • 2H$_2$O) or dicalcium-phosphate (CaHPO$_4$) to hydroxyapatite. It thus facilitates the repair mechanisms in enamel.

Fluoride is known to reduce the metabolic activity of bacteria by interaction with enzymes or with glucose uptake by the bacteria. This mechanism is probably of far less significance than the effect on the remineralization.

Fluoride is also assumed not only to increase the remineralization of enamel, but also directly to reduce the dissolution of enamel. This may be due to stabilization of surface enamel by surface adsorbed fluoride ions.

Conclusion – Calcium fluoride deposited on enamel or in plaque during topical application probably serves as a reservoir of fluoride, releasing fluoride ions during caries challenges. Fluoride increases remineralization in enamel providing a plaque fluid which is supersaturated with respect to fluorapatite during caries attacks. This phase is deposited and replaces the enamel which was lost during the caries challenge. Fluoride also reduces the demineralization of enamel, probably due to surface adsorption of F$^-$ and stabilization of the apatite surface. Fluoride furthermore catalyses the repair of demineralized enamel by transforming different acid calcium phosphates to hydroxyapatite.

A fairly good oral hygiene is a prerequisite for an optimal effect of topically applied fluoride.

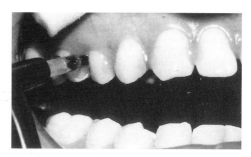

Fig. 9-5. Application of fluoride lacquer.

Practical aspects of topical application of fluoride

A variety of methods of topical application of fluoride have been developed.

The first method was by painting the fluoride solution, commonly 2% NaF, on the surface of teeth after proper cleaning. The solution is applied continuously to the teeth for 3-4 minutes. The schedule for application of the solution varied. In the original description of the method, four treatments were carried out at weekly intervals at the ages of 3, 7, 10 and 13 years. Other recommendations are annual or semi-annual applications.

Recently, fluoride-containing laquers have come on the market. These products are applied to the tooth surface after cleaning and drying (Fig. 9-5). Retention of the laquer on the tooth surface has been found to last several hours after application.

As an alternative to the application of fluorides as solution or laquer, fluoride may be applied as gels in mouth-trays. The advantage of gels over solutions is that they allow for a longer contact time between the fluoride preparations and the tooth enamel.

A number of different tray systems are available. One important aspect when selecting a system is the volume of gel used for filling the tray. In the case of some prefabricated trays, the total dose of fluoride which could be retained by a patient

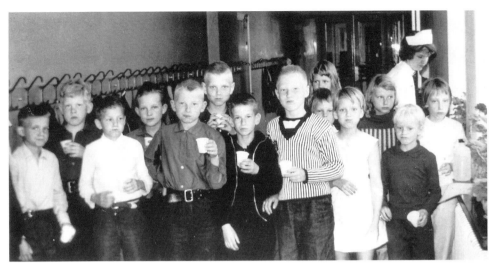

Fig. 9-6. Mouth rinses with 0.2% NaF-solution performed in school every 2 weeks.

during and after a gel treatment may exceed the dosage for initial toxic systemic reactions. Thus, individually fitted trays should be used. Mostly, the gels are applied annually or semi-annually. However, in some programs for highly caries-active children, daily application of fluoride-containing gels has been recommended.

Topical methods which can be used for self-application are fluoride mouth rinses and fluoride-containing toothpastes. These methods can be administered by the patient in a daily regime. Fluoride rinses are also used in programs where the rinses are performed under professional supervision, e.g. school-based mouth rinses every 2 weeks with 0.2% NaF-solution (Fig. 9-6). The advantages of these methods are that they require relatively few or no resources in terms of professional working hours. In such programs, careful planning has proved important in order to limit the interruption to classroom teaching.

In conclusion, caries prevention by fluoride in children should be based on the following recommendations:

– use fluoride-containing toothpaste twice daily

– in entire populations where toothpaste is not used or where large minorities show this behaviour pattern, water fluoridation should be considered as an alternative

– in schoolchildren with a reasonably high caries activity, school-based fluoride mouth rinsing programs should be instituted

– high dental caries risk patients should be treated individually with gels or laquers containing fluoride. The effect of such treatments is better the more often they are repeated. Combinations of antibacterial agents and fluoride should be tried in particular severe cases

– pre-eruptive use of fluoride (tablets, drops) is a valuable adjunct to topically applied fluoride in children if acceptable cooperation can be expected.

ORAL HYGIENE

Even if caries is a multifactorial disease, it has never been rejected that the dental plaque with its microflora plays a most central role in the development of dental caries. The importance which has been placed on oral hygiene in caries control is evident by the often presented statement "a clean tooth never decays". It is therefore understandable that a major measure in the prevention of caries is removing relevant microbial accumulations from teeth and surrounding areas (Chapter 8). There are basically two ways of achieving plaque control, mechanical and chemical.

Mechanical plaque control

Toothbrushing – Brushing of the teeth has for a long time been one of the basic components in programs aiming at prevention of dental caries. Today, about 90% of individuals in industrialized Western countries brush their teeth more or less regularly. As plaque removal today is the goal of toothbrushing, the beneficial effect on caries reduction should be obvious. Although several studies have investigated the relationship, the findings are still inconclusive. In some studies caries frequency correlates with the toothbrushing frequency or oral hygiene status prevailing when the clinical examination was performed. However, this is only static data and gives limited information about the effect of toothbrushing on caries increment. Only a restricted number of studies have followed toothbrushing habits and caries increment over several years.

Some studies have observed a correlation between frequency of toothbrushing and caries prevalence. It was found, for example, that in a group of 4-year-old children toothbrushing once a day reduced caries considerably compared with group with no regular toothbrushing habits. However, other studies were unable to demonstrate any correlation. Longitudinal studies have been carried out where children's toothbrushing habits were recorded by the use of questionnaires and the findings were related to new lesions developed during the study periods. Again results vary from almost no correlation to a slight reduction in new caries among children who brushed their teeth more than twice a day. From studies relating self-reported toothbrushing to dental caries, it can be concluded that brushing frequency bears little relation to caries prevalence. It is therefore reasonable, as several authors have, to look at the effect of brushing in terms of oral cleanliness rather than the brushing itself and relate the oral cleanliness to dental caries.

A more precise understanding has been obtained from longitudinal studies in which oral cleanliness was repeatedly recorded and related to caries increments during the same period. From these studies a clearer relationship emerged, particularly when looking at the extremes of oral cleanliness.

Mechanical oral hygiene in children involves several problems: when are children able to perform their own oral hygiene? How and when are they to be motivated for and trained in such procedures? Which methods and means are best suited in child populations?

It has been shown that parents have to brush their children's teeth at least until school age to ensure an acceptable oral hygiene.

The methods which have been used to interest children in regular oral hygiene have usually been lectures and demonstrations, audiovisal programs, or having children brush their teeth under supervision, to induce effective home practices. A number of studies aiming at achieving improved oral hygiene by increasing the children's knowledge of dental disease have been carried out. It was usually found that such approaches had only marginal effects, and slightly better results are obtained in older than in young children. Audiovisual instruction with tapes and colored slides had no effect in a study of 9-11-year-old children, as measured by plaque index in the participants 4 weeks after the instruction. To achieve a beneficial effect of toothbrushing on caries it seems important to continously repeat the information and motivate the child and the parents.

Many methods have been recommended to improve the effect of toothbrushing. In children with a limited capacity for concentration for extended periods and in whom normal dexterity is not yet highly developed, the simplicity of the method is essential. Parents will also appreciate a simple, straightforward brushing method, especially for use with small children.

The *scrub method* which involves a horizontal movement of the toothbrush along the outside and the inside of the dental arches has been shown to have a good effect performed both by children and by their parents. A convenient method by which a parent can brush the teeth of a child is illustrated in Fig. 9-7. A systematic brushing

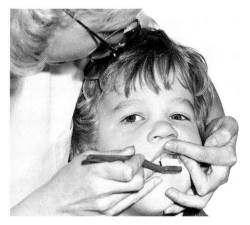

Fig. 9-7. Convenient method by which a parent can perform toothbrushing in a child.

of all toothsurfaces is important and a suitable program is presented in Fig. 9-8. It is imperative to train the parents and children in toothbrushing and monitor the procedure with *disclosing agent*s at regular intervals.

In some children the use of an electric toothbrush might stimulate interest in toothbrushing and also make the procedure

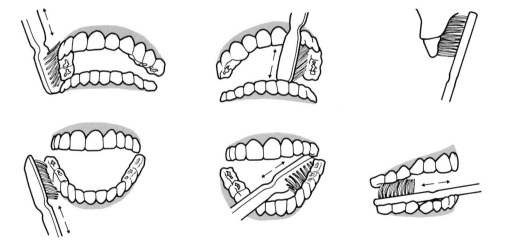

Fig. 9-8. Systematic toothbrushing. Place the toothbrush against the gingiva and cervical area of the tooth. Move the toothbrush with a scrubbing movement about 10 times in each area. When brushing the lingual surface of the incisors the toothbrush is held vertically. The occlusal surfaces are scrubbed. The sequence is shown in the picture.

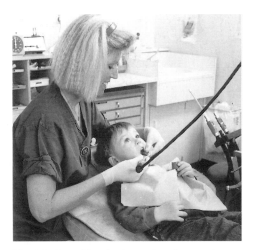

Fig. 9-9. Dental hygienist performing professional tooth cleaning.

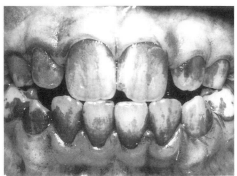

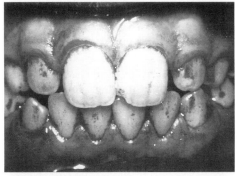

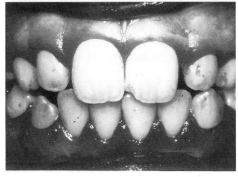

Fig. 9-10.
A. Stained plaque in situ
B. The effect of habitual toothbrushing
C. The effect of professional plaque removal

simpler for parent and child. Regular toothbrushing should be instituted in children not later than when the first primary molar erupts. It has been found that brushing once a day will control plaque accumulation. As mentioned earlier in this chapter the incorporation of fluoride in toothpastes is one of the most important measures to control caries. To maintain a desirable concentration of fluoride in the oral environment, it is recommended to brush the teeth with fluoride toothpaste twice a day, in the morning and before going to bed.

Flossing – Dental flossing has been found to be more effective than toothbrushing in reducing proximal gingivitis. As flossing is often recommended in oral hygiene programs directed against caries it is important to evaluate its effect on caries increment. In one study, based on the split mouth technique, daily professional flossing for two years in young individuals resulted in a substantial caries reduction. In other studies where the children themselves performed the flossing, sometimes under supervision, no additional effect on caries control was found. It seems justified to state that flossing if performed professionally or perfectly has a caries preventive effect on proximal tooth surfaces. Due to technical problems in performing effective flossing in children this measure should only be recommended in children with high caries activity and then as a part of a total oral hygiene and fluoride program.

Professional tooth cleaning – In children who are unable themselves or by help of their parents to achieve plaque removal to the level that high caries activity can be controlled, programs including professional tooth cleaning should be instituted, Fig. 9-9. The justification for this is a study where children every second week during a 2-year period received professional tooth cleaning and as a result showed 95% caries reduction. Even if other studies based on similar programs have not shown the same good results there is no doubt that professional tooth cleaning means good plaque control (Fig. 9-10). The intervals between professional tooth cleanings can gradually be increased to every second month as the patient's motivation and ability to perform oral hygiene increase.

Chemical plaque control

If the cariogenic part of the oral microflora can not be reduced to an acceptable level by either dietary sugar restrictions or oral hygiene measures, the use of topical antimicrobial agents effective against *S. mutans* should be considered.

The most thoroughly investigated substance is chlorhexidine, a basic multipurpose antibacterial agent which had been widely used for more than a decade before its astonishing ability to inhibit plaque formation in humans was observed. Further developments have mostly been achieved in Scandinavia, by a combination of clinical experiments and laboratory investigations. It appears that chlorhexidine and in fact a number of other cationic molecules are retained in the oral cavity and slowly released securing an antibacterial environment in the mouth for 6-8 hours after a single application. Knowledge concerning the nature of the retention and the chemical interaction taking place in the retention sites has also become available. Electrostatic interaction between negatively charged groups or the

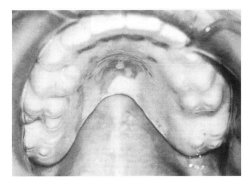

Fig. 9-11. Treatment with chlorhexidine gel in a mouth tray.

macromelecules present on the oral mucosa, in plaque and on the teeth, and the positively charged chlorhexidine molecules, seems to be the major mechanism involved. The electostatically bound chlorhexidine molecules are then slowly released, conceivably as a result of competition from calcium ions which are abundantly available in saliva.

S. mutans is highly sensitive to chlorhexidine. If high caries activity is combined with a high count of *S. mutans*, the following treatment is recommended: chlorhexidine gel 1% is applied in mouthtrays (Fig. 9-11) for 5 minutes every day for 2 weeks. The program is repeated after 3-4 months if the *S. mutans* count still is high which means more than 10^5/ml saliva. In children with low cooperation, the treatment with chlorhexidine gel can be performed in the clinic at two visits on consecutive days. At each apointment the gel is applied 3 times for 5 minutes. This program can also be used in preschool children.

The antimicrobial agents should always be used restrictedly and on an individual base. Repeated bacteria sampling of stimulated saliva should monitor the treatment program with microbial agents.

In conclusion, caries prevention by oral hygiene measures in children should be based on the following recommendations:

– brush the teeth twice daily with a fluoride toothpaste starting at eruption of
the first primary molar
– if there is high caries activity, supplement with programs including flossing
and professional toothcleaning
– with uncontrolled caries rates establish a
program of chemical plaque control.

DIET

Dietary counselling is an important part of
caries prevention. Firstly, because frequent
sugar consumption is one of the causal
factors in caries etiology, and secondly because food habits resulting in dental decay
may also lead to obesity which is a precon-
dition for more serious general diseases
such as diabetes and coronary heart disease.
Food habits learned in childhood will often
be difficult to change later in life. It is
therefore of great importance to modify
dysfunctional dietary habits, as well as to
induce positive health beliefs and attitudes
among childen and adolescents.

A child needs food for growth, development, heat production, and physical activity, but many factors other than physiological necessity influence the food habits of
children (Fig. 9-12). This is a challenge to
dental health personnel in that mere dis-
semination of information about diet and
dental health cannot be expected to influence dietary habits significantly. To do so,
other factors should be taken into account.
The different physical and psychological
stages in a child's development require different approaches. That is why this chapter
will consider each age group separately
with respect to physical and psychological
characteristics, dietary characteristics,
health risks, and target groups for counselling.

Infants (0-1 year)

Infancy is a period when the child's diet is
gradually changed from breast milk or prepared formulas to solid foods. Breastfeeding
is recommended when possible for the first
4-6 months for psychological and nutritional reasons. Breast milk contains a wide
range of antibodies which protect the child
against infections. Breast milk also seldom
causes allergy.

Because the infant's nutrient demands
are met by breastfeeding there is no benefit

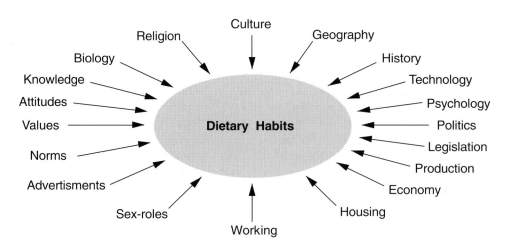

Fig. 9-12. Factors influencing dietary habits.

in introducing solid foods early in infancy. Until the child is 4 months old he sucks and swallows in one moment. At 5 months he gains control over the function of the lips and is then able to eat from a spoon. From 6 months of age the child can drink from a cup without choking on it. Thus, the introduction of solid foods to the diet should follow the child's motoric development.

Health risks – Iron deficiency is the most common nutritional disorder of infants. Breast milk or prepared formulas, however, usually prevent it. Breast milk and prepared formulas also eliminate the need for fruit juices as a source of ascorbic acid and the need for supplemental vitamins. Thus, fruit juices can be delayed until cup feeding begins.

If a child is allowed to suck frequently on a nursing bottle (containing sucrose in liquid or fruit juice) or a sweetened pacifier after tooth eruption, there is a risk of developing rampant caries (Chapter 8).

Since treatment of carious lesions is difficult at this age because of poor child cooperation, prevention is necessary. Topical fluoride application can be effective both in preventing and treating rampant caries. But of course the most important prevention is to inform the parents about the risks associated with bad breast and bottle feeding practices in order to establish sound eating patterns from the very first day of a child's life.

Target groups – The target groups for nutritional counselling in relation to infants are primarily expectant mothers and fathers. The advantages of breastfeeding should be stressed, but also the risk of nursing caries. Many new parents are confused by the contradictory suggestions they get from relatives, neighbors or friends. In modern society the health threat is very complex and scientific knowledge changes very fast. It is therefore important for the dental health profession to inspire confidence in matters concerned with dietary practice and dental health.

Toddlers (1-3 years)

The accelerated growth of the child decreases after the first year. Accordingly, the caloric needs of toddlers are less per kilo body weight than are those of infants. This may lead toddlers to refuse foods simply because they are not hungry. Another characteristic of toddlers is their need to assert their independence, which can be done by refusing certain foods. In both situations it is very important not to overfeed the child since the roots of obesity may lie in this age group, and insisting that they eat may lead to their rejection of certain foods later.

Health risks – From one year of age most children eat the same diet as the rest of the family, which often has a high content of fat and sugar. Apart from leading to overweight and dental caries, a sweet and fat diet also decreases the appetite for nutritious foods. Nutrition surveys indicate that the nutrients most often lacking in the diet of toddlers are iron and vitamin D. If a child is a heavy milk consumer the risk of iron deficiency increases because of the low iron content in milk. Therefore, milk consumption should be restricted to ½-¾ liter per day; the supplementary drink should be water. Vitamin D is essential for Ca-metabolism. Lack of this vitamin may lead to malformation of bones and teeth (rickets). In the northern countries, where lack of sunshine limits the supply of vitamin D, it is extra important to ensure a diet containing this vitamin (fatty fish, eggs, margarine, butter, milk).

Target groups – During working hours most children in modern Scandinavia are taken care of by persons other than the parents. To ensure a balanced diet for these children it is very important to coordinate the diet offered to the child during the day.

Often candy and other sweets are given to children by grandparents and other relatives in an attempt to communicate love. Also parents use or withhold sweet foods as reward or punishment. Besides the cariogenic effect of sweet foods, such practices may influence children's attitudes toward sweet consumption, relating it to good or bad emotions. Therefore, adults should be made aware of this perspective and encouraged to express their emotions in a more appropriate way, and to limit candy consumption to once a week followed by tooth brushing.

The children of immigrants from southern countries are at high risk of developing rickets, partly because they move to an area with less sunshine and partly because immigrant children often adopt the habits of sweets and soft drink consumption very quickly. Apart from the risk of vitamin D deficiency these practices are very dangerous for the children's dental health, since these families often have very little knowledge about oral hygiene and use of fluoride toothpaste or fluoride tablets. It is the responsibility of the health authorities to draw attention to this specific problem.

Preschool (3-6 years)

Preschool children are in an age group of growth spurts and increased activity, which may lead to fluctuating appetite and changing food preferences. Refusal to eat regular meals during preschool age is common. It is, however, important that the parents are not too concerned about food refusals. If a child knows that more popular food is available after a regular meal, of course it will eat less during the meal. Thus, some structure in eating practices is beneficial to preschool children, because otherwise they will lose the opportunity to experience hunger.

Health risks – The health risks of preschool children are the same as those of toddlers (dental caries, overweight, and malnutrition).

Target groups – Like toddlers, many preschool children spend the day in day-care centers or preschools. The dietary practices at these institutions are, of course, very important. People employed in child care are an important target group for dietary advice. Consciousness of candy consumption is normally high in institutions, but often knowledge about other sources of sugar is very low. Especially drinking practices need attention. Many grown-ups offer sweetened soft drinks to children instead of fresh water. Water is an excellent way of coping with thirst and has the advantage of being non-cariogenic and non-caloric.

Another challenge to children's eating habits is television advertising. Parents are advised to be aware of what children are watching and not to succumb to the child's insistence on certain foods that may be low in nutrients and high in sugar content.

School-age (6-12 years)

The appetite of school-children is usually good because of physical activity and growth. Due to a more structured food environment at school, frequency of food consumption is reduced, and snacking is usually limited to after school hours. At this age children have more access to money than preschool children, allowing for less influence from parents and more dependence on peer groups, at least with respect to snacking habits.

Health risks – Most often the energy needs of this age group are met, and even exceeded. Overweight among children is an increasing problem in many countries. Overweight children tend to withdraw from social and physical activities because of teasing. Obviously, this results in a vicious circle if help is not offered at an early stage. Overweight children frequently retain their weight into adolescence, taking with them the same food selection patterns. They can benefit from dietary counselling and weight control to avoid problems later. From a dental health perspective, focus should be on the eruption of permanent teeth. During this period (from 6-12 years) the permanent dentition erupts. When a tooth is newly erupted it is more susceptible to caries because of a low degree of maturity of the enamel. At this age children also feel that they have full control over their toothbrushing, making them refuse any assistance. Therefore, sugar consumption between meals is especially risky in this age group.

Target groups – The parents of school children still exert the greatest influence over main meals. Therefore, they should be encouraged to ensure a balanced diet to minimize the need for snacking. School teachers can contribute to establishing healthy group norms by their personal eating practice and by rules negotiated in class concerning snacking. Both teachers and students benefit from nutrition education offered by dental health personnel.

Adolescents (12-19 years)

Early adolescence is characterized by a marked increase in physical energy accompanied by an increase in appetite. The peer group becomes more important and influential while adult standards and patterns of behavior may be questioned and challenged. Less time spent at home, more time spent with friends, and easier access to money contribute to an increase in snacking behavior and less regular eating patterns. The fast food and confectionary industries aggressively target a large segment of their advertising efforts toward this age group, equating food and beverages with fun, sociability, and peer acceptance.

Health risks – Erratic eating practices include frequent snacking of high carbohydrate and/or fat and salty foods. The health risks of these practices are obesity and dental caries.

Young girls are also at risk of developing iron deficiency because of blood loss during menstruation. Iron supplements can be necessary, since iron is not usually found in the popular food items of this age group.

Anorexia nervosa is a complex syndrome mostly affecting adolescent girls. It is a psychiatric disorder characterized by refusal to eat or retain food. The dental symptoms can be erosions caused by gastric acid from repeated vomiting. If dental personnel become aware of such signs they should alert the family physician, because untreated, the condition can lead to absence of the menarche and suppression of the development of the secondary sexual characteristics. In addition, the dietary pattern and changes in the salivary composition can result in a dramatic caries development.

Target groups – Adolescents are usually very concerned about their appearance, particularly skin problems and body weight. Dental caries may, however, not be considered as a motive for dietary changes, since many adolescents do not feel susceptible to dental caries and the perceived severity of it is low. Therefore, dietary counselling and health education should be directed to food intake relative to appearance.

Since much adolescent snacking takes place during leisure time, the subculture of sports clubs and recreation centres plays a significant role. In most sports and recreation centres a wide range of unhealthy products are sold (soft drinks, sweets and snacks). Specially formulated "sports drinks" containing glucose are also pro-

Instructions for filling in the food diary

1. Use one hole page per day

2. State of time

3. Remember to note all products entering the mouth (i.e. soft drinks, fruit or sweets, dried fruit, chewing gum, throat pastilles)

4. Only absolute honesty and exactly filled in diaries makes it possible to evaluate the dietary intake

Example

Time	Thursday 1989-05-01
7.30	Cornflakes with milk and 1 spoonful of sugar 1 slice of white bread with butter of jam 1 glass of orange juice
8.50	1 orange
9.40	2 pieces of candy
11.50	1 piece of black bread with 2 slices of salami 1 piece of black bread with liverpaste 10 g of cucumber, 1 tomato
11.15	1 chocolate bar
14.30	1 glass of lemonade, 2 buns
18.00	3 meat balls, 2 potatoes, 2 carrots 1 glass of milk, 1 apple
20.00	1 glass of lemonade, 1 sandwich with cheese

Fig. 9-13. Instructions for filling in the food diary and an example.

moted for their beneficial effects on sports performance. The way they are consumed is, however, relevant to dental health. In this context, the youth leader is of great importance since he/she may play a significant role as a model.

It is very difficult for a young person to change snacking practices when under group pressure. Therefore, the most effective means of health education for this age group is to influence peer group norms. This can be done either by a direct approach to the pre-established peer groups (e.g. school classes, sports clubs) or by an attempt to influence group norms via mass media (e.g. television, movies, youth magazines).

Dietary counselling

The objectives of dietary counselling are to:

– direct attention to the influence of dietary intake on dental health and disease,

– help modify food selection patterns for better dental and general health,

– direct attention to the environmental influence on dietary habits, and to

– facilitate healthy choices.

Diet Analysis
Use the chart below to record number
of servings each day

Food group	Suggested no. of daily servings (school children)	No. of servings			Portion considered for 1 serving
		Day 1	Day 2	Day 3	
Milk, milk products	2 - 3*				250 ml milk; 10 g cheese
Meat, fish, poultry, egg	2+				50 g cooked lean, meat, poultry or fish; ¼ egg
Fat	1 - 2 (max)				20 g butter, margarine or fat
Fruit, vegetables	4 - 5				50 g vegetables or fruits;
Breads, cereals, potatoes	3 - 5 ·				1 slice of bread; 1 medium-sized potato

* Adolescents and pregnant and nursing women: 3 - 4 servings
+ Preschoolers 1½ serving
· Preschoolers 2 - 3 servings

Fig. 9-14. Form for evaluation of the appropriate number of servings and examples of one serving in the different food groups.

How to implement the dietary counselling depends on many factors, among which are the age of the children and the character of the dental health problem.

Individual counselling – When clinical examination reveals high caries activity, relevant information about the child's food habits must be collected to identify those dietary factors believed to be of major importance for the uncontrolled progress of caries, and to explore the norms and expectations of the parents and child. Various techniques have been devised to determine an individual's food intake. One technique is to let the child or parents record the dietary intake during the preceeding 24 hours, called 'the 24-hour recall'. This method has the disadvantage of not being representative of an individual's diet. Another technique is to obtain a written food record, where the parent or child is asked to write down in detail everything he or she eats and drinks during three to seven consecutive days. To clarify how detailed this book keeping has to be, the patient is shown an example of such a dietary record (Fig. 9-13). The weakness of this method is that it is rather demanding on the patient. A third method is to interview the patient about his/her usual dietary habits, using a technique called dietary history interview, where one can choose to ask about the dietary pattern during the last week. The usefulness of this method depends on the interviewer's neutrality and the memory and honesty of the patient. Neither of the methods are applicable to children below 10-12 years. Here, the parents should complete the records.

The suitability of the various methods is dependent upon the context, the patient, and the dentist. Despite the weaknesses of the different methods, they are, however, valuable for tailoring the dietary advice to the life-style and particular needs of the individual child. Special attention should be given to children with a special diet (allergies, medication, vegetarian). It is recommended that dietary counselling should always start by letting the patients (be it children or parents) evaluate their own recorded diet. It reveals their knowledge and attitudes toward the problem and gives the dentist an opportunity to adjust the message to each individual.

Following facts should be stressed:

– frequent sugar intake is the most important caries-inducing dietary factor

– the composition of meals determines the state of satiety and, thereby, affects the need for between-meal nibbling.

A special form can be used to evaluate the dietary intake (Fig. 9-14). The servings of each food group are recorded, one mark for each serving, and the total intake for each day is compared with the recommended amount. For evaluation of sugar intake a separate form can be used (Fig. 9-15). The child or the parents can be asked to circle all the foods on the record that contain sugar; this teaches where hidden sugar can be found, and often the frequency of sugar intake is considerably larger than anticipated. Another way is to use the sugar clock (Fig. 9-16), which is an excellent aid, because it causes the patient to realize for how many hours of the day acid production takes place in the mouth.

The long-term goal of individual dietary counselling is to starve the acid-producing bacteria in the oral cavity by a reduced sugar intake. The amount of these bacteria (*S. mutans* and lactobacilli) can be monitored by tests, which can also be used to motivate the patients. The changes should be negotiated and realistic goals defined in agreement with parents and child. Remember that stepwise inprovements are better than ambitious efforts in changing a life style totally. Any dietary counselling should be followed up during the course of treatment to evaluate the outcome and reinforce positive results.

Each positive inclination to change should be taken seriously and encouraged.

Group strategies – It is very hard to change behaviour without support. Small children need support from their parents, parents need support from family members, big children from their parents and peers, and peer groups from the school teachers and youth leaders. That is why it is very important to create positive group norms in order to support positive eating habits. Several psychological theories have been put forward to explain how social norms are influenced. One way is through group discussions, where pre-existing groups (e.g. expectant parents at a maternity course, parents to children in a kindergarten, teachers at a school, school classes, members of a sports club) discuss their attitudes toward diet as a prohealth measure in order to reveal their own attitudes and to come to an

Frequency of Sucrose Exposures

	Day 1	Day 2	Day 3
At meals			
Between meals			
Total			

Fig. 9-15. Form for evaluation of the sucrose intake.

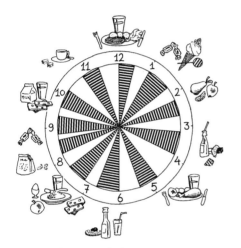
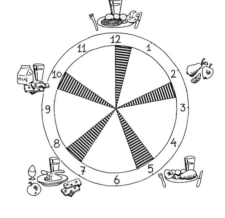

Fig. 9-16. The sugar clock.

understanding of the norms shared by the group. Here, the dentist can play a significant role as an initiator and introducer of such group activities.

Conclusion

The objective of diet counselling is to help people to maintain or to develop healthy habits. The multitude of factors influencing dietary habits (Fig. 9-12) makes this a very challenging task. As pointed out in this chapter the approach can be individually oriented and/or group oriented. There is also a third approach which is political.

Governmental influence on availability and accessibility of food products is high. Therefore, it can be concluded that the parents and children have a personal responsibility for their food selection, while society has the responsibility of making healthy choices easy.

PREVENTIVE DENTAL CARE

During the last decade preventive measures have been extensively introduced in the field of children's dentistry. Today, it is a well-documented fact that reparative dental care as such has very limited value if treatment is not also directed against the cause of the dental diseases. Our knowledge of the mechanism underlying the development of carious lesions and gingival inflammation is sufficiently well established to recommend prophylactic programs for all age groups and individuals. However, in spite of all our knowledge it has often proved difficult to implement practical methods of optimal prophylactic dental care adapted to both the individual and the community. The reasons may be several: deficient education of the dental team, attitudes among children and patients, and in particular the basic difficulty of changing the pattern of dental care from reparative to prophylactic. Another problem might be to find a suitable organizational form for functioning preventive dental care.

It is important to realize that preventive dental care must be integrated with other dental care and is, therefore, the responsibility of all members of the dental team. Preventive dental care is not only the application of prophylactic measures to the child patient, but also activities directed to such key groups around the child as parents, teachers, hospital personnel, etc.

The objectives of preventive dental care of children and adolescents are to keep the dental disease activity to an acceptably low level. Programs aiming at eliminating caries and gingivitis completely are unrealistic if they are to be applied to groups of children.

Epidemiologic studies have shown that the distribution of dental diseases among children is skewed. This means that in a small number of children we have to expect a very high disease activity compared with other children in the group. Preventive dental care, therefore, should be planned as a *basic program* for all children and an *additional program* to be applied to childen with high disease activity and children belonging to certain risk groups: children with bleeding disorders, heart and kidney diseases, etc.

The preventive capacity of the *basic program* should give sufficient control of the disease activity in 80-90% of the children, e.g. the children who are most easily influenced and also often have a low or more moderate disease activity.

For the rest of the children, about 10%, additional programs have to be used. It is uneconomical and, therefore, inappropriate to apply a dental health care program intended for children showing the highest disease activity to the whole child population.

Basically, all preventive dental care should be adapted individually to the needs of each patient. In most child populations, however, it has proved most beneficial from a cost-benefit aspect to run the preventive programs as a combination of collective and individual measures. When systems of preventive dental care are developed they may differ somewhat according to the dental delivery system in the respective region, but they will have the same approach.

Prerequisites for accomplishment

Team approach – Without a well-educated and motivated dental team a preventive dental care program will fail. It is therefore important to educate the team in recognition of early stages of lesions that can be controlled by prophylactic measures, etiology of dental diseases, measures of plaque control, use of fluorides, dietary counselling and psychology involved in applying preventive dental care in children.

The successful outcome of a prophylactic program is based on close co-operation between the various members of the dental team, i.e. the dentist, the dental hygienist, the preventive dentistry assistant (a dental assistant with special training in preventive dentistry) and the dental assistant. It is therefore essential that they are all well aware of what each member of the team does and what responsibilities they have, and that all are trained in working as a team to carry out the various preventive programs.

Epidemiology: evaluation – Another important prerequisite for the practice of effective preventive dentistry is the knowledge of the distribution of diseases in the child population so that a reasonable selection of children can be made for exposure to the various programs. Therefore, epidemiologic systems where the disease distribution is shown and where the effect of the prophylactic program can be monitored, analyzed and presented to the dental team are of great importance. The use of specially adapted dental charts, which enables the dental team to follow closely the individual response of children exposed to the differentiated preventive programs is also of decisive importance.

Dental health care programs

In the following, some examples of how basic and additional programs could be performed are presented.

Basic program – This program is applied to all children and includes measures of an individual, as well as a collective, character. The basic program consists of an information section, a plaque control section and a fluoride section all adapted to the needs of the various age groups. The information concerns the etiology and prevention of dental diseases and dietary counselling. It is given initially to the expectant mother and continues thereafter at the child health center and throughout the school years. Information during the school years takes the

form of motivational lectures at school and individual information in connection with dental treatment. The recommendations are simple: promote good dietary habits (which means sugar control), achieve good oral hygiene, and use fluorides.

Plaque control is based on information and instruction to give an understanding of the need for good oral cleanliness and ways of achieving it.

When the child is 12 months of age toothbrushing should be established. From the age of three years there is at least one instruction session every year when disclosing solution may be used to guide the parents in carrying out effective toothbrushing for the child. From the age of seven when the school program starts, oral hygiene is checked twice a year using a disclosing solution and at the same time instruction and training is given based on the degree of plaque. Occasionally, instruction in flossing for proximal cleaning is given. Most of these activities are performed by specially trained dental assistants at school or clinic.

Fluoride program – This is mainly based on topical fluoride applications. Fluoride tablets can be recommended and prescribed when the child visits the child health centre. This is reinforced during preschool age at yearly visits to the dental clinic from the age of 3 years. The use of tablets can be prolonged up to the age of 8-12 years.

From the age when the first primary molars erupt, daily toothbrushing with fluoride toothpaste is recommended. Topical fluoride applied at the yearly dental treatment sessions may consist of sodium fluoride solutions or fluoride varnish.

From 6-7 years of age children often take part in organized, collective weekly or fortnightly mouth rinsings at school with a 0.2% sodium fluoride solution. Such regimens have been routine since the 1960s. However, the frequent and increasing use of fluoride toothpastes has questioned the via-

TABLE 9-1

Additional preventive program for children with high caries activity. Each appointment requires 30-45 minutes

Appointment	Procedure	Comments
1	Information	Aims at presenting the reasons for performing an additional preventive program and gives condensed information about the etiology and prevention of caries.
	Salivary tests: secretion rate and buffering capacity	These tests are mostly used in teenagers. Simple methods have been developed for clinical use. A secretion rate below 1 ml/min and a buffering capacity below pH 4.5 should be looked upon as low and indicate high caries risk.
	Bacteriological tests: lactobacilli and S. mutans counts	A simple clinical method of determining the number of lactobacilli in saliva has been developed. A high number of lactobacilli indicates frequent consumption of carbohydrates and the test could be used as a basis for the dietary recommendations. S. mutans count may be indicated in severe cases in order to monitor the use of antibacterial agents (see p. 126).
	Dietary and medication history	24-hour recall in order to find a basis for dietary counselling (See appointment 2).
	Gingival index: according to gingival bleeding index system	
	Oral hygiene control	Bacterial plaque visualized with disclosing solution.
	Oral hygiene instructions and recommendations	Toothbrushing training. In cases with several proximal carious lesions in permanent teeth flossing is demonstrated.
	Professional tooth-cleaning including topical fluoride application	

Appointment	Procedure	Comments
2. One week later	Oral hygiene check	See Appointment 1
	Dietary counselling	Based on the dietary habit history taken at Appointment 1 recommendations are given in an attempt to reduce the number of consumptions to 5-6 per day. Special habits such as frequent intake of sweetened beverages, extensive snack and candy consumption, cough syrup, etc., are noted and recommendations made in an effort to change the habits.
	Audiovisual program	AV-program about etiology and prevention of caries, adapted to the age of the child, is presented.
	Professional tooth-cleaning including topical fluoride application	
3. One week later	Gingival index	To check the oral hygiene measures recommended. An improvement of at least 60% is required.
	Dietary habit check	
	Institution of intensified fluoride program	A fluoride gel program can be carried out at home. A 0.2% NaF gel applied in trays is used for 5 minutes every day for one month. As an alternative daily mouthrinsing and in yonger children toothbrushing with an 0.2% NaF solution can be performed.
4. One month later	**Evaluation** Gingival index	See Appointment 3
	Dietary habit check	See Appointment 1
	Oral hygiene check Bacteriological tests	Exceptionally, lactobacilli test may be used to control the change of dietary habits.
	Professional tooth-cleaning including topical fluoride application	Fluoride varnish application
5. Six months later	Follow-up	See measures (appointment 4)

bility of the additional caries preventive effect of fluoride mouth rinsings.

Additional programs for children with high disease activity – These are intended for individuals who, although exposed to the basic program, continue to exhibit a high disease activity. Children showing a great number of active initial carious lesions, several manifest proximal carious lesions, gingivitis or marginal bone loss should be included in such programs.

An additional program consists fundamentally of an *intensive* period of 3-5 appointments at intervals of one or two weeks and thereafter a *follow-up* period. The individualized program aims at investigating causal factors in the light of the clinical findings. Additional preventive programs imply analysis, motivation, education, demonstration, instruction and evaluation.

The practical application of the program is mostly carried out by preventive dentistry assistants or dental hygienists. Table 9-1 gives a schematic presentation of the procedures which may be performed at the different appointments when a child shows high caries activity.

If the evaluation reveals that the program has had an acceptable effect, the child should go back to the basic preventive program. At the next yearly visit to the dental clinic the findings will determine whether the child should again be subjected to an additional preventive program. However, if the effect of the intense prophylactic period is not substantial, it is important to analyze the situation in order to find out if the measures applied have to be changed or if the co-operation of the patient is lacking. This will be done in discussion where the dentist and the preventive dentistry assistant together plan the further approach and decide whether complementary tests or examinations (e.g. medical examination) have to be carried out. In some cases it may then prove useful to repeat the intensive period with some few modifications and in other cases it might be necessary to change the program completely, e.g. if the child has an uncontrolled disease activity and co-operation is considered very low and is difficult to improve. In such cases it is important to put the child on a more controlled program, for example weekly professional tooth cleaning and topical fluoride applications or chemical plaque control. In this way it is possible to keep the disease activity under control until co-operation has improved. It can be argued whether this is a justified use of prophylactic resources. However, these children are very few, often less than 5% of the child population, and experience has also shown that most of them will show increased motivation and co-operation within a year. The obligation of the dental team must include enforced activities to help children overcome critical periods in their dental disease.

Background literature

Ekstrand J, Fejerskov O, Silverstone LM, (eds). *Fluoride in dentistry.* Copenhagen: Munksgaard, 1988.

Granath L, McHugh WD, (eds). *Systematized prevention of oral disease:* theory and practice. Boca Raton, Florida: CRC Press, 1986.

Krasse B. *Caries risk.* A practical guide for assessment and control. Chicago: Quintessence, 1985.

Randolph PM, Dennison CJ. *Diet, nutrition, and dentistry.* St. Louis: Mosby, 1981.

Thylstrup A, Fejerskov O, (eds). *Textbook of cariology.* Copenhagen: Munksgaard, 1986.

CHAPTER 10

DENTAL CARIES: ANALYSIS OF DISEASE FACTORS

Dental caries: a multifactorial disease
Interpretation of data on caries prevention
Interaction of factors in disease
Estimation of effects of preventive measures
Prediction
Cost/value of preventive measures

DENTAL CARIES: A MULTIFACTORIAL DISEASE

Biological aspects

Dental caries is commonly described as a result of exposure of the teeth to easily fermentable carbohydrates and bacterial plaque. The etiology of the disease is, however, more complex than that, as is apparent from Chapter 8.

In addition to the composition of food, the pattern of intake, quantity and quality of dental plaque, quantity and quality of saliva, age and composition of the tooth and the fluoride concentration of saliva are factors of importance.

These biological variables interact in a complicated system by creating various combinations that influence the outcome of disease in the individual. Our knowledge about the effect of these various combinations is limited and requires further development. What is known today, should, however, be taken into consideration when preventive programs are planned and implemented. Knowledge of these interactive processes is also important as a basis for prediction of new disease. Further, cost/value considerations should be included at an early stage of planning of preventive programs.

Statistical methods

The above-mentioned interaction phenomena are studied statistically mainly through 1) subgroup analysis and 2) multivariate methods. With the first, results of the influence of single or combined variables are interpretable in terms of a reduction of the total amount of disease. The most common of the second type of method is multiple regression analysis. With this method, percentage explanatory values of single or combined independent variables are obtained with due consideration of the impact of the remaining variables under study.

INTERPRETATION OF DATA ON CARIES PREVENTION

The absolute effect of a caries-preventive measure tested in a specified population is mostly expressed as the difference between the mean values of disease of a control group (C) and an experimental group (E). To be able to apply the results on other populations, the absolute difference is converted to relative difference, according to the expression {(C-E)/C}100. This is termed "the percentage reduction". Such figures obtained from experimental clinical trials (the so-called clinical effectiveness) are expected to be higher than those obtained under more realistic conditions, for instance in a community clinical trial where the community effectiveness is established(12). This is assumed to be due to field attenuation, which means that optimal conditions for the preventive agent cannot be maintained under everyday conditions. Further, the final impact of the preventive measure, i.e. the net effectiveness, is influenced by the degree of public acceptance(7).

Percentage reduction is an acceptable way to describe the preventive effect, given that an adequate number of studies covering various levels of disease are available for calculation of "the average percentage reduction". Unfortunately, little attention has been paid to the concept of estimating statistically valid average reduction figures. Relevant methods are available, based on principles of interaction. These will be described in the next section of this chapter.

One of several problems when different preventive methods are to be compared is that some studies report prevalence data,

others are based on incidence data. Examples of the former group are observational (field) studies of the caries-preventive effect of water fluoridation and many of the early studies of fluoride tablets. Randomized clinical trials of, for instance, the effect of mouthrinse programs are examples of the latter. Prevalence and incidence data cannot be compared, and no method has been devised for converting the one measurement to the other.

INTERACTION OF FACTORS IN DISEASE

Principles

Interaction between factors in a process of disease means the reciprocal actions between disease-provoking and disease-preventing factors as they relate to the disease. These phenomena are of great importance in analytical epidemiology. In a practical sense, interaction results in effect-modification(9).

Table 10-1 shows dental caries, diet and oral hygiene in a group of 3-year-old children. Interaction is present, since subgroup mean caries values ($\bar{x}$) vary with different levels of one factor at different levels of the other factor (subgroup analysis). The most pronounced expression of the interaction phenomenon is found when moving diagonally from combination D1/O1 to combination D3/O3. This and similar results from many other studies have created the basis of a fundamental rule of interaction, which says that the absolute effectiveness of a preventive measure increases with the adversity of other factors in the disease process. This should be held apart from relative effectiveness, which will be dealt with later on.

What can be learned from the above? Different people have different habits, often

TABLE 10-1

Mean caries values in 143 3-year-old children in relation to dietary and oral hygiene habits for demonstration of interaction between the habits. From(15).

Oral hygiene	Dietary habits		
	D3	D2	D1
O3	9.2	4.6	2.6
O2	2.9	2.0	0.1
O1	0.8	0.1	0.1

D3 ≥ 2, D2 = 1-2 and D1 ≤ 1 regular unsuitable eatings per day; O3 = general gingivitis with bleeding on probing, O2 = partial or general gingivitis without bleeding on probing and O1 = practically without clinical signs of gingivitis.

related to their life-style. It is probably easier to alter the level of disease of an individual with a high caries activity, as a result of unsatisfactory diet and insufficient oral hygiene, than that of an individual who is already controlling his caries activity quite well, by practising one good habit. To further reduce the disease can be rather difficult. This applies also at the community level and should be considered, when preventive programs are planned so we do not grant success on a routine basis. Relevant background factors should always be taken into account.

Confounding

A particular type of effect-modifier is the confounder(9,10). A confounder is a factor that on one side is associated with the exposure under study, on the other it is in itself a risk indicator of the disease. It is moreover a risk indicator in absence of the association in question, which means that it is also a risk indicator for non-exposed individuals. A positive confounder is a factor that exag-

TABLE 10-2

Caries-preventive effect in 4-year-old children of chewing NaF tablets from 2-3 years of age, before and after correction for the confounding effect of diet. From(5).

Diet	Non-tablet group		Tablet group		$\bar{x}_1 - \bar{x}_2$
	n	% $\bar{x}_1$	n	% $\bar{x}_2$	
Very unsuitable	90	(57) 8.3	30	(37) 6.7	1.6
Unsuitable	47	(29) 3.2	29	(35) 3.8	-0.6
Suitable	22	(14) 2.1	23	(28) 1.3	0.8
Group mean		5.9*		4.1	1.8
Weighted subgroup mean difference					0.6**

n = number of children in groups previously matched for toothbrushing; $\bar{x}$ = subgroup mean value of smooth surface caries in posterior teeth; difference between groups on distribution in dietary subgroups: $\chi^2 = 20.2$, d.f. = 2, P < 0.001.

$$* \; \frac{90 \times 8.3 + 47 \times 3.2 + 22 \times 2.1}{90 + 47 + 22}$$

$$** \; \frac{30 \times 1.6 - 29 \times 0.6 + 22 \times 0.8}{30 + 29 + 22}$$

gerates the effect of the exposure, a negative confounder masks the effect. Confounding is one of the major systematic errors in epidemiology and can be controlled by, for instance, sampling restrictions, subgroup or multivariate analysis and by randomization in controlled clinical studies.

Table 10-2 gives an example of how the relationship between smooth surface caries in posterior teeth in a group of 4-year-old children (40 surfaces per individual) and chewing of fluoride tablets is corrected for the confounding effect of diet. For simplicity, the two groups had been matched

TABLE 10-3

Average effects on posterior smooth surface caries in 4-year-old children of practising diet, oral hygiene or chewing fluoride tablets at a more favourable level with the other habits kept constant, studied by means of subgroup analysis. From(5).

	Buccal and lingual caries			Approximal caries		
	m	P	% diff	m	P	% diff
D3 vs D1	2.9 (2.7)	< 0.001	86 (84)	3.3 (3.7)	< 0.001	68 (71)
O3 vs O1	1.3 (2.0)	NS	39 (54)	4.1 (3.4)	< 0.01	43 (51)
F3 vs F1	-0.1 (1.3)	"	46 (57)	1.0 (2.9)	< 0.01	51 (69)

The data were computed from caries values in combinations of habits comprising more than 5 individuals; D1 ≤ 6 regular consumptions per day with suitable between-meal eating and D3 ≥ 6 consumptions per day of which at least 1 unsuitable snack; O1 = children whose teeth were brushed at least once a day by an adult and O3 = children who seldom or never brushed their teeth; F1 = children who had started to chew tablets before the age of 2 years and F3 = children who had not chewed tablets; m = mean of dmfs differences; % diff = weighted mean percentage differences; figures within parenthesis based on uncorrected group mean values.

for oral hygiene in advance. The table shows that diet was a positive confounder. As an example, suitable dietary habits were found in 28% in the tablet group, while the corresponding figure for the non-tablet group was only 14%. Good habits do obviously go together. The crude difference in caries prevalence was 1.8 surfaces, which dropped to 0.6 surfaces after correction for confounding. The new mean difference was weighted proportionally to the number of individuals in the smallest component of each of the three comparisons. Without the correction procedure, a false picture of the caries-preventive effect of chewing fluoride tablets had been achieved.

Examples of studies of diet, oral hygiene and fluoride

Given the above circumstances one would expect that a great number of comparable data on the caries-preventive effects of die-

tary, oral hygiene and fluoride measures were available. Unfortunately this is not the case. General statistical problems of interpretation of data have already been touched upon. Dietary studies vary often so much in methods and criteria that generally applicable reduction figures can hardly be derived even though we know a great deal about the principal importance of different dietary factors. The situation is somewhat better for oral hygiene measures, however, not to the extent prevailing for fluoride measures. The effects of fluorides is mostly evaluated in highly standardized controlled clinical studies where, for instance, the problem of bias is met by randomization.

The results of two studies using different analytical approaches in order to correct for confounding and other effect-modifying factors are described here. In the first(5), based on subgroup analysis, diet expressed as the number of consumptions per day with or without unsuitable snacks was found to be a strong cariogenic factor

TABLE 10-4

Relationship between food frequency consumption, dental and socioeconomic variables, studied by means of multiple regression analysis. From(6).

Regressors* including variation in age from 3 years 10 months to 4 years 11 months	Regressands**	Regressors entering at a significant level of ≤ 1 %	R^2 in %***
Food variables	deft	Sweets	
Toothbrushing		Age	11.97
	defs	Sweets	
		Age	8.78
	GI	Soft drinks	
		Buns and cakes	7.52
Socioeconomic variables	deft	Father's education	13.71
Between-meal consumption	deft	Sweets	8.66
	defs	Sweets	4.70

* Independent variables, ** dependent variables, *** the amount in percent of the variation of the regressand explained by the regressors.

among 4-year-old children, irrespective of the type of smooth surface (Table 10-3). Chewing fluoride tablets had a significant, but not so strong, effect on approximal surfaces, and oral hygiene in terms of toothbrushing with or without help of an adult had even less effect on these surfaces. When comparing the uncorrected percentage differences (the figures within parenthesis in the table) with the corrected, it is found that the strongest variable in a system of interacting factors, in this case diet, is much less influenced by the correction procedure than the weakest variable, in this case chewing fluoride tablets.

In the second study(6), likewise in 4-year-old children, multiple regression analysis showed the relationships at the individual level to be quite modest (Table 10-4). A model specifying sweets and age as independent variables could explain about 9% of the variation in defs, sweets alone as

between-meal consumption about 5%. Dental variables of oral hygiene and fluoride supply did not enter at the 1% level of significance.

Apart from these examples, which have proved correction for effect-modifying factors is a highly relevant issue, several other examples can be found in the dental literature.

ESTIMATION OF EFFECTS OF PREVENTIVE MEASURES

Single measures

Estimation of effects of preventive measures concerns percentage reduction figures. As was said earlier, such values should be gen-

Disease

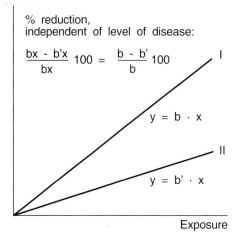

% reduction, independent of level of disease:

$$\frac{bx - b'x}{bx} 100 = \frac{b - b'}{b} 100$$

I

$y = b \cdot x$

II

$y = b' \cdot x$

Exposure

Fig. 10-1. Model for optimal function of a basic preventive measure. I = regression line for controls, II = regression line for individuals provided with basic prevention; refer to text.

erally applicable and thus be valid over a wide range of levels of disease. Single studies are not sufficient to provide such data. A greater number of similar studies are required to obtain a reasonable estimate of the effect of a preventive measure.

The model in Fig. 10-1 is one way to illustrate the effect of a single measure(3), as follows: two assumptions have to be made, 1) that non-exposed subjects do not get the disease and 2) that a linear relationship exists between disease and exposure. Regression line I is the line for controls, regression line II represents groups provided with basic prevention. The difference in slope between the two lines expresses the reduction of disease resulting from the prevention. The relative reduction is thus the same over the whole range of levels of disease. The figure also demonstrates the previously mentioned fundamental rule of interaction, namely that the absolute effectiveness of a preventive measure increases with the adversity of other factors in the process of disease.

TABLE **10-5**

Estimation of the combined effect of mouthrinsing with a fluoride solution and toothbrushing with a fluoride toothpaste in 12-year-old children regularly participating in a 2-year clinical trial(1).

	Mean base-line DMFS	Mean incremental DFS		Reduction in %
		reported	corrected*	
Controls	10.76	6.00		
Toothpaste group	10.03	4.75	5.10	15
Mouth-rinse group	10.20	4.95	5.22	13
Combined group	10.22	4.46	4.70	

Combined preventive effect in %:
15 + 0.13 (100 - 15) = 13 + 0.15 (100 - 13) = 26

Estimated residual DFS: 0.74 x 6.00 = 4.44

Observed residual DFS: 4.70

* correction for variation in baseline DMFS, i.e. the ratio control group value/experimental group value.

Combined measures

The basis of estimation of the effect of combined preventive measures was described in detail by Granath & McHugh(3) and applied on literature data.

The effect of combining a measure A, whose effect when used alone is known, with another measure B, whose effect is also known, can be estimated simply, assuming the previously described linear relationship between disease and exposure. Let us assume that the sole effect of measure A is 40% and that of measure B 30%. If A is at full effect, the additional effect of B can be calculated as $(100 - 40) \times 0.3 = 18$, where 100 represents the original amount of disease. The reduced effect of A when B is fully effective is accordingly $(100 - 30) \times 0.4 = 28$. The combined effect is obtained by adding the reduced effect of one measure to the sole effect of the other, in the above examples $18 + 40 = 58$ or $28 + 30 = 58$. If this did not apply, and if the full effect of each preventive measure was achieved in addition to that of other preventive measures, it would be easy to eliminate a disease completely by combining a number of different measures.

In 1984, with a somewhat different approach, Marthaler(8) suggested a formula leading to the same result.

The interested reader may use the data in Table 10-5 in order to check the applicability. The data are derived from a 2-year clinical testing of a mouthrinse and a dentifrice containing fluoride(1). The combined preventive effect of regular use of the rinse with a sole effect of 15% and of the dentifrice with a sole effect of 13% was calculated to 26%. The estimated remaining amount of disease should then be 4.44 DFS. The observed value was 4.70 DFS, in other words quite a good agreement.

PREDICTION

With the declining caries prevalence over the past 15–20 years in industrialized countries in the Western hemisphere, there has been an increasing interest in predicting disease in the remaining afflicted group. This group, of various size and disease seriousness in different countries, is well known from epidemiological studies.

Principles

The advocated model for prediction, among others discussed by Vecchio(18) and widely used in medicine and dentistry, is based on the following fourfold table.

Attribute or screening (test) value	Condition or disease		Total
	Present	Absent	
Positive	a (true positives)	b (false positives)	a+b
Negative	c (false negatives)	d (true negatives)	c+d
Total	a+c	b+d	a+b+c+d

The sensitivity {a/(a+c)} is the proportion of diseased subjects whose test value is positive and the specificity {d/(b+d)} the proportion of healthy subject whose test value is negative. The predictive value of a positive test {PV⁺, a/(a+b)} is the probability that an individual with a positive test is diseased and the predictive value of a negative test {PV⁻, d/(c+d)} the probability that an individual with a negative value remains healthy.

It is understood that sensitivity and specificity are not dependent on the prevalence of disease, while the predictive values are. For that reason, a model based on the so-called Bayes' theorem has been developed.

Test	Diagnosis	
	Diseased	Healthy
Positive	sens x p	(100-spec) (1-p)
Negative	(100-sens) p	spec (1-p)

The expression **sensitivity x p**, where p is the disease prevalence, is based on probability theory. With this as a fact, the other expressions follow from the first fourfold table. Sensitivity and specificity are expressed in percent, p from 0 to 1. The predictive power (PV⁺) is then:

$$\frac{\text{sens x p}}{\text{sens x p} + (100 - \text{spec}) (1-p)}$$

It is evident that high predictive values are dependent on high values of both sensitivity and specificity. Furthermore, prediction is of most interest at low disease prevalences, which explains its fame over the last 10 to 15 years of declining caries prevalence. At low prevalences, PV^+ is particularly dependent on a high specificity.

It is easy to be familiar with the system by simulating different quantities of a certain number of subjects in the cells of the four-fold table.

Past research has tried to identify epidemiological as well as caries etiological variables which could be used for screening. Some data are presented here.

Epidemiological variables

Past caries history has been used in a few studies. Among the best results were those of Poulsen & Holm[14] for a group of 151 children in Northern Sweden. The criterion of risk was > 0 dmfs at the age of 3 to predict caries in the permanent dentition at 9. The sensitivity was 0.54 and the specificity 0.87. The coefficient of correlation (r) was 0.42, which means that about 18% ($r^2 = 0.176$) of the variation in caries in the permanent dentition could be explained by the variation in caries in the primary dentition.

Granath & McHugh[4] made a regression analysis of the inter-relationship between caries incidence during 1 year and the incidence in the immediately prior year in 144 children, 12 to 13 years of age at the start of the observation period. The r-value was 0.49.

Caries etiological variables

Schröder & Granath[15] used dietary and oral hygiene habits as predictors in a retrospective study on 143 3-year-old children. The habits had been the same over the past 2 years. Disease was defined as > 0 carious lesions. The most discriminating border

TABLE **10-6**

Distribution of 143 non-diseased (-) and diseased (+) 3-year-old children in nine classes with regard to dietary and oral hygiene habits for prediction purposes. From(15).

Oral hygiene	dmfs > 0	Dietary habits		
		D3	D2	D1
O3	+	8	6	2
	-	1	2	3
O2	+	21	11	1
	-	9	12	14
O1	+	2	2	1
	-	10	26	12

D3 ≥ 2, D2 = 1-2 and D1 ≤ 1 regular unsuitable eatings per day; O3 = general gingivitis with bleeding on probing, O2 = partial or general gingivitis without bleeding on probing and O1 = practically without clinical signs of gingivitis; ———— = screening level at which the highest possible values of sensitivity (0.89) and specificity (0.70) were reached simultaneously; refer to text.

was searched for by stepwise pooling classes of habits until the screening level was obtained at which the highest possible values of sensitivity and specificity were reached simultaneously[13]. The screening level in Table 10-6 indicates that children with clean teeth, irrespective of dietary habits and those with less than one regular unsuitable intake per day, provided they do not have general gingivitis with bleeding, might be regarded as at no caries risk. The sensitivity was 0.89 and the specificity 0.70, which are among the best values reported.

Microbiological variables have been of particular interest. Some of the best results were obtained by Crossner(2) and Stecksén-Blicks(16). Crossner(2) used a screening criterion of ≥ 10⁵ lactobacilli per ml saliva in the study of 14-year-olds over 64 weeks and obtained a sensitivity of 0.50 and a specificity of 0.96. Disease was defined as ≥ 2 new lesions during the period. Stecksén-Blicks(16) combined lactobacilli and *S. mutans* (screening criteria ≥ 10⁵ lbc and > 20 CFU of *S. mutans* on plate) for prediction in 8-year-olds over 1 year. The sensitivity was 0.38 and the specificity 0.91. Disease was defined as ≥ 3 new lesions during the period.

The most thorough analysis of the ability to predict caries in the primary dentition with the aid of a number of caries-related factors was performed by Sullivan & Schröder(17) in a group of 105 children from 5 to 7 years of age. The variables were gingival state as an expression for oral hygiene, *S. mutans* and lactobacilli in saliva, saliva secretion rate and buffer capacity of saliva. Disease was defined as > 0 new lesions during the period. All available screening levels for the variables were analyzed systematically by stepwise testing consecutive scale values of the individual variable and for the combinations of variables to find the level where the highest possible values of sensitivity and specificity were reached simultaneously. For every screening level with the combinations of variables there were two alternatives to test: the group with only favourable values against the remaining group, and the group with only unfavourable values against the remaining group.

The best combination of sensitivity (0.41) and specificity (0.83) for a single variable was obtained with *S. mutans* (screening level > 5 CFU on plate). The best combination of two variables were gingival state and *S. mutans* (screening levels general gingivitis with bleeding on probing and > 5 CFU) with a sensitivity of 0.53 and a specificity of 0.74. With three variables, the best combina-

tion was gingival state, *S. mutans* and lactobacilli (screening level for lbc > 10⁵, the others as above). Sensitivity and specificity were the same as with two variables.

Unfortunately, it has to be concluded that our present possibilities to predict caries development are rather limited, probably due to measurement difficulties associated with the methods used and unknown confounding or modifying effects of the system. Perhaps it might be needed to tread quite new paths.

COST/VALUE OF PREVENTIVE MEASURES

Planning of health and care activities should be based on 1) disease prevalences, 2) objective treatment needs, 3) public demands (subjective treatment needs, consumption of care resources), and 4) the costs, which requires a strict epidemiological support. The cost-effectiveness ratio (CRE)(7) can for instance be expressed as

$$\frac{\text{average cost of the preventive procedure per person per year}}{\text{costs for the operative treatment of the mean number of surfaces saved per person per year through the preventive measure.}}$$

It is obvious that such calculations have to be based on careful estimations of the effect of the preventive procedure. With regard to basic preventive measures, aimed for the whole population or group, strict cost-effectiveness principles can be applied and decisions may not be controversial. When it comes to additional or individualized prevention, a cost-benefit or cost-value perspective should also include the value of being healthy.

In a study by Petersson et al (11), the costs to select patients for individualized caries preventive programs as well as the implementation of such programs were calculated. Three different ways to select and two different programs were evaluated. None of the screening and preventive programs were profitable in the sense that they would offer a public saving, as all of them turned out to be more expensive than the alternative restorative care.

The following modified example from the paper by Petersson et al(11) can be used as an illustration. Lactobacillus test (Dentocult®-LB, Orion Diagnostica, Espoo, Finland) can be used to select patients with a high risk for caries (cut point $\geq 10^5$/ml saliva). The caries increment during one year in a group of 107 children was predicted to be 89 cavities. Twenty children were likely to be at high risk for caries. Four annual sessions of oral prophylaxis were assumed to give a 50% caries reduction.

Cost

Screening material	1 400 SEK
Four prophylactic sessions for 20 children	4 100 SEK
Costs for children's time	500 SEK
Costs for failure to turn up	300 SEK
Total costs	6 300 SEK

Savings

Costs for restorations	4 500 SEK
Costs for children's time	200 SEK
Costs for failure to turn up	400 SEK
Total saving	5 100 SEK
Savings minus costs	-1 200 SEK

However, costs and savings were calculated for only one year, and thus no prices set on the long-term value of healthy teeth, the lowered risk of periodontal problems, less risk of recurrent decay or the value for the individual to avoid discomfort and trouble, factors that should be considered when similar screening and preventive programs are planned and implemented.

Literature cited

1. Ashley FP, Mainwaring PJ, Emslie RD, Naylor MN. Clinical testing of a mouthrinse and a dentifrice containing fluoride. A two-year supervised study in school children. *Br Dent J* 1977; **143**: 333-8.

2. Crossner C-G. Salivary lactobacillus counts in the prediction of caries activity. *Community Dent Oral Epidemiol* 1981; **9**: 182-90.

3. Granath L, McHugh WD. Basic prevention for the individual. In: Granath L, McHugh WD, eds. *Systematized prevention of oral disease: Theory and practice.* Boca Raton, Florida: CRC Press, 1986: 129-44.

4. Granath L, McHugh WD. Individualized prevention. In: Granath L, McHugh WD, eds. *Systematized prevention of oral disease: Theory and practice*.Boca Raton, Florida: CRC Press, 1986: 161-79.

5. Granath L-E, Rootzén H, Liljegren E, Holst K, Köhler L. Variation in caries prevalence related to combinations of dietary and oral hygiene habits and chewing fluoride tablets in 4-year-old children. *Caries Res* 1978; **12**: 83-92.

6. Holm AK, Blomquist H K-son, Crossner C-G, Grahnén H, Samuelson G. A comparative study of oral health as related to general health, food habits and socioeconomic conditions of 4-year-old Swedish children. *Community Dent Oral Epidemiol* 1975; **3**: 34-9.

7. Horowitz HS, Heifetz SB. Methods for assessing the cost-effectiveness of caries preventive agents and procedures. *Int Dent J* 1979; **29**: 106-17.

8. Marthaler TM. Explanations for changing patterns of disease in the Western world. In: Guggenheim B, ed. *Cariology today: International congress in honour of Professor Dr Hans R Mühlemann*. Zürich, September 2-4, 1983. Basel: Karger, 1984; 13-23.

9. Miettinen O. Confounding and effect-modification. *Am J Epidemiol* 1974; **100**: 350-3.

10. Norell S. *Epidemiologisk metodik*. Studieuppläggning, tillförlitlighet, effektivitet. Lund, Sweden: Studentlitteratur, 1987.

11. Petersson T, Löfgren C, Holm A-K. Selektering av riskpatienter inom barn- och ungdomstandvården. En modell för samhällsekonomisk lönsamhetsberäkning. *Tandläkartidningen* 1983; **75**: 885-91.

12. O'Mullane DM. Efficiency in clinical trials of caries preventive agents and methods. *Community Dent Oral Epidemiol* 1976; **4**: 190-4.

13. Poulsen S, Granath L, Gustavsson K-H. Selektering av cariesrisikoindivider. In: Grahnén H, Granath L, eds. *Epidemiologisk forskning inom barn- och ungdomstandvården*. Rapport från internordiskt seminarium. Umeå: 1980; 37-42. (in Danish)

14. Poulsen S, Holm A-K. The relation between dental caries in the primary and permanent dentition of the same individual. *J Public Health Dent* 1980; **40**: 17-25.

15. Schröder U, Granath L. Dietary habits and oral hygiene as predictors of caries in 3-year-old children. *Community Dent Oral Epidemiol* 1983; **11**: 308-11.

16. Stecksén-Blicks C. Salivary counts of lactobacilli and Streptococcus mutans in caries prediction. *Scand J Dent Res* 1985; **93**: 204-12.

17. Sullivan Å, Schröder U. Systematic analysis of gingival state and salivary variables as predictors of caries from 5 to 7 years of age. *Scand J Dent Res* 1989; **97**: 25-32.

18. Vecchio TJ. Predictive value of a single diagnostic test in unselected populations. *N Engl J Med* 1966; **274**: 1171-3.

CHAPTER 11

DENTAL CARIES: OPERATIVE TREATMENT

The relation between preventive and operative dentistry

Treatment planning

Diagnosis and treatment of incipient enamel lesions

Treatment of deep lesions

Dental amalgam, composite resin, glass ionomer cement

Traditional restorative procedures

Special treatments in the primary dentition

Special treatments for pits and fissures

The 1960s was the decade when prevention was recognized as an integral part of caries therapy in many Western countries, over the past 20 years this has resulted in a dramatic decrease in the reported incidence of caries. During the 1970s this led some prophets to prognosticate the downfall of operative treatment, now ranked lower than preventive treatment. This disappointed many clinicians and created a basis for passive resistance to further preventive activities. In the 1980s it has been quite evident that for practical, psychological, social and economical reasons the total extinction of dental caries is a utopian dream. Simultaneously, the literature reveals an increased interest in the advancement of operative dentistry. Biomechanics and toxicology are in focus, exemplified by the search for alternatives to dental amalgams.

From these premises, the purpose of this chapter is to present a comprehensive view of the modern operative treatments of caries in primary and mixed dentition, bearing in mind generally accepted principles of operative dentistry and the necessary modifications due to the anatomy and physiology of primary dentition and the continuous somatic and mental development of children.

THE RELATION BETWEEN PREVENTIVE AND OPERATIVE DENTISTRY

Much knowledge has been gathered about potential sequelae of operative dentistry, i.e. indirect factors in the development of new disease. Such factors are defective margins, insufficient extension for prevention, insufficient obturation and adverse effects of restorative and luting materials in the etiology of new carious lesions, periodontal diseases and pulp damage. How this knowledge can be efficiently utilized was expressed in three statements by Granath & McHugh(11).

1. By ensuring that the operative treatment is an integral part of the individual's preventive program.

2. By performing restorative dentistry according to biomechanical principles, i.e., balancing requirements for effective use of the restorative material against biologic factors, preserving tooth substance as far as possible.

3. By avoiding any form of overtreatment.

While primary prevention has a long history, very little has changed in operative dentistry in the same period, and even less attention has been paid to coordinating preventive and operative therapy. As a basis for evolution in this area, two further statements were made.

1. Prevention is the foundation of virtually all operative measures. This includes primary, secondary, and tertiary prevention, i.e., the prevention of diseases *per se,* the discovery and treatment of early injuries, and the rehabilitation of advanced damage.

2. There is no conflict between preventive and operative care. Both forms are essential components of a coordinated system. The effect of primary preventive measures will never be fully achieved unless established injuries are also dealt with. By analogy, the treatment of established injuries has little chance of yielding lasting results unless it is combined with primary prevention.

New developments of operative dentistry should be linked to secondary and tertiary prevention. This chapter takes such aspects into account.

Accepting the above statements, some questions of apparently great impact on the treatment of children and adolescents could be asked.

1. Is the therapy in an objective sense (the dentist's) and/or a subjective sense (the patient's) justified from a) a physiologic point of view, and b) a psychologic and esthetic point of view?

2. Will the therapy involve a direct or an indirect risk of further disease or damage?

3. Does the therapy prevent further disease or damage?

Given that these questions are properly answered, the therapy will focus on the concepts of *risk* and *prevention* and be planned according to physiological, psychological and esthetic principles with due regard to the patients' subjective opinions and to avoidance of overtreatment.

TREATMENT PLANNING

General guidelines for operative dentistry in the primary dentition

The dentist is often faced with the question of why primary teeth, which are to be shed, should be treated. This is particularly applicable when the level of disease is low and during periods of economic restraint. The answer is founded on a number of related facts, whose fundamental meaning is that a pathological condition should not be left unheeded.

1. The child should be protected from toothache and be able to eat and drink

without pain from the teeth. The reasons are of broadly humane and nutritional nature. As a matter of fact, a grossly destroyed dentition seldom or never leads to functional disturbances of the masticatory apparatus. However, extensive carious lesions might influence the child's dietary habits far more than reduction of the number of teeth. Among those with painful open lesions, one can find children who refuse to eat and, occasionally, are undernourished.

2. Untreated carious lesions can impair medical (general) illness and cause dental (local) complications. Children, for example, with a bleeding disease or a disease that causes decreased resistance against infection run a greater risk of general complications in connection with infections in the pulp or jaw-bone than others. Inflammatory conditions in the jaw also create a potential risk of disturbances to the developing tooth germs.

3. Treatment of carious teeth is a part of, and prerequisite for, maintenance of good oral hygiene. If bacterial foci such as proteolyzed dentin in open cavities and retention places difficult of access are not removed, the patient will not fully benefit from oral hygiene measures.

4. The risk of caries attacks in the permanent dentition should be diminished through preventing newly erupted teeth from contact with carious primary teeth. Susceptibility to caries is lower in teeth which for a longer period have been exposed to saliva supersaturated with calcium phosphate and its content of trace elements, compared with that in newly erupted teeth. This is ascribed to a posteruptive increase of minerals in the superficial enamel with formation of phosphates difficult to dissolve due to their content of fluoride, but also of such metals as tin and lead. It is obvious that contact with carious primary teeth is particularly critical for permanent teeth immediately after eruption, which is why it should be avoided.

5. Horizontal bite dimensions should be preserved in order to secure space in the arches for the permanent teeth. In certain cases, this is also valid for vertical dimensions. The value of restorative procedures in the traditional sense is, however, related to the actual developmental stage of the bite. The need to restore a reduced vertical height in the primary dentition is only called for in connection with interceptive orthodontic interventions.

6. There are also psychological reasons for treatment. A child will be as well satisfied as any adult, with nice teeth and a nice smile.

Treatment priorities in primary dentition

It is a common opinion among pedodontists that treatment of the primary dentition should be complete. This is, in the main, correct, if by "complete" is understood that all parts of the bite should be taken care of in some way, in case of disease or other change. However, to advocate treatment principles applicable to the permanent dentition would not be wise on all occasions. This is simply because the value of the single primary tooth varies with the stage of bite development. Therefore, priorities are realized through differentiated operative dentistry that, in principle, aims at *giving the single primary tooth a treatment no more advanced than is required with regard to its value at the actual stage of bite development.* This means that the goal is not *maximum* but *optimum* treatment.

Given the self-evident prerequisite that a carious lesion is taken care of, the priorities are governed by the need for preventing unsuitable, and/or provoking suitable, migration of primary teeth. Two stages of bite development are crucial: 1) when the primary dentition is complete (about 2-2½ years of age); and 2) when occlusion of the permanent first molars has been established. The first stage marks that the primary incisors are no longer so important, the second that the value of the primary molars decreases.

It has not been shown, under otherwise normal conditions, that loss of primary incisors, after the primary dentition is fully developed, decreases the arch perimeter, nor that loss of primary molars after the age of 7 does so(17,18,36). This means that the requirement of maintaining the arch perimeter within the incisor and molar regions by means of traditional operative dentistry comes to an end at about the ages of 3 and 7, respectively. Thereby, prerequisites for differentiated operative dentistry are created.

Departure from normal bite development may make it of interest to extend the period of traditional treatment. It could be a case with a small maxilla and a tendency to anterior crossbite. The length of the upper tooth arch has to be carefully supervised during the time necessary for consolidation of the bite, while a shortening of the lower arch is probably desirable to the extent allowed by the difference in mesiodistal width between the primary molars and their succedaneous permanent teeth. Another example is the case of a deep bite, where the lower permanent incisors lack the vertical support of the upper incisors and, therefore, are forced lingually during the growth of the mandible. Loss of the horizontal support that a primary first molar of normal mesiodistal width offers the primary cuspid might impair the situation.

Choice of treatment alternatives

Primary teeth – The treatment alternatives for primary teeth are traditional restorations, stainless steel crowns, modified (atypical) restorations, disking and extraction. At cavity preparation in primary teeth, the operator is faced with problems not so pronounced in permanent teeth. Primary teeth are smaller than permanent ones, but have a comparatively larger pulp chamber and consequently thinner enamel and dentin layers, which provides less space for restorations. This is of particular interest with regard to Class II cavity restorations for which traditional concepts of cavity form and size are preferentially maintained. Extended use of acid etch-retained composite resins has led to modifications of cavity preparation for Classes I, III and V cavity restorations, which are described in connection with treatment of permanent teeth.

There are indications for stainless steel crowns where modified restorations or disking, as described below, are not good enough as substitutes for traditional restorations. Practically, such situations occur in connection with restoring of the height of the bite as part of interceptive orthodontics. Sometimes it might also be necessary to restore the mesiodistal width of a tooth by means of a stainless steel crown.

A carious lesion has to be moderate, if a Class II cavity is to be prepared according to traditional norms. The more extensive the damage, the more the result departs from a standard cavity. Often the retention possibilities are insufficient after excavation. Remaining walls might be undermined with risk of fracture, which is why the restorative design has to be modified. It is particularly complicated in teeth with a clinically healthy pulp, but with extensive carious lesions. It can be difficult to maintain the mesiodistal width of the tooth. The surplus of arch space in the posterior regions after

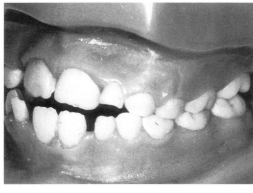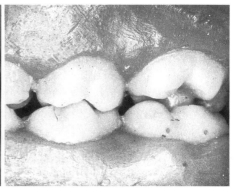

Fig. 11-1. Angle Class I occlusion with a flush terminal plane in a 7-year-old child with risk of anterior crossbite.

shedding is therefore made use of in advance.

Disking as a substitute for, or in combination with, a restoration implies a further step of simplification. The benefit of disking is best elucidated by means of a case illustrating the relation between preventive and operative dentistry on one hand, and preventive orthodontics on the other, taking the physiology of the mixed dentition into account(11). Fig. 11-1 shows the mixed dentition of a 7-year-old child with an Angle Class I occlusion, belonging to the subdivision that has a flush terminal plane which causes a cusp-to-cusp relationship between the 6-year molars. The upper jaw was comparetively small, with a potential risk of developing into an anterior crossbite. There were several approximal carious lesions in the primary molars.

As the horizontal arch space in the upper jaw clearly had to be preserved in order to avoid an anterior crossbite, conventional Class II cavity restorations were needed in the upper primary molars. In the lower jaw, however, some reduction of arch length was desirable. Since the total mesiodistal width of the mandibular primary molars in a quadrant is about 3 mm greater than the total width of their successors and 1 mm should be saved for the larger width of the

permanent cuspid, appropriate use can be made of the remaining 2 mm. Normally, nature is so wise as to shed the primary second molars in the lower jaw before those in the upper jaw, which leads to a neutral occlusion between the 6-year molars through slight mesial drifting of the mandibular teeth. So to conform with nature, instead of making a Class II disto-occlusal restoration in the primary second molar, therapeutic disking was performed.

This measure has several advantages. The possible sequelae of recurrent caries and amalgam fracture are avoided. The caries-preventive effect on the mesial surface of the 6-year molar is substantial. A newly erupted tooth has a higher caries susceptibility than later in life. Further, if a Class II cavity restoration has to be inserted in the permanent molar shortly after conventional treatment of the primary molar, the height of the approximal portion has to be adapted to the low clinical crown. Later, the cervical border of the amalgam will be located in the contact area to be formed with the second premolar, with a subsequent high risk of recurrent caries. The primary molar also received the treatment, which would facilitate development of a sound occlusion. A practical approach was synthesized from many theoretical compo-

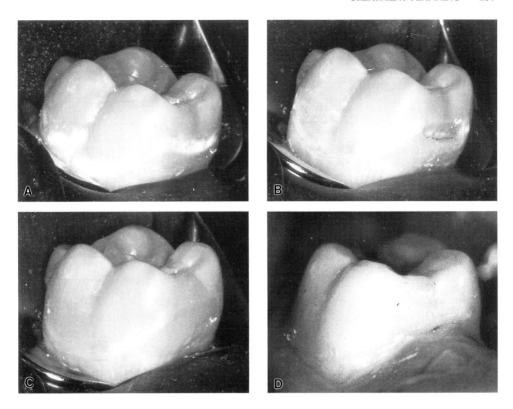

Fig. 11-2.

A. Lower permanent first molar with cavities in demineralized areas mesially and buccally;
B. Enamel with surface demineralization and cavities ground away and cavity borders bevelled;
C. Removed enamel replaced with composite resin after acid etching;
D. Follow-up after 2 years with remineralization of the subsurface lesion in the mesiobuccal angle.

nents, which is a sound basis for successful clinical practice.

On the basis of what was said about priorities, extraction might be an alternative, particularly in connection with pulp exposure in grossly damaged teeth.

Permanent teeth – There was a time when the floor of an occlusal cavity should be placed in the dentin. While such an approach is relevant for a Class II cavity restoration exposed to masticatory forces causing bending stresses that can lead to isthmus fracture, this is not true for the Class I restoration. Fractures are rare, mainly be-

cause optimal occlusion is easy to achieve and since the embracing tooth matrix does not allow bending stresses to occur. The extension of the Class I cavity depends therefore on the anatomy of the fissure system and the carious lesions, while its depth is solely determined by the lesion, irrespective of which restorative material is used.

As a principle, the border of a restoration should not be located in a fissure prone to new caries attack, i.e. extension for prevention should be exercised, which means that a lot of sound tooth substance is removed in many cases. This problem has lately been overcome through the introduction of the concept of preventive resin restorations(33, 37), which is a combination of a composite resin filling restricted to the carious area and a fissure sealing.

Indications for a traditional Class II cavity restoration prevail for caries in approximal surfaces of molars and premolars, where the contact with neighbouring teeth does not allow a more simple cavity design. Basic principles according to *GV Black* have to be acknowledged (retention, resistance, outline and convenience form and extension for prevention). Approximal extension for prevention should be minimal in case of low caries activity in order to preserve sound tooth substance. Conversely, when the patient is not suited to causal and resistance-increasing therapy, the cavity has to be extended to easily accessible areas.

A modified treatment of approximal lesions in molars and premolars can be tried, where there is no contact with a neighbouring tooth or where the contacting tooth is prepared for a Class II cavity restoration. If the lesion is limited and does not undermine the marginal ridge, the surface can be treated according to the acid etch composite resin technique which provides minimum risk and maximum prevention in combination with modified cavity preparation (Fig. 11-2). In case of a more advanced lesion with little risk of fracture of the marginal ridge, glass ionomer cement is preferable.

Traditional Class III and V cavities were based on the concept that the walls should follow the direction of the enamel prisms with the floor and retention grooves located in dentin. Since acid etch composite resin and glass ionomer cement are the restorative materials of choice for treatment of lesions in smooth surfaces not to be included in Class II restorations, cavity preparation today takes a more biologic course, with preservation of sound tooth substance. The technical aspects on these and other treatments mentioned above are presented later in this chapter.

Treatment order

After the choice of treatment alternatives has been settled, crude interventions are first performed, which means that necessary extractions, excavation of teeth with extensive lesions and application of temporary filling material are made. This aims at facilitating the effect of oral hygiene measures. One should, however, be aware of that psychological conditions may modify this treatment order.

The teeth are then treated with priority for those which require endodontic procedures, whereafter primary teeth are restored in order of importance for further bite development. In the mixed dentition, permanent teeth have precedence unless extreme orthodontic conditions require another course.

DIAGNOSIS AND TREATMENT OF INCIPIENT ENAMEL LESIONS

Caries in smooth surfaces

Demineralized enamel, i.e. an incipient (white spot) lesion without a cavity in the adopted sense, can be remineralized as described in Chapter 9, and must be acknowledged during treatment planning. The first clinically detectable stage is the subsurface lesion with a relatively well-preserved surface layer, 25-30 μm(42), under which the main mineral loss is located. The depth of the lesion is probably at most 300 μm(22). The porosity in the subsurface enamel explains the loss of translucency and the appearance of the white spot. The surface itself is still lustrous. At the second clinical stage of caries development, the growing body of the lesion involves deeper parts of the ena-

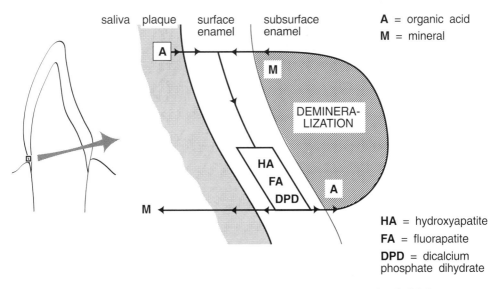

Fig. 11-3. Model for subsurface demineralization according to Moreno & Zahradnik(28).

mel, as well as the surface layer. The surface is now lustreless and chalky with a roughness that can be detected with an explorer.

A congenial, experimentally supported explanation of the occurrence of a subsurface lesion was given by Moreno & Zahradnik(28), as shown in Fig. 11-3. At a certain acid concentration and initial pH, a slight dissolution of the superficial enamel occurs, followed by precipitation of fluorapatite and dicalcium phosphate dihydrate which is favoured by the mediating action of fluoride present in the surface enamel. Together with the original hydroxyapatite, these two phases are in some kind of equilibrium with the solution in the pores of the surface layer. Concomitant with further diffusion of acid from the plaque into the surface layer, acid diffuses from this layer into the inner enamel. The acid constituents in the inner enamel are neutralized by dissolution of mineral, which makes basic constituents diffuse in the opposite direction. In this way, the equilibrium in the surface layer is maintained because the loss of mineral in this layer is compensated by the transport of mineral from the inner enamel.

Thus, the model acts as a pumping mechanism, the surface enamel is continuously regenerated, and a subsurface lesion is created.

As the lesion progresses, the rate of precipitation decreases because the rate of dissolution in the body of the lesion decreases and the diffusion path increases. When the transfer of mineral from the surface layer to the saliva is greater than the rate of precipitation in the surface layer, the system collapses and the second clinical stage of caries lesion develops, eventually yielding a cavity as the end result.

The thin surface layer covering an enamel subsurface lesion is vulnerable and should, therefore, be treated gently. Cautious cleaning of the surface precedes treatment with fluorides in order to facilitate remineralization. The more advanced lesion with a demineralized surface is given a similar treatment. However, after remineralization which makes the surface layer mechanically more stable, the surface should be polished with a mild abrasive paste in order to smooth the surface, thereby decreasing the propensity for retention of plaque.

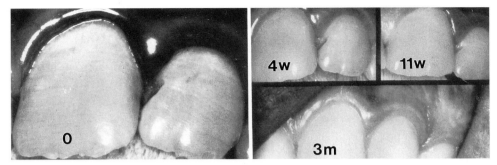

Fig. 11-4. Upper permanent incisors with subsurface demineralization in the gingival third of the buccal surfaces (Day 0); remineralization with disappearance of white spots after 4 and 11 weeks of good oral hygiene and topical treatment with fluoride; results after 3 months; note improved gingival state.

Remineralization of subsurface lesions is visible by the disappearance of white spots, which gives an optical impression of healing (Fig. 11-4). The opaque appearance of the demineralized surface remains after remineralization, which causes uncertainty whether it actually has happened. Since there often are subsurface lesions in the vicinity of a demineralized surface area, visual remineralization of the subsurface lesions may indicate an effect on the whole (Fig. 11-5).

The remineralization of the more advanced lesion (the second clinical stage) does for different reasons only reach a certain depth. After a long period, such an arrested lesion can appear as a white spot covered with a hard and shiny surface layer (Fig. 11-6). A second type of subsurface lesion has then developed, the shiny surface probably also being a result of abrasion.

What has been described above is, at first hand, relevant for buccal and lingual surfaces. When it comes to contacting approximal surfaces, the situation is somewhat different.

In case of a macroscopic cavity in a contacting approximal surface, the choice of treatment is simple. The cavity has on principle to be restored, if progression of the carious lesion shall be stopped. Progression is inevitable and may be rapid unless the

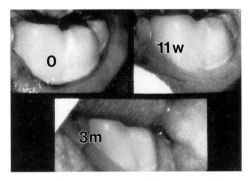

Fig. 11-5. Lower permanent first molar with subsurface and surface demineralization in the gingival third of the buccal surface (Day 0); remineralization with partial disappearance of the white spot after 11 weeks of good oral hygiene and topical treatment with fluoride; result after 3 months; note improved gingival state.

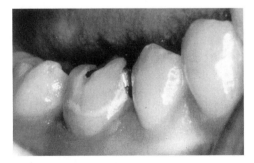

Fig. 11-6. Arrested lesion with hard and shiny enamel in the buccal surface of a lower permanent first molar; note the distance of the lesion from the gingival border.

TABLE 11-1

Percentages of progression of approximal radiographically detectable caries lesions. From(9).

Gröndahl et al 1977(13)		1974				
		01	02	03	F	
1971 (16-year-olds)	01	37.8	26.8	12.9	22.5	n = 770
	02		18.1	18.8	63.1	n = 469

Gröndahl & Hollender 1979(14)		1977				
		01	02	03	F	
1971 (16-year-olds)	01	25.9	22.6	11.9	38.7	n = 333
	02		13.5	7.6	77.8	n = 284

Granath et al 1980(10)		1977					
		01	02	03	F	R	
1975 (12-13-year-olds)	01	29	43	11	13	4	n = 236
	02		35	10	48	7	n = 160

Modèer et al 1984(27)		After 3 years					
		01	02	03	F	R	
Start (14-year-olds)	01	32	30	8	23	7	n = 306
	02		21	11	66	2	n = 82

01 = radiolucency in the outer half of the enamel
02 = radiolucency in the inner half of the enamel
03 = radiolucency into the dentin
F = restored surface
R = reversal
n = number of diagnosed surfaces

supply of the bacteria in the cavity with fermentable carbohydrates is interrupted, which is an exception. The problem with contacting approximal surfaces is, however, that it can be difficult to diagnose a small cavity, and this problem is of particular interest where the corresponding radiolucency in the x-ray picture approaches the dentin. Studies in Scandinavia have shown that with the radiolucency visible only in the enamel, there is a clinical cavity in 15% (1) to 60%(24) of the surfaces. These contrasting results may be explained by different techniques for exploration of the presence of a cavity and different age of the children under study. There is evidence that the approximal surfaces of young permanent premolars and molars with a radiolucency in the inner half of the enamel more often show a clinical cavity compared with the corresponding surfaces of older teenagers(25). This observation is in agreement with the observed higher rate of caries progression in young permanent teeth compared with older (Table 11-1).

The clinical x-ray picture has insufficient ability to image small mass differences. An approximal subsurface lesion is not visible. Therefore, a radiolucency represents at least the second clinical stage of demineralization. Further, keeping in mind the conical lesion, the buccolingual cross-section of the lesion decreases towards the dentin, while at the same time the total cross-section of the tooth increases. This leads to an inevitable underregistration. Moreover, the rate of progression is rather high in young teeth as seen in Table 11-1. All these conditions elucidate the complexity of carious lesions in contacting approximal surfaces and have resulted in the following recommendations (39).

1. A clinical cavity should be restored.

2. A carious lesion visible as a radiolucency in the x-ray picture without a distinct extension into the dentin and without a clinically detectable cavity is treated according to principles for remineralization.

3. A carious lesion in the x-ray picture with a distinct extension into the dentin should be treated with restoration irrespective of whether a clinical cavity can be detected.

Pit and fissure caries

Pits and fissures constitute areas where microbial deposits are hardly accessible to oral hygiene measures. They are therefore caries-prone, particularly in molars, many of which show signs of early caries shortly after eruption. The diagnosis of early pit and fissure caries is difficult and is related to the shape and sharpness of the explorer, the pressure exerted and the fissure anatomy. As for the anatomy, it has been shown that deep fissures are more prone to caries than shallow fissures(16).

The start is usually in the walls underneath the entrance of the pit or fissure. The pattern of spread is primarily towards the dentin and along the enamel-dentin border, which explains why considerable dentin caries and undermined enamel can be revealed when seemingly innocent carious pits or fissures are opened. It is obvious that early preventive treatment of pits and fissures is of paramount importance in caries-susceptible individuals. It has, however, been indicated that erupting teeth are more likely to develop caries and that many such lesions are arrested when the teeth come into function(2).

TREATMENT OF DEEP LESIONS

In case of an extensive carious lesion, undermined enamel is first ground away to create a good view of the area of operation. Proteolysed dentin is then removed with a spoon excavator and underlying softened dentin with a round bur of a size fitting the cavity in order to avoid accidental exposure of the pulp. At low progression of the lesion, the pulp of primary teeth can produce irritation secondary dentin to a large extent. This can result in great differences in level of the floor of the cavity and is why excavation has to be undertaken with caution.

After the cavity is clinically cariesfree, the preparation is completed according to principles described in a subsequent section. The deep cavity is cleaned with water spray, eventually also with a cotton pellet soaked in a mild detergent, and dentin canals connected with the pulp are covered with a liner or an insulation cement. In deep cavities, it is recommended to apply a pure calcium hydroxide-water mixture or a recognized calcium hydroxide cement over the deepest parts. The liner is covered with a phosphate or glass ionomer cement to create a firm base. The reason for employing calcium hydroxide is its ability to reduce pulpal irritation from restorative materials and the oral environment; through its antibacterial effect, probable capacity to precipitate the contents of dentinal tubules which may reduce diffusion of noxious agents, and eventual ability to stimulate the pulp to produce secondary dentin when applied close to the pulp(30,43).

If there is a risk of exposing the pulp when the innermost layer of softened dentin is removed, the operation should be interrupted. The tooth is treated with calcium hydroxide, as above, and a temporary filling of zinc oxide-eugenol cement, in order to await formation of secondary dentin for a period of 6-8 weeks. Then the cavity is opened again, remaining carious dentin removed and the restorative treatment completed.

If the dentin at the first instance is insignificantly softened, it can be left. Such dentin contains few microorganisms(4). The pulp of primary, as well as young permanent, teeth has a remarkable ability to recover with formation of secondary dentin when the irritant is removed. It is then supposed that the tooth does not exhibit signs and symptoms of chronic pulpitis as described in Chapter 12.

DENTAL AMALGAM, COMPOSITE RESIN, GLASS IONOMER CEMENT

Over the last 5-10 years, the use of dental amalgams have been widely questioned from a toxicological point of view. While the possibility of acquiring allergy against mercury should not be denied, it has been shown to be rather uncommon. Chronic poisoning has only been found among dental personnel, probably as a result of inefficient handling of the material(38). One positive side of the debate is that extended use of alternative materials, which are plastic at the time of insertion, has been discussed and tried in combination with modified cavity preparations. The alternatives are composite resins and glass ionomer cements.

Even if the alternative materials are less suited than amalgam for restorations exposed to masticatory forces because of their insufficient resistance to wear and permanence of form in combination with their chemical degradation in saliva, there are situations where they can be utilized(40).

1. For Class I restorations of limited size and where the mechanical stress exerted on the occlusal surface is moderate.

2. For Class II restorations, as under 1, and where accessibility and possibilities for observation are good, i.e. where the risk factors are judged insignificant and defects can be detected at an early stage.

3. For restoration of minor cusp fractures, as under 1, and where the restoration can be given a sufficient retention.

The selection between glass ionomer cements and composite resins should be based on the following considerations:

1. Composite resins are superior to glass ionomer cements with respect to strength, surface texture and aesthetic appearance, and the bond strength to acid-etched enamel is far above that of glass ionomers to enamel and dentin. This implies that composites should be preferred in stress-bearing areas and when aesthetic considerations are important, supposing that the restoration may be bonded to acid-etched enamel.

2. In vital teeth the dentin must be lined underneath composite resin, while glass ionomer cement is only irritating to the pulp in very deep cavities. The accessibility for a safe lining procedure, as well as the depth of the cavities, may therefore be factors to consider.

3. In patients with high caries activity, glass ionomer cement should be preferred due to its fluoride-leaching effect and since composite resin is known to retain more plaque.

4. The caries-preventive effect of glass ionomer cement may be utilized in certain contact areas, e.g. when caries develops in the approximal surfaces of a primary second and a permanent first molar. A glass ionomer cement restoration in the primary molar may prevent progression of the caries process in the permanent molar.

TRADITIONAL RESTORATIVE PROCEDURES

Class I cavity restorations

The Class I cavity for amalgam is prepared with a cylindrical diamond with a semicircular top. Width and depth are determined by the size of the carious lesion. Occlusal convergency for retention is brought about by slightly tilting the diamond. All caries-prone fissures are included in the preparation.

The procedures are the same for cavities for composite resin or glass ionomer cement except that there is no need for the special retention form, because of the bonding ability of glass ionomer cement, and that the enamel of the cavity walls is acid-etched with use of composite resin.

Class II cavity restorations

The modifications of *GV Black's* principles for the Class II cavity that modern research has advocated can be expressed so that a cavity of a given size should have a form, which gives rise to the most suitable stress distribution in the remaining tooth substance, as well as in the restoration at different clinical loadings(7). The best shape from a mechanical point of view has, if necessary, to be modified according to morphological conditions.

The optimal biomechanical design for primary molars is described below. The nomenclature is given in Fig. 11-7.

The most typical example of an unsuitable cavity design is the sharp internal angles of the occlusal box. The difference in fracture-inducing effect between a sharp and a rounded-off configuration is elucidated in Fig. 11-8.

For retention, and to satisfy requirements of strength of the restoration, the cavity has to be prepared down into the dentin. In cases where first molars in the lower jaw and second molars in the upper jaw have an intact transverse ridge and where sufficient retention can be obtained without inclusion of the ridge in the preparation, extension is restricted to the fissures. The extension is shown in Fig. 11-9 that also demonstrates how the occlusal part of the cavity smoothly continues into the approximal part.

The thickness of the occlusal part of the restoration should be 1.5 - 2 mm. It must, however, be acknowledged that the depth from the orifice of the fissure to the floor of the cavity does not amount to this measurement. Antagonistic cusps have mostly therefore to be reduced in order to let the restoration have enough thickness. By filling the cavity with softened wax and having the patient close the bite, a good perception of the occlusion and need for reduction of antagonising cusps may be achieved. The occlusal width of the cavity, i.e. the isthmus

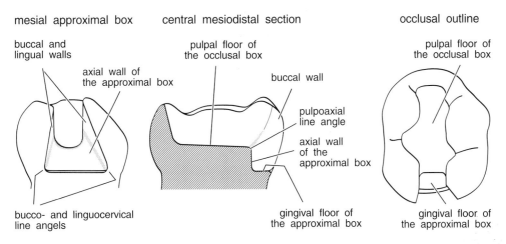

mesial approximal box   central mesiodistal section   occlusal outline

buccal and lingual walls

axial wall of the approximal box

pulpal floor of the occlusal box

pulpal floor of the occlusal box

buccal wall

pulpoaxial line angle

axial wall of the approximal box

bucco- and linguocervical line angels

gingival floor of the approximal box

gingival floor of the approximal box

Fig. 11-7. Principle drawings of a Class II cavity in a lower primary second molar. From (8).

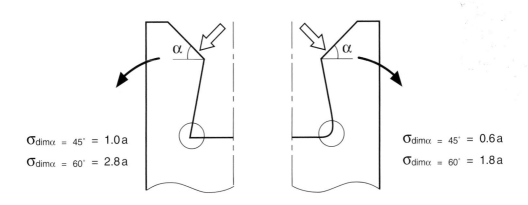

$\sigma_{dim\alpha\ =\ 45°} = 1.0\,a$

$\sigma_{dim\alpha\ =\ 60°} = 2.8\,a$

$\sigma_{dim\alpha\ =\ 45°} = 0.6\,a$

$\sigma_{dim\alpha\ =\ 60°} = 1.8\,a$

Fig. 11-8. Comparison of the effects of sharp and rounded-off internal angles on stress concentration as a result of loading of separated buccal and lingual cavity walls in photoelasticity model experiments; tensile stresses expressed as dimensionless stress for different cusp inclinations. From(8).

region of the restoration, is approximately one fourth of the buccolingual width of the tooth or half of the intercuspal distance.

The most suitable shape of the cross-section of the occlusal part of the cavity comprises a semicircular floor and, towards the occlusal surface, slightly converging walls (Fig. 11-10), corresponding to the course of the enamel prisms. An alternative, appreciating the same cross-sectional area, is a cavity combing a plane floor at slightly less depth

with rounded-off internal angles and similarly converging walls. From a clinical point of view, the two alternatives are equivalent with regard to outward bending of buccal and lingual cavity walls during loading(12). A continuous retention form gives a better support to the enamel compared with localized undercuts in the dentin, which may have an undermining effect because of the modest depth of the cavity. As long as the cavity follows the course of the fissures and

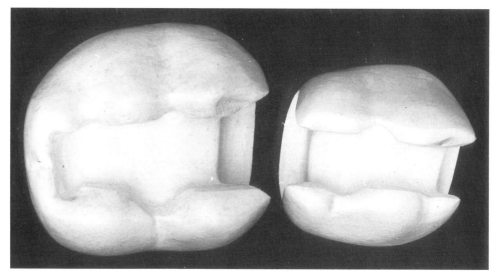

Fig. 11-9. Occlusal outline of Class II cavities in models of lower primary molars. From(8).

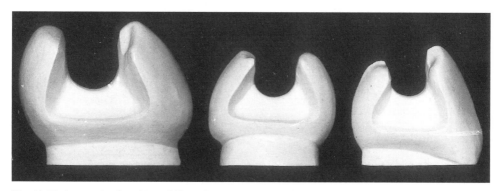

Fig. 11-10. Approximal outline of Class II cavities in models of lower primary molars. From(8).

the recommendations for depth and width are maintained, the restoration becomes well adapted to the anatomy of the pulp chamber. In particular, the extension of the mesiobuccal pulp horn should be taken into account.

The buccal and lingual walls of the approximal box should form 90° cavosurface angles with the approximal surfaces of the tooth. The reason is that otherwise the enamel will not be supported by dentin or a flap of the restorative material will prevail, which in both cases may result in fracture. Extension for prevention is required. The extension is, however, a relative concept, as previously mentioned. By allowing the buccal and lingual walls of the approximal box to converge towards the axial wall of the box and also occlusally, so that the outer border is more or less parallel with the contour of the tooth, the enamel becomes supported by dentin in the long direction of the prisms. Such a cavity shape is further promoted by the fact that the caries-suscep-

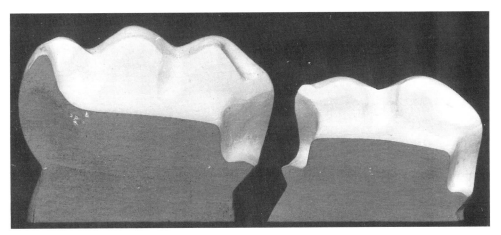

Fig. 11-11. Central mesiodistal sections of Class II cavities in models of lower primary molars. From (8).

tible part of the approximal surface is located between the cervical border of the box and the area of contact with the neighbouring tooth, while a new lesion seldom occurs in the area above the contact. The requirement of extension for prevention is therefore very limited in the latter area (Fig. 11-10). The bucco- and linguocervical angles should be rounded off.

The gingival floor of the approximal box is located slightly below the gingival margin. From a caries-preventive point of view, the contact with the neighbouring tooth has to be removed. An area between the border of the cavity and the gingival margin inaccessible to cleaning should not be left behind. However, the floor should not be prepared deeper because of the cervical curvature of the molar tooth crowns and the risk of damage to the periodontal tissues. Further, it is a misleading conception that the occlusal and approximal parts of a Class II cavity must, at any cost, be located at different levels. Finally, the floor should be sloped inward-downwards by 5-10° (Fig. 11-11). This so-called Bronner-inclination aims at preventing the restoration from sliding out of the cavity as a result of plastic deformation during loading. The mesiodis-

tal depth should be about 1 mm for primary first and 1.5 mm for primary second molars.

The pulpoaxial line angle should be moderately rounded off (Fig. 11-11) in order to reduce its wedging effect at loading of the marginal ridge of the restoration(8a). A too-pronounced rounding off might lead to fracture-inducing movements of the restoration.

Instrumentation: In case of a limited carious lesion, it is recommended to start the intervention by preparing the occlusal box, which gives a good overview and reduces the risk of traumatic exposure of the pulp. With a cylindrical diamond with a flat top and suitable size, the fissures are opened down to the dentin. With the same instrument the approximal box is prepared to correct upper width and vertical and mesiodistal depths. Bronner-inclination is brought about by tilting the diamond without removing tooth substance in the axial wall. The occlusal box is completed, as described in connection with the Class I cavity. With a thin diamond or carbide bur with a semicircular top, the final outline of the approximal box is prepared. The same instrument is used for preparation of the angle between the inclined gingival floor

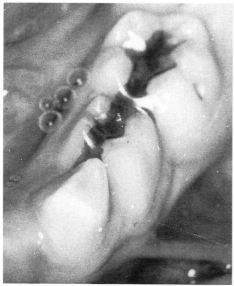

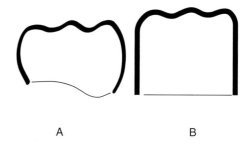

Fig. 11-13.

A) precontoured (crimped) stainless steel crown; B) standard (uncrimped) crown.

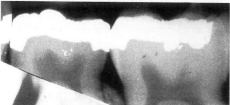

Fig. 11-12. Class II cavity restorations in lower primary molars.

and the axial wall. Rounding off of the pulpoaxial line angle is performed with a chisel.

The application of the above principles is demonstrated in Fig. 11-12.

Class III, IV and V cavity restorations

Smooth surface caries is removed with round burs. Access to carious approximal areas is provided from the buccal or lingual side, where the slightest loss of sound tooth substance will be caused. The size of the cavity is determined by the extent of the lesion.

Bevelling of the cavosurface margin with

a small tapered diamond is recommended, if composite resin is to be used as restorative material. This gives an increased area for acid etching utilizing the direction of the enamel prisms. The bevel should be 30 to 45° throughout.

Composite resin is the material of choice for Class IV cavity restorations in both dentitions and for Class III and anterior Class V cavity restorations in permanent teeth. Glass ionomer cement is the alternative for Class III and V cavity restorations in primary teeth and could also be used in patients with high caries activity in permanent teeth.

SPECIAL TREATMENTS IN THE PRIMARY DENTITION

Stainless steel crowns

Stainless steel crowns are superior to restorations of amalgam and alternative materials in many respects, particularly in heavily destroyed primary molars. Retrospective studies have shown that the frequency of revisions of such crowns is low compared to traditional multi-surface restorations(3, 5,

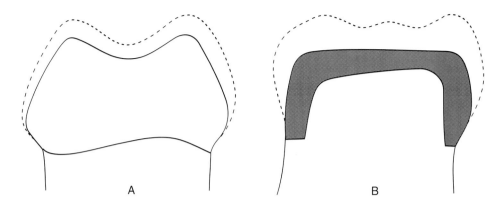

Fig. 11-14.

A) retention of a stainless steel crown in the cervical area;
B) extensive carious defects initially restored with glass ionomer cement and the crown subsequently adapted to the restoration.

32). The use of crowns may, therefore, be more cost-efficient.

The crowns are made of austenitic stainless steel, i.e. comprised of Fe as the main element in addition to Cr and Ni. In one product, nickel is the main element. It has recently been reported that the prevalence of sensitivity to nickel is increased among children with such crowns(6).

Two types of crowns are available, precontoured and standard, dependent on whether the cervical margins are crimped inward or not (Fig. 11-13). The precontoured crowns are usually easier to adapt gingivally.

Indications

1. Primary molars with extensive caries where the prognosis for other types of restorations is poor.

2. Hypomineralized molars, particularly permanent first molars where the steel crown may be an excellent intermediate restoration in the mixed dentition.

Technique – The preparation should be conservative in reducing sound tooth substance. Small undercuts may be advantageous for the retention of the crown. In particular, the gingival contour of the buccal and lingual surfaces should be preserved (Fig. 11-14A). All carious tissue is removed, and deep areas are lined with a biocompatible liner. The occlusal surface is reduced according to the occlusion and the approximal surfaces sliced just enough to let the crown pass the contact points. The preparation should not be extended into the gingival crevice, even if the margin of the crown is supposed to do so, because the elasticity of the crown permits it to be pressed over the preparation border and into the gingival pocket. In cases where the caries process has extended deeply underneath the gingival margin, it may be necessary to restore the defect before the crown is adapted to secure an adequate marginal fit. Glass ionomer cement is suitable for this purpose. The margin of the steel crown may then be adapted to the restoration rather than to the cavity margin (Fig. 11-14B).

Selection of the crown may be done by

measuring the distance between the contact points of the neighbouring teeth, or the distance from the mesial to the distal surface in the gingival area of the prepared tooth, using a divider. A crown with corresponding mesiodistal width is selected from the kit. If the precontoured crown is used, it may not pass the preparation border until it has been reduced in height. Irrespective of the type of crown, reduction is performed with a crown scissor or a stone. The edge of the crown should be in the gingival crevice without exerting pressure on the periodontal membrane. The crown must rest on the occlusal surface and the position be stable and repeatable, before the contouring process starts.

The purpose of contouring is mostly to obtain a nice fit at the gingival margin in order to prevent gingival irritation. It may also be necessary to adapt the crown into the bite by altering the contact points and the occlusal surface. Different pliers are available for these purposes (Fig. 11-15).

Finally, the margin of the crown is polished with a rubber wheel and cemented with phosphate, polycarboxylate or glass ionomer cement. The latter two adhere to the tooth substance and may therefore be

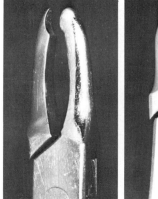
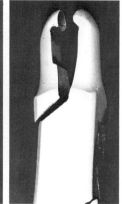

Fig. 11-15. Pliers for adaptation of stainless steel crowns. *Left.* No. 114. *Right.* No. 112.

preferred. A clinical case is shown in Fig. 11-16.

Modified restorations

As was discussed under treatment planning, the grossly destroyed primary molar can be difficult to restore both with regard to horizontal and vertical dimensions unless a stainless steel crown is used. Thin walls have to be reduced in height in order

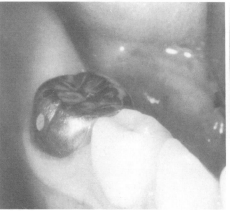
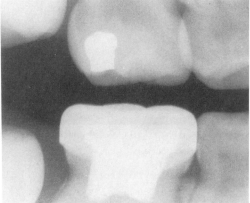

Fig. 11-16. Stainless steel crown on a pulpotomized lower primary second molar with an amalgam filling in the buccal surface contributing to the retention.

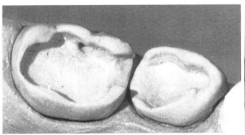 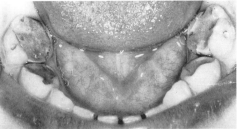

Fig. 11-17. Modified (atypical) Class II cavity restorations in lower primary molars.

to minimize the risk of fracture of tooth substance and the restoration modified in height and width in order to reduce the effect of masticatory forces. The atypical restoration is therefore a plane sloped filling of amalgam or glass ionomer cement (Fig. 11-17).

During the 1980s, other modified treatments for approximal lesions in primary molars have been discussed, i.e. tunnel preparations extending from the occlusal to the approximal surface and so-called minimal cavities (bowl-shaped approximal cavities including the marginal ridge area). Glass ionomer cement is the restorative material. Since long-term results are lacking, these treatments are not further elaborated on.

Disking

Disking of a carious lesion was previously described as an integral part of interceptive orthodontics and also as a further simplification of the atypical restoration. After separation from the neighbouring tooth through wedging, the carious approximal surface is rounded off in the buccolingual and occlusocervical directions so that the largest mesiodistal width is located centrally and cervically. The procedure is performed with a thin, tapered diamond so that the approximal surface continues stepless in the occlusal surface. If any carious tooth substance remains after the disking, a

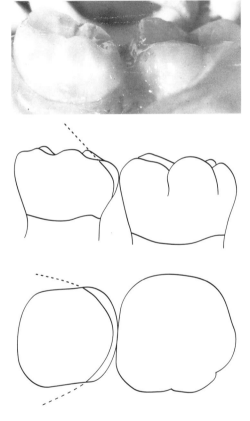

Fig. 11-18. Therapeutic disking of the distal surface of a lower primary second molar; refer to discussion of the case in Fig. 11-1.

Class I cavity restoration of amalgam or glass ionomer cement is performed (Fig. 11-18).

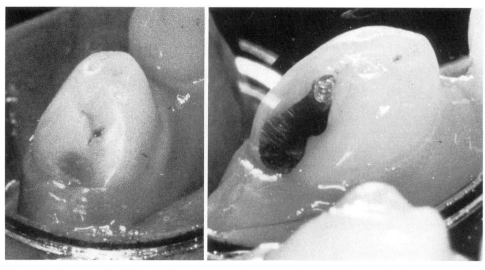

Fig. 11-19. Therapeutic disking (left) and one-surface restoration (right) as modified treatment of an approximal carious lesion in a lower primary first molar instead of a Class II cavity restoration when the primary second molar is extracted.

A special case, where disking is indicated, is when the second primary molar is extracted and the primary first molar has an approximal lesion that undermines the marginal ridge. Normally a Class II cavity restoration should be made. Since a Class III cavity restoration is not suitable, the approximal surface is sloped and a modified Class I cavity restoration of amalgam or glass ionomer cement performed (Fig. 11-19). The treatment is quick and simple. The risk of fracture of a conventional Class II cavity restoration can be tangible as a result of changed occlusion after extraction of the primary second molar.

Treatment of advanced lesions at an early age

Rapidly developing carious lesions during early childhood constitute problems of a psychological nature. The child does not cooperate, if it has not reached an age at which it is mature enough to accept operative treatment. First the incisor region is affected, but often also primary first molars. The lesions are mostly extensive and irregular and include all surfaces of incisors and the occlusal surface of first molars. All enamel caries, proteolysed and most of the softened dentin is removed with a spoon excavator. Undermined enamel is left for mechanical retention and glass ionomer or zinc oxide-eugenol cement inserted (Fig. 11-20). The floor of very deep cavities might be covered with calcium hydroxide paste. To secure the retention of the lining and restorative material, an orthodontic band may be adapted to the tooth and cemented with a glass ionomer cement (Fig. 11-21). When the child has matured, the treatment can be completed in a more ordinary way.

Prosthetics

Many kinds of prosthetic therapy may be relevant in pedodontics, e.g. dentures, acid-etched retained bridges, cast crowns and laminate veneers. This section deals with

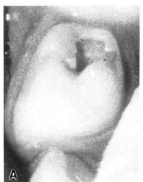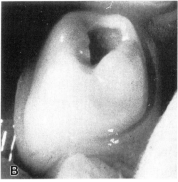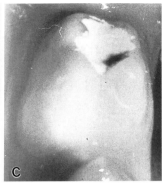

Fig. 11-20. Temporary treatment of an advanced carious lesion in a lower primary first molar at an early age.

A) before treatment;
B) after excavation of proteolysed and most of the softened dentin;
C) after application of temporary filling material.

dentures in the primary dentition. Treatments with crowns and bridges in the permanent dentition are described in Chapters 14 and 15.

The causes for need of prosthetic treatment in preschool children may be loss of teeth due to caries, trauma, or developmental disturbances. The reasons that they should be replaced by prostheses are their influence on aesthetics, speech function, function of lips, tongue and cheeks, chewing and swalloving functions, position of the remaining teeth and relationship between the jaws(21). Among these factors, the two first-mentioned constitute the strongest indications. Very early in childhood, people become conscious of the importance of aesthetics, related to clothing, hairdressing, jewelry and so on, and even a sound dentition is one of the important factors. Therefore, the psychological effect of missing teeth should not be underestimated, even in preschool children. The dental profession should be proud of this attitude, since it is a result of successful preventive care. The correct pronounciation of the S and T sounds is dependent upon the presence of the upper incisors. In absence of these teeth,

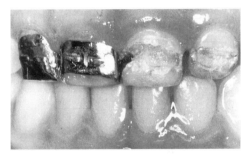

Fig. 11-21. Temporary treatment of advanced carious lesions in upper primary incisors at an early age; orthodontic bands used for retention of lining and temporary filling material after excavation.

the child has to compensate by establishing wrong habits, which may be difficult to treat later on.

Dentures are usually made in 3- to 4-year-old children with loss of incisors and first molars due to rampant caries (Fig. 11-22). The cuspids and second molars are less prone to early caries, and since these teeth are the most important for a normal development of the occlusion, efforts are usually made to preserve them. In addition to aesthetic and functional motives, the denture

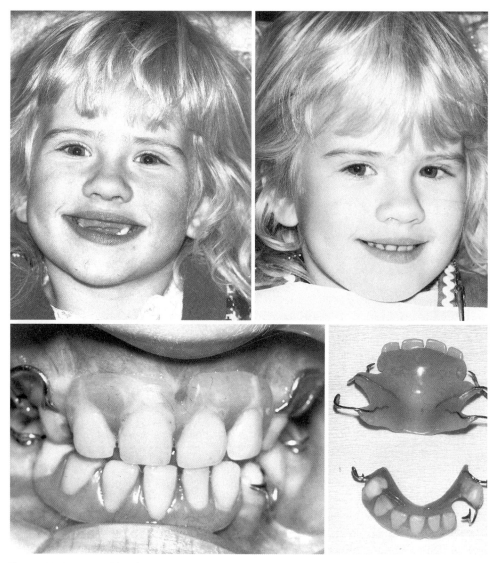

Fig. 11-22. A 4-year-old girl with upper and lower partial dentures.

acts as a space maintainer for the premolars. Impressions of both jaws are taken in alginate, and a wax bite for positioning of the models in an occludator. The base of the denture is fully supported by the gums and follows the gingival margins of the teeth to obtain sufficient stability. The posterior extension is usually the distal surface of the second molar. The cuspids and second molars are supplied with either Adam's clamps or finger clamps. Artificial primary teeth are usually made by contouring resin teeth originally aimed for the permanent dentition. They must be extremely white and mounted in a vertical position with small diastema to give a convincing representation of the primary dentition.

It is important to maintain good oral hygiene in patients with dentures so that caries and periodontal diseases are prevented. The denture must be cleaned after each meal and kept in a glass of water during the night, and the remaining teeth must be properly cleaned twice per day, usually after breakfast and the evening meal.

The denture is usually finally removed at the time for eruption of the permanent teeth at the age of 6. In this age group, children normally lack incisors so the aesthetic need is reduced. There is also an increased growth of the jaws in this period, which may interfere with the adaptation of the denture. It is recognized that dentures do not impair the growth, the problem is rather that they do not fit any more, if the period of wearing is prolonged.

Children seem to accept dentures very well, if they have been motivated. Their ability to adaptation is better than adults, they have a good tonus of the muscles which facilitates retention, and the distance between the jaws is short and favourable for stability. And, as in adults, aesthetic motives seem to be very relevant to them.

SPECIAL TREATMENTS FOR PITS AND FISSURES

Aspects on the occlusal surface of permanent molars

While caries reduction among children in Scandinavia in general has been substantial during the last 20 years, the occlusal surface of the permanent molars has still to be considered caries-prone. The reasons for this are that their mostly complicated fissure anatomy makes them difficult to clean properly and that fluorides in toothpastes and mouthrinses seem to be less effective on these surfaces(19). Therefore, special preventive measures are widely used, such as application of fluoride varnish and fissure sealing.

Factors that should be considered when deciding on preventive measures are: 1) the overall caries activity of the child; 2) the anatomy of the fissures; and 3) the time the tooth has been erupted.

If the child has no or little caries at the time of eruption of the permanent molars, it can be questioned if it is necessary to apply special preventive measures to these teeth. In a child population with low prevalence of caries, the cost-effectiveness of such measures has to be estimated.

To benefit best from preventive measures, the tooth should be treated as soon as possible after eruption. It should be considered that a tooth, which has been erupted for some years and still has not become carious, is less likely to develop caries and therefore in general does not need any additional prevention besides daily fluoride supply through toothpastes.

During eruption, the molars may be covered distally by a gingival flap, a so-called operculum. This may be an obstacle for obtaining a dry operation field necessary for effective fissure sealing. In such cases, treatment with a fluoride varnish is the alternative.

Use of fluoride varnish

The most commonly used varnish is Dura-phat® (Woelm ICN Pharmaceutical, Esch-wege, FRG). It has been shown to give a caries reduction of between 30 and 75% in occlusal surfaces of permanent first molars(1,29). The varying results depend on different experimental designs, such as time of application after eruption, number of applications, procedures at application and the caries activity of the children. The reason for the caries-preventive effect in fissures has been explained by the extended time of exposure compared with other kinds of topical fluorides and the formation of calcium fluoride, which serves as a slow-release system for fluoride ions(45). In a

TABLE 11-2

Indications (+) for fissure sealing stated at a Nordic conference in 1983.
Modified from(23).

Individual caries risk	Anatomy of the fissures	
	Shallow fissure (no caries disposition)	Deep fissure (narrow entrance, disposition for caries)
Low	– (*)	+ (**)
High	+	+

* Indications for fluoride varnish
** Alternative: fluoride varnish

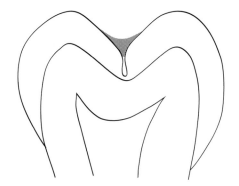

Fig. 11-23. Fissure sealing blockades the entrance to the underlying fissure.

study of Swedish children(16), where newly erupted permanent first molars were treated three times at 6-month intervals, the reduction was 56% after an observation period of 2.5 years. It should be noted that the prevalence of caries in the occlusal surfaces in the control group amounted to 80%. The study also showed that the effect was higher for surfaces with narrow entrances of the fissures compared with those with easily accessible entrances as judged clinically.

The advantage of using a fluoride varnish instead of a sealant is that the procedure is not as sensitive to saliva contamination as that of sealing. The best effect can be expected for newly erupted teeth.

Procedure – The surface is cleaned and dried before application. Gentle scraping with an explorer may be necessary to clean the entrances of the fissures. In order to get the varnish in close contact with the enamel surface, a blunt explorer can be used to force the varnish into the fissure entrances. A few drops of water on the varnish after applica-tion make it harden faster. The child is told not to eat hard food and not to brush the varnished surfaces during the same day. The procedure is preferably repeated 1-2 times at 6-month intervals.

Indications for use of fluoride varnish in relation to fissure anatomy and caries activity are given in Table 11-2.

Fissure sealing

Fissure sealing is accepted as an effective and safe method for the prevention and treatment of initial caries in pits and fissures (31). The method is based on the acid etch technique, in which resins are bonded to the enamel so effectively that leakage into the underlying fissure is prevented and that the microflora will suffer from lack of nutrients for the caries process (Fig. 11-23).

Technique – It is necessary to remove plaque and pellicle to obtain the best possible etch pattern of the enamel. A pumice-water slurry and a rubber cup may be used, or an air-abrasive instrument (e.g. Prophy Jet, De Treys Dentsply, Wiesbaden, FRG) which has been shown to give better cleaning in the deeper parts of the fissures(41). The slurry must be removed by an air-water spray. The isolation of the tooth may ideally be done with a rubber dam, but since the teeth frequently are newly erupted, the clamp may be harmful to the gingiva and painful for the child. Use of cotton rolls or absorbent pads in combination with a saliva ejector is recommended, and it is important to have close control on any movements of the tongue and cheek, which may displace the cotton rolls and ejector. The etchant is applied with a small cotton pellet or a brush and must be extended sufficiently to ensure that the margin of the sealant is placed on etched enamel. The etching time is approximately one minute. The acid is then washed away with excessive water spray, and a high-volume aspirator tube should be held close to the tooth to prevent swallowing reflexes, which may interfere with the isolation of the tooth. The acid-etched surface must not be contaminated with saliva. After drying the etched surface with compressed air, the sealant is applied with an instrument, brush or applicator dependent on the type of sealant and experience of the operator. All areas with pits and fissures must be covered, and the margins must be firmly bonded to etched enamel to prevent marginal leakage (Fig. 11-24). The time needed for isolation is dependent on the type of sealant, light-cured being faster than chemically cured. Before the patient is dismissed, the sealant must be controlled in respect of retention and occlusion.

The sealant should be checked at regular intervals for retention, and reapplication may be done according to the original procedure in cases where it is missing or partially missing.

Effectiveness – In order to evaluate the effectiveness of fissure sealing, two parameters are used: 1) retention and 2) the caries-preventive effect. There are a number of studies reporting on both these aspects, and the results vary within wide ranges(34,35).

A complete retention of the sealant in all areas of the fissure is necessary for effective caries prevention. Even if it has been experimentally shown that residual resin tags in the enamel after a lost sealant may prevent caries, the clinical significance of this is unknown. It is observed that caries may arise in cases with lost or, in particular, partially lost sealants. The frequency of total retention of the sealants is therefore a measure of their potential capacity for preventing caries. All studies show decreasing rate of retention with increasing observation period. After 2-8 years, the results vary between 3 and 97%, with the majority between 40 and 80 %. The main reason for the wide range is probably the different clinical conditions under which the sealants have been applied. Some of the surveys have been done as field service programs using transportable and primitive equipment. In a Swedish study, however, the frequency of total retention after 8 years was 80%, and after 10 years 95% of the sealed surfaces were still sound(44).

Most studies of the caries-preventive effect of fissure sealants have been done according to the split mouth technique, in which one of the teeth in a homologous pair is sealed and the contralateral used for control. The basis for the trials is the fact that the individual caries pattern is usually symmetric. By comparing the number of carious unsealed and sealed teeth after different observation periods, the caries-reducing effect is expressed as the difference in percent of the number of carious unsealed teeth. Among reported studies, it varies between 12 and 90 %, with an average of about 50 % after 4 years. Several factors influence the effect, among them the retention and the caries prevalence in the population. If the frequency of total retention and the prevalence of fissure caries in the studied population are high, the caries-preventive effect is usually excellent.

The caries-preventive effect may also be expressed as the *net gain*, which is the number of teeth that have been saved from being

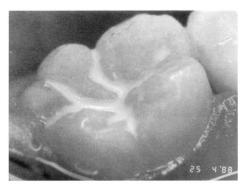

Fig. 11-24. Fissure sealing blocking the entrance to all parts of the fissures.

carious, related to the number of teeth that have been sealed. Among the reported studies, this varies between 8 and 48%, with an average of 27% after 4 years, indicating that 27 teeth are saved when 100 are sealed. Since the net gain takes the number of teeth that have been treated into account, it gives relevant information for the discussion of the cost/effectiveness of sealing programs.

Indications – Many authors recommend that all teeth with pits and fissures are routinely sealed without judging the risk of their becoming carious. Due to the decreasing caries prevalence in the Scandinavian countries this approach may be unnecessary and expensive since the net gain obviously will be very low. Particularly the pits and fissures of premolars show low caries activity, and if all of them are sealed, most of the sealants will be superfluous. The permanent first and second molars are more prone to fissure caries. When judging the risk of these teeth becoming carious, the individual caries activity, as well as the anatomy of the fissures, should be estimated. At a Nordic conference(23), the indications in Table 11-2 were suggested.

Sealing of primary molars is used less frequently, even if it has been shown that the retention may be good, if the fissures are sufficiently cleaned and dried. But since fissure caries in these teeth usually develops when the children are very young and uncooperative, the clinical procedure may be difficult.

In handicapped patients and patients with general diseases, the need for preventive care is of more importance than for others, and sealing should be used more routinely than indicated above. The same is the case for teeth with certain developmental defects, e.g. invaginations where early sealing may prevent the invasion of microbes into the pulp.

Sealing over caries – The anatomy of the fissures makes it impossible to clean the deepest parts of them before sealing, and there is always a microbial flora left underneath the sealing (Fig. 11-23). The diagnosis of early caries is also difficult, and active caries processes are frequently unconsciously sealed.

Many studies have dealt with the problem of what happens, when caries is sealed in this way. Most experiments have been done by placing sealants over obvious caries processes, in enamel as well as dentin, and after different observation periods the sealant has been removed and the focus examined clinically and by microbiological methods. Observation periods up to 5 years have been used, and the results are convincing that sealants are capable of arresting such lesions(26,15). The number of viable bacteria is reduced to a minimum, and the caries process has changed its character into the typical dry and leatherlike appearance of an arrested process.

In conclusion, sealants may be indicated for the prevention of caries in intact fissures, as well as for arresting initial caries lesions. The latter indication is disputable, since many dentists prefer to remove carious tissue before sealing a fissure (see next section), but the safety of sealing over initial caries lesions is first of all a matter of diag-

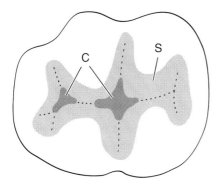 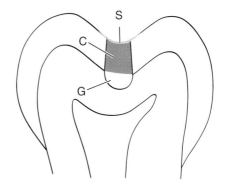

Fig. 11-25. Preventive resin restoration; C = composite resin, G = glass ionomer cement, S = sealant.

nostic and technical standards. If the lesion is small, and the clinical procedure for placement of the sealant is followed strictly, there are minimal chances for progression of the lesion.

Preventive resin restorations

The term preventive resin restoration has been adopted for treatment of early carious lesions in pits and fissures, including the removal of carious tissue and insertion of a resin filling material followed by the application of a sealant, which covers all pits and fissures (Fig. 11-25). The rationale behind this is a limited intervention in sound dental tissue in cases with limited caries lesions (33,37).

The technique consists of removal of fissure caries only, including any dentin caries using a rotating instrument. Use of slowly rotating burs results in more conservative preparations than high-speed equipment. Only as much enamel is removed as is necessary for access. There is no need for undercuts, since retention is based on the acid etch technique. The sound part of the fissure is not involved in the preparation. If dentin is exposed, it must be lined with a biocompatible material, e.g. a calcium hydroxide or glass ionomer cement. The latter

may be preferred in normal cavities, since it adheres both to dentin and the subsequent resin material, while calcium hydroxide preparations should be used close to the pulp. After the acid etch procedure, the cavity is lined with a thin layer of fluid resin (enamel bonding agent), filled with a posterior composite restorative material, and finally covered with a sealant, based on the same type of polymer as the composite resin, to ensure that all adjacent pits and fissures are sealed. If a light-cured material is used, curing is done after each step. In small cavities, as in cases with enamel caries only, the procedure may be simplified by using a diluted composite resin as a combined filling and sealing material(33). For more extensive cavities with dentin caries, a filling material with improved physical qualities is needed, and the posterior composite resins are most suitable.

The preventive resin restoration is an alternative to the amalgam restoration, and the main advantages are the conservative cavity design and more pleasing aesthetics. It should, however, be remembered that the technique is demanding with respect to patient management and moisture control, and the method should not be instituted if the operator can not master these factors.

Literature cited

1. Bille J, Thylstrup A. Radiographic diagnosis and clinical tissue changes in relation to treatment of approximal carious lesions. *Caries Res* 1982; **16**: 1-6.

2. Carvalho JC, Ekstrand KR, Thylstrup A. Dental plaque and caries on occlusal surfaces of first permanent molars in relation to stage of eruption. *J Dent Res* 1989; **68**: 773-9.

3. Dawson LR, Simon JF, Taylor PP. Use of amalgam and stainless steel restorations for primary molars. *J Dent Child* 1981; **48**: 420-2.

4. Edwardsson S. Bacteriological studies on deep areas of carious dentine. *Odontol Revy* 1974; 25: Suppl. **32**: 1-143.

5. Eriksson A-L, Paunio P, Isotupa K. Restoration of deciduous molars with ioncrowns: retention and subsequent treatment. *Proc Finn Dent Soc* 1988; **84**: 95-9.

6. Feasby WH, Ecclestone ER, Grainger RM. Nickel sensitivity in paediatric patients. *Pediatr Dent* 1988; **10**: 127-9.

7. Granath L-E. Photoelastic model experiments on Class II cavity restorations of dental amalgam. *Odontol Revy* 1965; 16: Suppl. **9**: 1-38.

8. Granath L-E. Operativ kariesterapi. In: *Nordisk lärobok i pedodonti*. 3rd ed. Stockholm: Sveriges Tandläkarförbunds Förlagsförening u p a, 1976; 191-224.

8a. Granath L-E, Edlund J. The role of the pulpoaxial line angle in the origin of isthmus fracture. *Odontol Revy* 1968; **19**: 317-34.

9. Granath L, Holm A-K, Matsson L, Schröder U. Tidiga approximala kariesskador i permanenta tänder. Ett diagnostiskt och terapeutiskt problem? *Tandläkartidningen* 1985; **77**: 68-72.

10. Granath L, Kahlmeter A, Matsson L, Schröder U. Progression of proximal enamel caries in early teens related to caries activity. *Acta Odontol Scand* 1980; **38**: 247-51.

11. Granath L, McHugh WD. The relation between preventive and operative dentistry. In: Granath L, McHugh WD, eds. *Systematized prevention of oral disease*: Theory and practice. Boca Raton, Florida: CRC Press, 1986; 9-16.

12. Granath L, Svensson A. Elastic outward bending of loaded buccal and lingual premolar walls in relation to cavity size and form. *Scand J Dent Res* 1991; **99**: 1-7.

13. Gröndahl H-G, Hollender L, Malmcrona E, Sundquist B. Dental caries and restorations in teenagers. II. A longitudinal radiographic study of the caries increment of proximal surfaces among urban teenagers in Sweden. *Swed Dent J* 1977; **1**: 51-7.

14. Gröndahl H-G, Hollender L. Dental caries and restorations. IV. A six-year longitudinal study of the caries increment of proximal surfaces. *Swed Dent J* 1979; **3**: 47-55.

15. Handelman SL, Leverett DH, Espeland M, Curzon J. Retention of sealants over carious and sound tooth surfaces. *Community Dent Oral Epidemiol* 1987; **15**: 1-5.

16. Holm GB, Holst K, Mejàre I. The caries-preventive effect of a fluoride varnish in the fissures of the first permanent molar. *Acta Odontol Scand* 1984; **42**: 193-7.

17. Høffding J, Kisling E. Premature loss of primary teeth: I. The overall effect on occlusion and space in the permanent dentition. *J Dent Child* 1978; **45**: 279-83.

18. Høffding J, Kisling E. Premature loss of primary teeth: II. The specific effects on occlusion and space in the permanent dentition. *J Dent Child* 1978; **45**: 284-7.

19. Koch G. Effect of sodium fluoride in dentifrice and mouthwash on incidence of dental caries in schoolchildren. *Odontol Revy* 1967; **18**: Suppl. 12: 57 and 83.

20. Koch G, Petersson LG. Caries preventive effect of a fluoride-containing varnish (Duraphat®) after 1 year's study. *Community Dent Oral Epidemiol* 1975; **3**: 262-6.

21. Krasse M. Prosthetic rehabilitation in preschool children. *Odontol Revy* 1957; **8**: 37-56.

22. Mannerberg F. The incipient carious lesion as observed in shadowed replicas ('en face pictures') and ground sections ('profile pictures') on the same teeth. *Acta Odontol Scand* 1964; **22**: 343-63.

23. Mejàre I, Koch G, Axelsson P, Sundström F. Symposium om fissurförsegling. *Tandläkartidningen* 1983; **175**: 1015-32.

24. Mejàre I, Malmgren B. Clinical and radiographic appearance of proximal carious lesions at the time of operative treatment in young permanent teeth. *Scand J Dent Res* 1986; **94**: 19-26.

25. Mejàre I, Malmgren B. Clinical tissue changes in advanced proximal lesions related to age. *J Dent Res* 1987; **67**: 756 (ScADR Abstr. No. 29).

26. Mertz-Fairhurst EJ, Schuster GS, Fairhurst CW. Arresting caries by sealants: results of a clinical study. *J Am Dent Assoc* 1986; **112**: 194-7.

27. Modèer T, Twetman S, Bergstrand F. Three-year study of the effect of fluoride varnish (Duraphat) on proximal caries progression in teenagers. *Scand J Dent Res* 1984; **92**: 400-7.

28. Moreno EC, Zahradnik RT. Chemistry of enamel subsurface demineralization in vitro. *J Dent Res* 1974; **53**: 226-35.

29. Murray JJ, Winter GB, Hurst CP. Duraphat fluoride varnish. A 2-year clinical trial in 5-year-old children. *Br Dent J* 1977; **143**: 11-7.

30. Möller B. Reaction of the human dental pulp to silver amalgam restorations. The modifying effect of treatment with calcium hydroxide. *Acta Odontol Scand* 1975; **33**: 233-8.

31. National Institutes of Health. Dental sealants in the prevention of tooth decay. NIH Consensus Development Conference Statement. *J Dent Educ* 1984; **48**: No. 2 suppl: 126-31.

32. Nielsen LA, Daugaard-Jensen J, Ravn JJ. En klinisk-radiologisk evaluering af praefabrikerede stålkroner. *Tandlaegebladet* 1978; **82**: 183-6.

33. Raadal M. Follow-up study of sealing and filling with composite resins in the prevention of occlusal caries. *Community Dent Oral Epidemiol* 1978; **6**: 176-80.

34. Raadal M. Fissurforsegling. Kariesprofylakse og terapi. *Nor Tannlaegeforen Tid* 1986; **96**: 51-8.

35. Rock WP. The effectiveness of fissure sealant resins. *J Dent Educ* 1984; **48**: No. 2 suppl: 27-31.

36. Rönnerman A, Thilander B. A longitudinal study on the effect of unilateral extraction of primary molars. *Scand J Dent Res* 1977; **85**: 362-72.

37. Simonsen RJ. Preventive resin restorations: three-year results. *J Am Dent Assoc* 1980; **100**: 535-9.

38. Socialstyrelsen. Kvicksilver/amalgam, hälsorisker. Rapport från socialstyrelsens expertgrupp med uppgift att utreda effekter av lågdosexponering för kvicksilver (With an English summary.) Stockholm: *Socialstyrelsen redovisar* 1987: **10**.

39. Socialstyrelsen. *Socialstyrelsens allmänna råd om diagnostik, registrering och behandling av karies.* Stockholm: SOSFS 1988: 30.

40. Socialstyrelsen. Val av tandfyllningsmateial för tuggytor. Stockholm: *Meddelandeblad* 1989: **8**.

41. Strand GV, Raadal M. The efficiency of cleaning fissures with an air-polishing instrument. *Acta Odontol Scand* 1988; **46**: 113-7.

42. ten Cate JM, Arends J. Remineralization of artificial enamel lesions *in vitro*. III. A study of the deposition mechanism. *Caries Res* 1980; **14**: 351-8.

43. Warfvinge J, Rozell B, Hedström K-G. Effect of calcium hydroxide treated dentine on pulpal responses. *Int Endod J* 1987; **20**: 183-93.

44. Wendt L-K, Koch G. Fissure sealant in permanent first molars after 10 years. *Swed Dent J* 1988; **12**: 181-5.

45. Ögaard B, Rölla G, Helgeland K. Uptake and retention of alkali soluble and alkali insoluble fluoride in sound enamel in vivo after mouthrinses with 0.05% or 0.2% NaF. *Caries Res* 1983; **17**: 520-4.

CHAPTER 12

ENDODONTICS

Diagnosis of pulpal conditions
Healing
Tissue reactions of importance
Treatment of primary and young permanent teeth with pulp exposure
Complications

Pedodontic endodontics means pulpal treatment of primary and young permanent teeth. The aim in primary teeth is to keep them healthy and functional until exfoliation, or at least as long as they are important to occlusal development. Treatment of young permanent teeth aims to maintain continuing root development, if possible, and to keep the tooth functional in the dentition. Pedodontic endodontics has its own characteristics which demand special handling and consideration.

Background factors of psychological, medical, orthodontic or cariologic character, may influence the choice of therapy and wound dressing. Treatment of primary teeth is usually restricted to vital pulps, either by covering the pulpal wound directly, or by excising a pulp horn or the entire coronal pulp. Conditions in tissue left behind should be normal or close to normal, since no medicament has any healing effect on chronically inflamed pulpal tissue. Successful treatment thus depends on a correct pulpal diagnosis. A differentiation is, therefore, required, not only between vital and non-vital pulps, but also between healthy and inflamed pulpal tissue, and between partial and total chronic pulpitis. In young permanent teeth, the recognition of pulpal necrosis after trauma often requires special consideration, as does root treatment of the immature tooth.

DIAGNOSIS OF PULPAL CONDITIONS

Pulp is healthy when exposed by trauma or accidentially during cavity preparation and can be kept healthy if properly treated.

Cariously exposed pulp is always chronically inflamed, partly or totally, or necrotic.

Pulp suffering injury to apical vessels sometimes becomes necrotic.

Diagnostic problems may arise in the child patient due to inadequate communication. Furthermore, primary teeth clinically judged to be free of pulpitis and without any history of subjective symptoms may actually have profound pulpal changes.

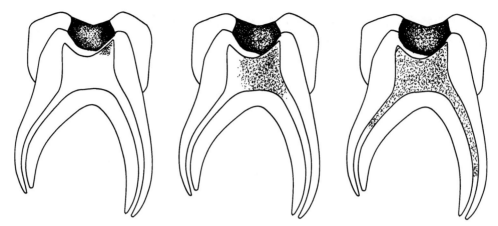

Fig. 12-1. Extent of chronic inflammation in the pulp of deep carious lesions (left), in partial chronic pulpitis (centre) and in total chronic pulpitis.

A correct diagnosis may be particularly difficult in cariously exposed pulp. A meticulous diagnostic procedure should, therefore, be followed, including all anamnestic, clinical and X-ray information. This would allow for a proper diagnosis in most cases.

Factors to consider are presented in Table 12-1. The diagnosis *partial chronic pulpitis* in a cariously exposed pulp is when there are no symptoms or signs of total chronic pulpitis. These diagnostic criteria are listed in Table 12-2. If there are negative/question-

TABLE **12-1**

Factors to consider in clinical diagnosis of pulpal conditions.

Case history

Pain, shooting or persisting, precipitated by cold, heat or sweets when chewing, or spontaneous pain at night

Tenderness

Bad taste or foul odours from the mouth

Recent orofacial trauma

Past medical and dental history

Status

Swelling, fistulae, sensitivity

Tenderness to palpation or percussion

Increased tooth mobility

Breakdown of marginal ridge, broken, missing or old restorations

Site and extent of pulpal exposure

TABLE **12-2**

Diagnostic criteria for partial and total chronic pulpitis.

Diagnostic factors	Diagnostic criteria for	
	partial chronic pulpitis	total chronic pulpitis
Mobility	+	–
Percussion	+/–	–
Sensitivity	+	+
X-ray	+	–
Exposure level	coronal	coronal/ cervical
Bleeding	+	–
Toothache	+/–	–

+ = Normal/positive diagnostic factor

– = Pathological/negative diagnostic factor

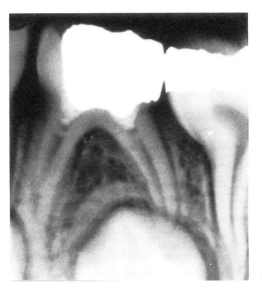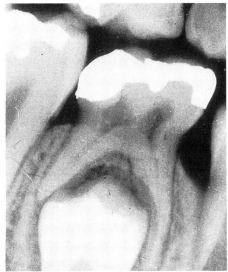

Fig. 12-2. Clinically successful coronal pulpotomy (left) and partial pulpotomy (right). Hard tissue barrier in relation to the pulp wound and no periradicular pathology.

able symptoms, the diagnosis is *total chronic pulpitis* (Table 12-2). Agreement of 80% has been shown between accumulated clinico-radiographic evaluation and histological findings(19).

Diagnostic criteria are, in general, the same for primary and permanent teeth, but a young permanent tooth in good communication with well-vascularized periapical tissue may cope better with both inflammation and trauma.

Partial or total necrosis may be the consequence of untreated caries, invagination of enamel, or traumatically exposed pulp.

If the necrosis is liquefactious, as observed after infection, it causes great irritation to the adjacent tissue with the sequelae of apical periodontitis or external root resorption. Necrosis may also develop following a luxation injury to the tooth where the apical circulation has been compromised or disrupted.

A sudden cessation of the blood supply to the pulp, as may be the case after luxation, results in pulpal infarct, firm necrosis, which in contrast to the liquefaction ne-

crosis is only slightly irritating. Such necrotic pulp tissue may be restored by ingrowth of tissue which eventually may become mineralized. This type of necrosis can be seen in primary, as well as permanent teeth.

Clinically the non-vital tooth usually shows no sensitivity. Colour changes towards grey support the diagnosis of pulpal necrosis. X-rays are important adjuncts and often more than one is necessary. Such pathological radiographic changes as widened periodontal space with diffusely lined or broken cortical bone, are indicative of necrotic pulp. Other radiographic indications are lack of narrowing of the pulpal lumen compared with earlier observations and/or discontinued root development of the immature tooth.

In connection with luxation injury, with pulp necrosis as a consequence, *external root resorption with osteolysis* may be seen. Irritation from the necrotic pulp tissue in relation to the injured periodontal membrane is most probably the cause.

HEALING

Clinically, pulpal healing means absence of pathological clinical and radiographic findings, but these do not guarantee a healthy residual pulp. Biologically, *the criteria of healing are absence of chronically inflamed tissue or necrotic tissue in the residual pulp*. The prerequisites for healing are considered to be: healthy residual pulp, gentle surgical technique, correct wound treatment; appropriate wound dressing, and effective prevention of secondary infection of the pulp.

Bacterial contamination and infection are the prime threat to healing of the pulp. The formation of a hard tissue barrier may be regarded as an indication of wound healing. It is, however, not necessarily the same as healing of the residual pulp, which is why it is necessary to distinguish between wound healing as such, and the healing of possible inflammatory changes in the residual pulp (Fig. 12-2).

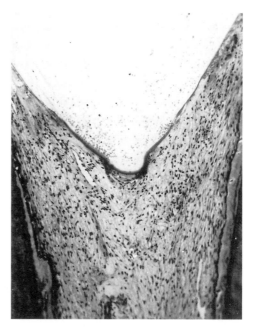

Fig. 12-3. Atraumatic pulp wound created with a spherical diamond in high-speed equipment and continuous flow of sterile saline.

TISSUE REACTIONS OF IMPORTANCE

Surgical technique

The recommended technique includes use of diamond burs on high-speed equipment and irrigation with sterile saline so as not to cauterize the vital pulp. This procedure has under experimental, as well as clinical, conditions been shown to be almost atraumatic to the residual pulp (Fig. 12-3).

Wound treatment - vital pulp

The presence of an intermediate layer of blood clot between the wound and the wound dressing has been shown in experimental as well as clinical studies(18,20) to interfere significantly with the ability of the pulp to heal and also to induce chronic

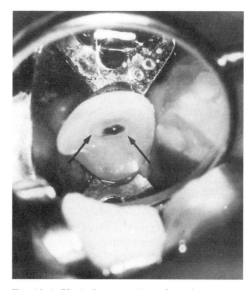

Fig. 12-4. Clinical appearance of gently amputated pulp; bleeding stopped. Note that the amputation also involves surrounding dentin.

inflammation in the residual pulp. The explanation of this might be that the coagulum acts as a bacterial substrate and, thereby, induces or enhances inflammation.

The wound should consequently be gently irrigated with sterile saline in order to achieve hemostasis and to get a clean wound without any extrapulpal blood clot (Fig. 12-4). If bleeding persists, the addition of calcium hydroxide to the saline might enhance hemostasis.

Wound dressing - vital pulp

The wound dressing should not induce any persistent pathologic changes of the residual pulp, but should favorably protect it by inducing a hard tissue barrier. Such a wound dressing is calcium hydroxide.

Calcium hydroxide – Calcium hydroxide is strongly alkaline with a pH about 12 and causes a chemical injury to the pulp. The initial caustic effect of calcium hydroxide on the exposed pulp is development of a superficial three-layer necrosis with a zone of firm necrosis adjacent to the vital pulp tissue.

The zone of firm necrosis causes slight irritation and stimulates the pulp to defense and repair. The tissue response is characteristic of wounded connective tissue. It starts with a vascular and inflammatory reaction to control and eliminate the irritating agent. Thereafter follows the repair process, including proliferation of cells and formation of new collagen. When the pulp is separated from the irritation by the first formed bone-like tissue, odontoblasts differentiate and the new-formed tissue assumes the appearance of dentin, i.e. the function of the pulp is restored(21). Mineralization of the barrier starts with dystrophic calcification of the necrotic layer leading to deposition of mineral in the newly formed collagen as well (Fig. 12-5). Hard tissue formation has been reported in direct contact with hard-setting calcium hydrox-

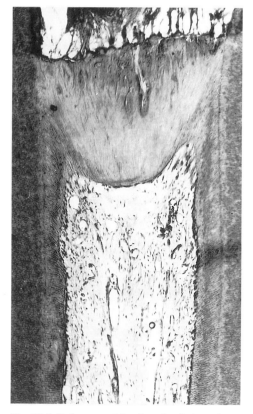

Fig. 12-5. Pulp wound healing, hard tissue barrier, following pulpotomy and capping with calcium hydroxide.

ide cements, indicating a less extensive initial chemical injury than that produced by calcium hydroxide *per se.* Such a difference might depend on factors such as variation in pH and rate of release of hydroxyl ions.

The pulp reaction to calcium hydroxide might be considered not as a specific characteristic of the medicament, but rather as a reaction to slight irritation. It is therefore most probable that any medicament or operative technique that induces the same degree of slight irritation will initiate similar pulp tissue reactions. This has been shown in experimental studies using other capping agents(8).

Formation of a hard tissue barrier as a

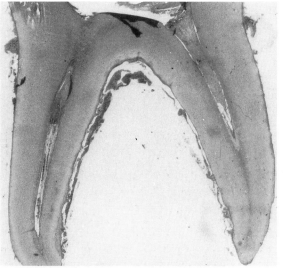

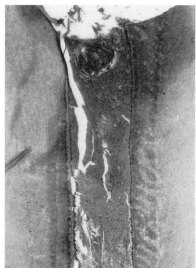

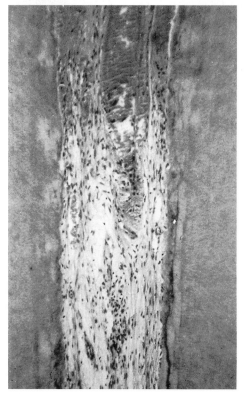

Fig. 12-6. Histological appearance of a pulpo-tomized primary molar, capped with formocre-sol and clinically without any pathological symptoms (left); devitalized (fixed) pulp tissue with loss of cellular distinction (right); border between devitalized and chronically in-flamed root pulp tissue (lower left).

criterion of wound healing must be re-garded favorable in an organ such as the pulp that lacks epithelium which normally contributes to healing. Even if the hard tissue barrier is not completely tight, it gives mechanical protection of the wound and is thus of great clinical importance.

Since the effect of calcium hydroxide on the pulp tissue is restricted to wound heal-ing by induction of a hard tissue barrier, it should only be used in cases with a clinically healthy residual pulp.

The main goal must be to choose a biologic wound dressing, but sometimes there are exceptions with primary teeth. For primary teeth of major importance to the dentition, but with a pulpal state that does not fulfill the criteria for partial chronic pulpitis, other wound dressings and endodontic therapies must be chosen. These might be devitalization of the residual pulp, or a pulpectomy and obturation of the pulp canals by a resorbable root-filling material.

Formocresol – The devitalizing ingredient in formocresol is formaldehyde. Formaldehyde, the aqueous solution of the gas formaldehyde, is used for fixation of tissue in histologic studies because it does not coagulate the tissue, which means that the tissue keeps its structure. The same process is considered to occur *in vivo*. The degree of penetration of formocresol is shown to be dose- and time-dependent(15). Clinical-histologic investigations, however, show that the effect of this medicament is more often chronic inflammation or even partial necrosis of the residual pulp(16) (Fig. 12-6). Animal studies have shown systemic absorption of formaldehyde. Formaldehyde has a known immunogenic, toxic, mutagenic and carcinogenic potential, which also makes it questionable as a wound dressing in primary teeth(13).

Several modes of therapy exist with variations of length of application and concentration of the drug. In spite of the tissue reactions observed histologically, formocresol treatment very seldom causes subjective or objective symptoms during a 2-3-year follow up.

In conclusion, formaldehyde-containing medicaments do not induce healing in a biological sense, but pathologic changes in the residual pulp. The use of formaldehyde-containing wound dressing should therefore be restricted.

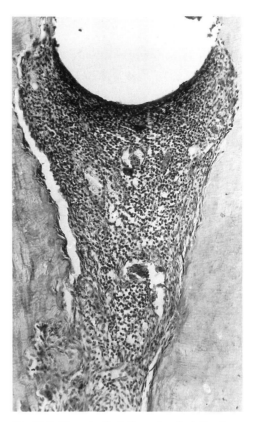

Fig. 12-7. Chronically inflamed pulp following pulpotomy and capping with zinc oxide eugenol.

Glutaraldehyde – Glutaraldehyde has been proposed as a substitute for formocresol. Similar tissue reactions and clinical results have been demonstrated(9). Because of its chemical structure, a larger molecule, it might be less diffusible but most probably it has similar disadvantages regarding immunogenic, toxic, mutagenic and carcinogenic potentials as formaldehyde-containing drugs.

Zinc oxide-eugenol – Zinc oxide-eugenol has been used as a wound dressing in relation to coronal pulpotomy of primary teeth and clinically-radiographically favorable results have been reported. Histological studies(14) have, however, shown chronic

Pulp therapy in the primary dentition

Therapy		Indication
Intermittent excavation	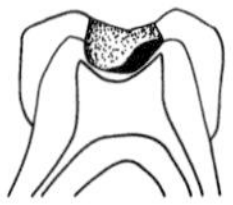	Deep carious lesion. Carious softened tissue close to pulp but presumably no exposure. No clinical or radiographic symptoms of pulpitis.
Direct pulp capping	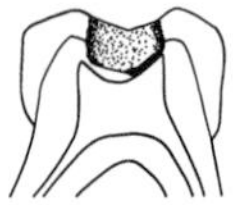	Accidental minimal exposure of healthy pulp during preparation or via trauma. Little or no contamination of the exposed area.
Partial pulpotomy	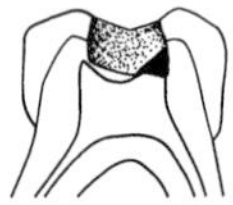	Accidental exposure - healthy pulp. Carious exposure - partial chronic pulpitis
Pulpotomy	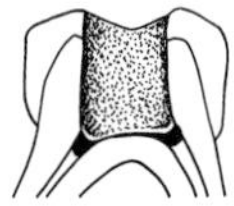	Carious exposure - partial/total chronic pulpitis

Fig. 12-8.

inflammation, internal resorption and also pulpal necrosis (Fig. 12-7). The medicament is not an ideal wound dressing in primary teeth, but may be used in cases of pulpectomy.

In the following the various forms of therapy will be discussed in relation to pulpal state and dentition, as well as to the etiological factors caries and trauma.

CHOICE OF TREATMENT

Definitions

Intermittent excavation is used in teeth with deep carious lesions but without any symptoms of pulpitis. Following removal of most of the carious substance, demineralized dentin is covered with calcium hydroxide and left temporarily under an intermediate filling. Intermittent excavation is not equivalent to indirect capping, where carious substance is left permanently under the restoration.

Direct pulp capping means no removal of pulp tissue, only covering the exposed pulp with a wound dressing.

Partial pulpotomy means excision of a superficial part of the coronal pulp, i.e. the wound surface is placed in coronal pulp tissue.

Pulpotomy, vital amputation, means in dentistry removal of the coronal pulp with the wound surfaces placed in the orifices of the root canals (Fig. 12-8).

Pulpectomy is removal of most of the pulp. The wound surface is placed in the apical part of the root canal 1-2 mm short of the apical foramen.

Root canal treatment means treatment of teeth with necrotic pulps.

Primary dentition

The value of keeping the tooth should first be established. The pulpal state will thereafter determine the choice of endodontic treatment.

Direct pulp capping, partial pulpotomy and pulpotomy are the most common endodontic therapies. Pulpectomy is more rarely performed because of the difficulty of instrumenting and obturating the root canals without causing injury to the underlying tooth germ.

Healthy pulp – Exposure of healthy pulps may occur accidentally during excavation of deep caries. To avoid accidental exposure in teeth without any signs of pulp involvement intermittent excavation may be performed. All softened carious dentin is removed, the floor of the cavity covered with calcium hydroxide and the cavity sealed with a temporary filling, for instance IRM. After 2-3 months the cavity is reopened, all residual carious dentin is removed and the tooth permanently restored. During this interval secondary dentin may have formed on the pulpal side of the cavity floor decreasing the risk of accidental exposure when removing the residual carious dentin.

Healthy pulp, in the sense that no chronically inflamed pulp tissue is suspected, might be a candidate for endodontic treatment in cases of accidental and traumatic exposures. In such cases direct pulp capping or partial pulpotomy is the therapy of choice and calcium hydroxide used as a capping material.

Direct pulp capping is used on minimal mechanical exposure, while partial pulpotomy should be done when contamination with infectious material or intrapulpal bleeding is observed. The wound area is then better controlled, securing a wound surface situated in healthy tissue. Furthermore, the wound dressing is placed more safely because of the better retentive capacity of the cavity. Both therapies have shown a favorable prognosis clinico-radiographically, about 80%. For the procedure of partial pulpotomy, see Appendix 12-1.

Traumatic exposures of primary incisors are rare. Partial pulpotomy might be performed. The value of the incisor for the occlusal development is limited, which is why extraction is most often the therapy of choice.

Partial chronic pulpitis – In primary teeth with carious pulp exposure and with a diagnosis of partial chronic pulpitis, a partial pulpotomy is the therapy of choice. The prognosis of coronal pulpotomy of primary molars with partial chronic pulpitis is less favorable than for partial pulpotomy(20,22), 67% and 83% respectively.

The reasons for this might be several. The histologic picture of partial chronic pulpitis shows in most cases that the chronic inflammation is restricted to the area adjacent to the exposure site. Furthermore, as partial pulpotomy does not involve any great vessels, bleeding is easier to control, which increases the possibility of avoiding an extrapulpal blood clot.

In cases where some symptoms point to coronal and some to total pulpitis, the wound surface must be placed deeper in the root pulp or pulpectomy might be considered. Calcium hydroxide could still be used as the wound dressing/temporary root-filling material. The prognosis might be expected to be favorable. For the procedure of pulpotomy, see Appendix 12-2.

Total chronic pulpitis – If the tooth is of great value for the occlusal development, pulpotomy might be attempted. Calcium hydroxide cannot be used, since neither it nor other medicaments have any healing effect on chronically inflamed pulp.

Devitalization of the root pulp with formocresol/glutaraldehyde may be used, but on very restricted indications. However, its deleterious potentials should be borne in mind. Whenever another therapy is available formocresol and glutaraldehyde should be avoided.

Zinc oxide-eugenol, which also induces inflammation, is recommended by some.

This medicament might help to keep the tooth long enough to avoid occlusal complications.

Preferably, however, a molar with total chronic pulpitis could be pulpectomized and a resorbable paste such as calcium hydroxide used as the root-filling material.

Extraction of the primary molar with total pulpitis and insertion of a space maintainer might also be considered.

Pulpal necrosis – In Scandinavia primary teeth with necrotic pulps are in general extracted and if necessary, for orthodontic reasons, a space maintainer is inserted. From a biologic standpoint there is no fully acceptable endodontic treatment for necrotic primary teeth. One of the difficulties involved is the fact that instrumentation of the root canals of a primary tooth always involves a risk of damaging the permanent tooth germ directly or indirectly. This is specially true when treating primary molars, their root canals being ribbon-shaped and curved. Another is finding a root-filling material which is resorbed in step with the physiological resorption of the root. Calcium hydroxide paste is to be recommended. In cases of aplasia of a second premolar, a conventional guttapercha root filling is in order.

To leave untreated a primary tooth with a necrotic pulp, perhaps out of a vague wish for space maintenance, is a serious omission. No orthodontic principle can alter the basic fact that necrosis of the pulp indicates either root canal treatment or extraction of the tooth.

Permanent dentition

The contents of this section will be focused on endodontic treatment of immature permanent teeth with pulpal involvement due to caries or trauma.

After clinical eruption of the tooth, the apical part of the root continues its growth for more than 3 years. The great width of the apical foramen during this period allows for a beneficial communication between the pulp tissue and the periodontal membrane and, consequently, for satisfactory vascularization of the pulp. These factors ensure favorable conditions for pulpal healing. However, any damage to the epithelial root sheath entails a risk of arrested root growth and a stunted root. Removal of pulp tissue also leads to an immediate arrest of dentin formation and cessation of the natural diminution of the pulp cavity in the corresponding area. This means reduced strength of the tooth and a greater risk of fracture in the event of trauma to the tooth.

Healthy pulp – The indications for intermittent excavation in young permanent teeth are the same as mentioned for primary teeth.

Direct pulp capping with calcium hydroxide may be performed in permanent teeth with minute accidental pulpal exposures. The cavity should immediately be sealed with a permanent restoration in order to avoid contamination from the oral cavity and infection of the wound. Under these circumstances direct capping has been shown to have a high success rate clinically/radiographically, 82% after 5 years (12).

If there is a risk of infection of the wound through leakage, a partial pulpotomy is preferred because it allows for more efficient sealing of the pulp-capped area. For procedure see Appendix 12-1.

Vital pulps affected by caries – Young permanent teeth with partial, as well as total, chronic pulpitis and incomplete root development are pulpotomized and calcium hydroxide used as wound dressing. The procedure is described in Appendix 12-2. Partial pulpotomy might be attempted, but if the bleeding is difficult to control, it is probably due to a more ad-

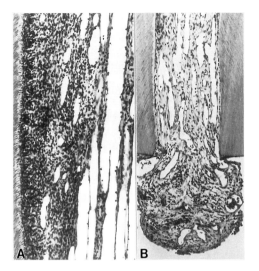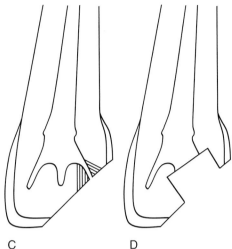

Fig. 12-9. Pulp exposure of monkey pulp by crown fracture; A) inflammation at pulpal end of exposed dentinal tubules; B) pulp polyp at the exposure site; C) schematic drawing showing the relationship between depth of pulpal reactions in relation to where exposed dentinal tubules reach the pulp; D) removal of affected tissue by partial pulpotomy.

vanced inflammatory state of the pulp than expected, and further amputation of the pulp should be performed. The wound surface should be situated in healthy pulp tissue.

Because of favorable nutritional conditions, healing might be expected even in pulps with total chronic pulpitis, followed by continued root development and diminution of the root canals.

However, obliteration of the root canals is often seen following coronal pulpotomy of immature permanent molars with total chronic pulpitis at the time of treatment, which makes future endodontic treatment, if required, very difficult to perform. Therefore, pulpotomy of young permanent molars should be regarded as a temporary treatment and followed by a pulpectomy as soon as the roots are mature and the root canal lumen developed to a normal size. Consequently, the root length of the tooth should be evaluated before treatment. If the length of the roots or any of the roots is almost complete, a pulpectomy should be performed. Calcium hydroxide is used as the temporary root filling material and is later replaced with guttapercha.

Pulpotomy and capping with calcium hydroxide of immature permanent teeth are successful treatments with respect to the continuation of the root development and physiological constriction of the root canal.

Traumatically exposed pulps (complicated crown fracture) – The pulp exposed by a complicated crown fracture is lacerated and in contact with the oral environment. Healing cannot be expected to occur spontaneously since infection leads to inflammation and necrosis. Histological studies show that the exposed pulp is chronically inflamed to a depth of about 2-3 mm but healthy beyond that(4,10). In most crown-fractured incisors a hyperplastic tissue reaction takes place and a pulp polyp is formed (Fig 12-9). Abscess formation or necrosis is very seldom observed. Why the proliferative reaction predominates might be explained by such factors as continuous

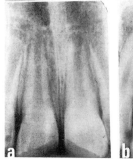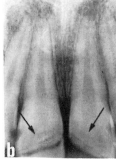

Fig. 12-10. 11 and 21 with complicated crown fracture; a) at the time of trauma; b) 3 years after partial pulpotomy showing hard tissue barrier and normal root development.

salivary rinsing of the exposed pulp and the frequently limited or no retentive capacity of the fracture which prevents infectious material from being kept in contact with the exposed pulp.

Partial pulpotomy is the preferred treatment, but in some cases direct pulp capping, pulpotomy or even pulpectomy may be considered.

Partial pulpotomy (Appendix 12-1) has a very high success rate, irrespective of the size of exposure, degree of root development and time interval between trauma and treatment(3). These results observed in a clinical-radiographic study are supported by results in experimental studies on monkey teeth(11).

A concomitant luxation of the tooth may interfere with healing following partial pulpotomy because that means a risk of injury to the apical vessels and thereby interference with the blood circulation of the pulp. An immature tooth is at an advantage compared with a mature tooth in this respect, and has a greater chance of overcoming such an injury, which is the reason why partial pulpotomy should always be considered.

The advantages of partial pulpotomy are several. In a young tooth it is essential that the natural tooth development should continue in order to obtain full root length and physiological diminution of all the pulp cavity. This will produce a mechanically stronger tooth, which better resists other trauma (Fig. 12-10). Histologic studies of partially pulpotomized incisors show relatively unaltered and healthy pulps(4).

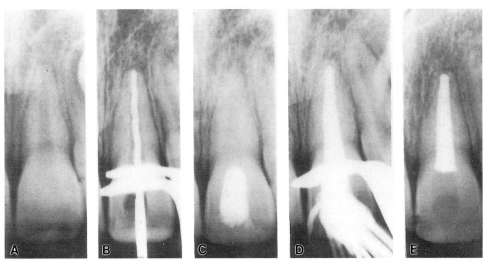

Fig. 12-11. Pulp necrosis due to trauma at 9 years of age; A) at the time of trauma; B) endodontic treatment; C) root canal filled with calcium hydroxide; D) at the time of root filling with guttapercha; E) 2 years follow-up.

Direct pulp capping might be performed if the pulp exposure is minimal and the tooth is treated immediately after trauma. The indication for direct capping is based on the assumption that the pulp injury is only superficial and will be overcome by the initial effect of calcium hydroxide. Failures observed following direct capping in complicated crown fractures mainly stem from infection of the wound due to insufficient wound sealing.

Pulpotomy does have some definite disadvantages. The pulp chamber cannot contract physiologically and testing the sensitivity of the tooth is virtually impossible. If root canal treatment is required locating the root canal might prove difficult.

Pulpectomy may be performed on mature teeth with concomitant luxation injury, but in immature teeth partial pulpotomy should always be tried initially.

In conclusion, partial pulpotomy is the superior pulp treatment in teeth with complicated crown fractures, and gives a favorable prognosis of 94-96%.

Pulpal necrosis – Root canal treatment is performed when infection/caries or trauma has caused pulpal necrosis with or without apical periodontitis.

The treatment is started in the conventional way by removing all necrotic pulp tissue. With immature teeth it is necessary to consider their anatomical features (Appendix 12-3). In immature teeth the root canal is tightly filled with calcium hydroxide in order to induce hard tissue formation apically, as well as to dissolve any pulp tissue accidentally left behind.

The treatment should be checked every 3-6 months. The calcium hydroxide filling, which has the same radioopacity as dentin, should be renewed when the calcium hydroxide has been resorbed from the apical part of the root canal. Usually 2-3 changes of calcium hydroxide are required before a hard tissue barrier is formed apically and

apical periodontitis and/or external resorption is healed (Fig. 12-11). Thereafter, permanent root filling is performed. Most often there is no pressing need to make a permanent root filling, since the crown usually is intact and does not need any crown restoration with anchorage in the root canal. Even in cases of apical periodontitis and/or inflammatory external root resorption the frequency of successful treatment has been shown to be very high, 95% after 4 years(1,2).

COMPLICATIONS

Internal dentin resorption in primary teeth

Internal dentin resorption is most frequently reported to occur in relation to pulpotomy of primary teeth (Fig. 12-12).

According to early reports the use of calcium hydroxide was considered the most probable cause of extensive internal dentin resorption. A more realistic explanation is that the internal resorption is due to the presence of chronic inflammation in the residual pulp, that had escaped the diagnosis at the time of treatment, and/or the presence of an extra-pulpal blood clot between the wound surface and the medicament(17,18). As mentioned before, a blood clot between the wound surface and the wound dressing prevents wound healing and induces chronic inflammation in the residual pulp even under optimal experimental conditions.

Furthermore, the occurrence of internal resorption some time between pulpotomy and extraction/exfoliation is observed histologically in practically all pulpotomized primary teeth without healing irrespective of type of wound dressing. Most failures due to internal dentin resorption following capping with calcium hydroxide appear within 6 – 10 months after treatment. Radio-

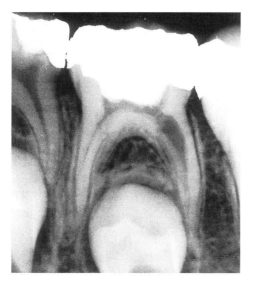

Fig. 12-12. Pulpotomized primary molar with internal dentin resorption in the distal root.

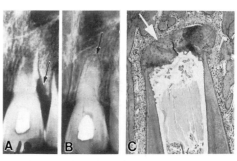

Fig. 12-13. Pulp necrosis in a very young tooth due to luxation; A) 2 months after initial root-canal treatment with calcium hydroxide; B) hard tissue formation apically and normal periradicular conditions, 1 year later; C) histologic picture of the hard tissue barrier. The tooth was lost due to another trauma causing cervical root fracture.

graphically diagnosed internal dentin resorption indicates chronic inflammation of the residual pulp and the tooth should be checked frequently or extracted, if the underlying permanent tooth germ is in any danger.

Complications in relation to traumatic injuries with special reference to endodontic treatment

External root resorption – External root resorption following luxation injuries can be surface resorption, replacement resorption (anchylosis) or inflammatory resorption related to pulp necrosis. In all cases the resorption depends on an injury to the periodontal membrane in connection with the trauma. In this context only the inflammatory resorption will be dealt with; for more information the reader is referred to Chapter 14.

External root resorption and osteolysis of the alveolar bone, a so-called inflammatory resorption, is observed as a consequence of a luxation injury that causes pulpal necrosis, as well as damage to the periodontal ligament. Toxins and bacteria from the necrotic pulp may, via dentinal tubules, cause inflammation in the injured periodontium and subsequent progressive external root resorption.

The treatment is the same conventional endodontic therapy, as for teeth with necrotic pulps.

Careful removal of all necrotic pulp tissue is imperative for healing. The choice of root-filling material is of less importance(2). In immature teeth, however, calcium hydroxide is preferred, since it dissolves any necrotic pulp tissue accidentally left and, thereby, eliminates further irritation of the periodontium and stimulates a hard tissue barrier apically. If the resorption has perforated the root, calcium hydroxide in contact with periodontal tissue stimulates hard tissue formation. For treatment procedure see Appendix 12-3.

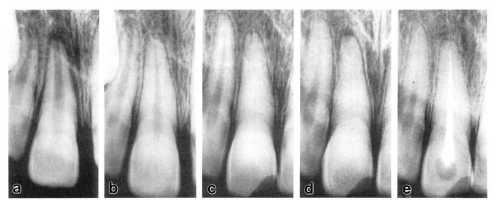

Fig. 12-14. Luxated and obliterating maxillary incisor; a and b) at the time of injury and 6 years later; c) at the time of an additional accidental injury in which the crown was fractured; d) 6 months later, periapical radiolucency; e) follow-up 4 years after endodontic treatment, periapical healing (Courtesy of Dr. M. Cvek).

Healing is highly frequent (96%) and characterized by cessation of resorption and a re-establishment of a radiographically normal periodontal membrane (Fig. 12-13).

Pulp obliteration with subsequent pulp necrosis – The most common type of obliteration following trauma is that of accelerated hard tissue deposition resulting in an even decrease and, sometimes, radiographic disappearance of the pulpal lumen. The vast majority of these teeth show no periapical pathologic complications, even after many years. Histologic studies of obliterated pulps have shown no pathologic changes that would indicate endodontic treatment. The frequency of apical periodontitis is very low, 13% after 16 years of follow-up.

Furthermore, in the event of periapical pathology, clinical-radiographic studies(7) have shown that endodontic treatment is possible and the outcome of the treatment is favorable, 80% success after 4 years (Fig. 12-14). Consequently, there is no need for any preventive endodontic treatment of incisors with obliterating pulps.

Teeth with discolored crowns - bleaching

Bleaching of teeth discolored by necrotic tissue is usually a successful procedure. The tooth may have become discolored before root canal treatment or by mistake after incomplete reaming-out of the pulpal horns. Prerequisite for bleaching is that the tooth has an adequate guttapercha root filling and is isolated from the oral cavity by a rubber dam, because the bleaching agents are extremely caustic. The procedure (Appendix 12-4) includes removal of all tissue and filling material of the coronal part of the pulp chamber. As much as possible of the discolored dentin is removed carefully without weakening the tooth crown too much. Thereafter, the root filling material is removed to the level of the cemento-enamel junction and isolated with a layer of 1-2 mm zinc phosphate cement to prevent seepage of the bleaching agent into the attachment area through the dentinal tubules.

The dentin is then carefully etched with buffered phosphoric acid and cleaned with chloroform or acetone. The bleaching medicament, 30% hydrogen peroxide solution is placed in the pulp chamber, but also applied externally to the enamel surface and the tooth is illuminated with UV-light or heat for 5-10 minutes, the procedure is repeated 3-4 times, whereafter a cotton pellet moistened with 30% hydrogen peroxide is placed in the pulpal lumen. The cavity is then carefully sealed with slow-setting zinc oxide eugenol and phosphate cement, and the tooth is left for 3-5 days. Sometimes the procedure must be repeated before a suitable result has been achieved. When a satisfactory result is achieved the pulpal chamber is acid etched and filled with composite of as light a color as possible. Another bleaching procedure using sodium perborate can also be used (Appendix 12-4).

Bleaching of teeth might be complicated by cervical external resorptions, which is why the treatment should be carefully followed up(5). Reasons for external resorptions might be several. Firstly, the bleaching procedure should be performed under as safe conditions as possible to avoid leakage of the etchant through the rubber dam. Secondly, after treatment the tooth should be very carefully rinsed to make certain no bleaching agents are left. There is also a possibility that the periodontium has been injured by the trauma, and that through the dentinal tubules, the bleaching agent might damage the cementum layer.

Literature cited

1. Cvek M. Treatment of non-vital permanent incisors with calcium hydroxide. I. Follow-up of periapical repair and apical closure of immature roots. *Odontol Revy* 1972; **23**: 27-44.

2. Cvek M. Treatment of non-vital permanent incisors with calcium hydroxide. II. Effect on external root resorption in luxated teeth compared with effect of root filling with guttapercha. A follow-up. *Odontol Revy* 1972; **23**: 343-54.

3. Cvek M. A clinical report on partial pulpotomy and capping with calcium hydroxide in permanent incisors with complicated crown fracture. *J Endod* 1978; **4**: 232-7.

4. Cvek M, Lundberg M. Histological appearance of pulps after exposure by a crown fracture, partial pulpotomy, and clinical diagnosis of healing. *J Endod* 1983; **9**: 8-11.

5. Cvek M, Lindwall A-M. External root resorption following bleaching of pulpless teeth with oxygen perixode. *Endod Dent Traumatol* 1985; **1**: 56-60.

6. Cvek M, Cleaton-Jones PE, Austin JC, Andreasen J. Pulp reactions to exposure after experimental crown fractures or grinding in adult monkeys. *J Endod* 1982; **8**: 391-7.

7. Cvek M, Granath L, Lundberg M. Failures and healing in endodontically treated non-vital anterior teeth with post-traumatically reduced pulpal lumen. *Acta Odontol Scand* 1982; **40**: 223-8.

8. Cvek M, Granath L, Cleaton-Jones P, Austin J. Hard tissue barrier formation in pulpotomized monkey teeth capped with cyanoacrylate or calcium hydroxide for 10 and 60 minutes. *J Dent Res* 1987; **66**: 1166-74.

9. Fuks A, Bimstéin E, Michaeli Y. Glutaraldehyde as a pulp dressing after pulpotomy in primary teeth of baboon monkeys. *Pediatr Dent* 1986; **8**; 32-6.

10. Heide S, Mjör I. Pulp reactions to experimental exposures in young permanent monkey teeth. *Int Endod J* 1983; **16**: 11-9.

11. Heide S, Kerekes K. Delayed direct pulp capping in permanent incisors of monkeys. *Int Endod J* 1987; **20**: 65-74.

12. Hørsted P, et al. A retrospective study of direct pulp capping with calcium hydroxide compounds. *Endod Dent Traumatol* 1985; **1**: 29-34.

13. Lewis BB, Chestner SB. Formaldehyde in dentistry: a review of mutagenic and carcinogenic potential. *J Am Dent Assoc* 1981; **103**: 429-34.

14. Magnusson B. Therapeutic pulpotomy in primary molars - clinical and histological follow-up. II. Zinc oxide-eugenol as wound dressing. *Odontol Revy* 1971; **22**: 45-54.

15. Mèjare I, Hasselgren G, Hammarström LE. Effect of formaldehyde-containing drugs on human dental pulp evaluated by enzyme histochemical technique. *Scand J Dent Res* 1976; **84**: 29-36.

16. Rølling I, Hasselgren G, Tronstad L. Morphologic and enzyme histochemical observations on the pulp of human primary molars 3 to 5 years after formocresol treatment. *Oral Surg* 1976; **42**: 518-28.

17. Schröder U, Granath L-E. On internal dentine resorption in deciduous molars treated by pulpotomy and capped with calcium hydroxide. *Odontol Revy* 1971; **22**: 179-88.

18. Schröder U. Effect of an extra-pulpal blood clot on healing following experimental pulpotomy and capping with calcium hydroxide. *Odontol Revy* 1973; **24**: 257-69.

19. Schröder U. Agreement between clinical and histologic findings in chronic coronal pulpitis in primary teeth. *Scand J Dent Res* 1977; **85**: 583-7.

20. Schröder U. A 2-year follow-up of primary molars, pulpotomized with a gentle technique and capped with calcium hydroxide. *Scand J Dent Res* 1978; **86**: 273-8.

21. Schröder U. Effects of calcium hydroxide-containing pulp-capping agents on pulp cell migration, proliferation, and differentiation. *J Dent Res* 1985; **64**(Spec Iss): 541-8.

22. Schröder U, Szpringer-Nodzak M, Janicha J, Wacinska M, Budny J, Mlosek K. A one-year follow-up of partial pulpotomy and calcium hydroxide capping in primary molars. *Endod Dent Traumatol* 1987; **3**: 304-6.

APPENDIX 12-1

PARTIAL PULPOTOMY

Prior conditions – The tooth has been anesthetized and isolated with a rubber dam. The treatment is performed with due observation of sterility.

Pulpal status – healthy/partial chronic pulpitis

Procedure	Method	Rationale - comments
Removal of pulp tissue	Starting from the exposure, 1-2 mm of the pulp tissue is removed with a high-speed rotating spheric diamond cooled with an ample flow of sterile physiologic saline.	As judged by histology, the least traumatic wound is achieved with this technique.
	The diamond should be big enough to work in the hard tissue concomitantly with the cutting of the pulp tissue.	To gain support for a smooth cut.
Control of hemorrhage	Rinse gently with sterile physiologic saline. Dry gently with a sterile cotton pellet.	A smooth-cut healthy pulp tissue will bleed moderately.
	Check that there are no residual tags of pulp tissue.	Residual tags may prolong bleeding.
	Lime-water (supersaturated solution of Ca(OH)$_2$) may be used as a hemostatic. If bleeding persists the pulp tissue must be considered chronically inflamed.	The calcium ions enhance coagulation. Avoid other hemostatics - they either damage the tissue or may induce after-bleedings. Remove more pulp tissue or reconsider choice of therapy.
Application of calcium hydroxide	Cover the pulpal wound with a 1 mm thick layer of calcium hydroxide. Check carefully that no bleeding has started.	A coagulum between the wound and the dressing will impair healing.
Placement of the base	Apply a layer of slow-setting zinc oxide-eugenol cement. Cover with a setting calcium hydroxide base.	Gives a bacteria-tight seal. The base prevents pressure on the pulpal wound.
	Proceed with restorative work.	

APPENDIX 12-2

PULPOTOMY

Prior conditions – The tooth has been anesthetized and isolated with a rubber dam. The treatment is performed with under sterile conditions. An x-ray of the tooth is available.

Pulpal status – partial/total chronic pulpitis

Procedure	Method	Rationale - comments
Gain access to the pulpal chamber	Establish an occlusal cavity corresponding to the size of the pulp chamber. Remove all decay.	There is no need to undermine or reduce the cusp tips. To minimize bacterial contamination.
	With a cylindrical diamond, preferably on a high-speed machine, penetrate the roof of the pulp chamber.	
	Remove the roof completely. Check with a probe that no overhanging ledges remain.	To gain maximum visibility and access to remove all coronal pulp tissue.
Remove the coronal pulp	The bulk of the coronal pulp is removed with a high-speed diamond cooled with sterile physiologic saline.	
	Use an efficient suction apparatus. Alternatively, the coronal pulp is removed with a sharp spoon excavator.	Bleeding may be profuse and impair visibility. Less risk of overextension of the cavity or accidental perforation.
	Identify the positions of the root canal openings.	In the lower jaw - one bucco-lingually elongated root canal opening in each root. In the upper jaw - three openings normally situated at the corners of a rightangle triangle with the right angle at the distobuccal canal.

Procedure	Method	Rationale - comments
Establish smooth wound surfaces	The root pulps are amputated in the orifices of the canals with a high-speed spheric diamond flushed with sterile physiologic saline. The diamond should have a diameter slightly greater than the width of the root canal.	Will result in the least traumatic wound. The technique requires a cooperative child.
	A smooth cut may also be performed with a small sharp excavator.	Eliminates risks for perforation, but involves a risk of the tissue being pulled from the canals.
Control hemorrhage	Rinse gently with sterile physiologic saline. Dry gently with a sterile cotton pellet. Check that there are no residual tags of pulp tissue.	A smooth-cut healthy pulp tissue will bleed moderately. Residual tags may prolong bleeding.
	Lime-water (supersaturated solution of $Ca(OH)_2$) may be used as a hemostatic.	The calcium ions enhance coagulation.
	If bleeding persists, the root pulp must be considered chronically inflamed.	Reconsider choice of wound dressing/choice of treatment!

A. Calcium hydroxide technique

Procedure	Method	Rationale - comments
Application of wound dressing	Place a calcium hydroxide paste in a 1 mm thick layer above each root canal orifice. Tamp lightly with a cotton pellet.	
	Check carefully that no bleeding has started from the pulp stumps.	A coagulum between the wound and the dressing will impair healing.
	Cover the entire furcation area with a 1 mm thick layer of calcium hydroxide compound.	
Placement of base	Cover the areas of root canal openings and then the furcation area with small portions of slow-setting zinc oxide-eugenol cement.	Small portions to ensure a tight seal and no empty spaces to avoid afterbleeding. Zinc oxide-eugenol cement gives a bacteria-tight seal.
	Proceed with the restoration or apply a temporary filling.	

Procedure	Method	Rationale - comments
B. Formocresol technique		
Application of formocresol	Cotton pellets are cut to a "pointed" shape. The pellet is moistened with formocresol and placed with slight pressure on the root canal openings for 5 minutes.	The formocresol will fix the pulpal tissue. No further bleeding is observed.
	Avoid "soaking" the furcation area with formocresol.	To avoid interradicular irritation. The furcation area may have accessory canals.
Placement of base	See above, calcium hydroxide technique. Wound dressing zinc oxide-eugenol cement with or without formocresol.	

APPENDIX 12-3

ROOT CANAL TREATMENT OF IMMATURE PERMANENT INCISORS

Prior conditions – The tooth has been isolated with a rubber dam. The treatment is performed with due observation of sterility. An x-ray of the tooth is available.

Pulpal status – pulp necrosis

Procedure	Method	Rationale - comments
	Use a cylindrical bur on high-speed equipment and place a triangular cavity into dentine.	The shape of the cavity corresponds to the outlines of the pulp chamber.
	Erect the bur and slope outwards the wall at the base of the triangle.	These two steps are to accomodate a direct-line access into pulp chamber and root canal in the long axes of the tooth.
	Erect the bur more and produce a groove in the enamel up to the incisal edge.	

Procedure	Method	Rationale - comments
	Perforate to the pulp with a round bur at low speed. Then move the bur incisally, from inside the pulp chamber and outwards down to the tip of the pulpal horn.	Perforation in apical direction omits compromizing the labial wall. Working from inside the pulp chamber restricts removal of dentine to the roof of the chamber.
	Shift to a round bur with a long shank. Place the bur apical to the lingual ledge of dentine and move the bur out to the cavo-surface.	The resulting groove in the ledge should be merely wide enough to allow passage into the canal of properly sized root canal instruments.
	Cleanse the access cavity. Use a precurved file and barbed broaches, around the periphery of the root canal.	To reach the irregularities of the root canal walls.
	Irrigate with 15-20 ml of 0.5% sodium hypochlorite or sterile saline. Dry the canal with coarse paper points.	For mechanical and chemical debridement.
	Fill the canal stepwise with calcium hydroxide paste, using a cartridge syringe. Be sure of contact with vital tissue apically.	For disinfectant and luting activity, and to promote apical closure. Necessary in order to achieve hard tissue barrier.

Procedure	Method	Rationale - comments
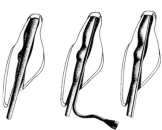	Pack the paste stepwise with the blunt end of a thick paper point. Seal the cleansed opening with 4 mm of IRM-cement.	To blot excess moisture. The radiodensity of a well packed canal is similar to that of dentine.
Control period	Check by x-rays every 3-6 months. If the apical one third of the canal appears empty, refill with calcium hydroxide paste.	Evidence of complete apical closure with hard tissue is checked radiographically and clinically after 12-18 months.
	Rootfill using an inverted, coarse guttapercha point and then lateral condensation with secondary points up to the apical barrier.	Be particularly aware of the wide labio-lingual dimension of the canal.
	Cover root filling with zinc phosphate cement, followed by composite, including the incisal groove.	Check with radiograph after 6-12 months, thereafter once a year for 4 years.

APPENDIX 12-4

BLEACHING OF NON-VITAL DISCOLORED TEETH

Prior conditions – The tooth has an adequate guttapercha root filling and has been carefully isolated with a rubber dam following careful cleaning with an aqueous slurry of pumice.
An x-ray should be available.

Procedure	Method	Comments
A. Bleaching with 30% hydrogen peroxide		
Gaining access to pulp chamber	Remove all restorative material and as much as possible of discoloured dentin without weakening the tooth unnecessarily.	Permits easier penetration of the bleaching agent.
Removal of root filling material	Remove the guttapercha to the level of the cemento-enamel junction. Apply a 1-2 mm thick layer of zinc oxide-eugenol cement.	To prevent seepage into the root canal and/or into the periodontium via dentinal tubules.
Pretreatment of the cavity	Carefully etch the dentin. Clean with chloroform or acetone. Blow the pulp chamber dry.	To dissolve any fatty material.
Bleaching	Place cotton wet with 30% H_2O_2 in the pulp chamber and on the buccal surface of the tooth. Illuminate with UV-light or heat for 5-10 minutes, keep the cotton moistened all the time.	Wipe off any excess in order to avoid leakage through the rubber dam.
	Repeat the procedure 3-4 times or until a satisfactory result is achieved.	It is recommended to overbleach because the bleached tooth tends to darken with time.
Rinsing of the cavity	Rinse with ethanol or chloroform.	
Temporary sealing of the cavity	A pellet moistened with 30% H_2O_2 is placed in the cavity and sealed with zinc-oxide cement and phosphate cement between appointments.	To prolong the bleaching procedure. To avoid leakage to the oral cavity.

Procedure	Method	Comments
Rinsing of the gingival crevice	Rinse carefully with water.	In order to avoid chemical injury to the soft tissue and thereby the risk of cervical external root resorption.
Final sealing	Remove all bleaching agents. Flush the cavity carefully with water and finally with chloroform. Acid etch the cavity, blow it dry and restore the tooth with the lightest composite available.	In order to enhance the result of the bleaching.

B. Bleaching with sodium perborate

Procedure	Method	Comments
The same as A until "bleaching"		
Preparation of the bleaching paste	Mix sodium perborate and 3% H_2O_2 to a thick paste.	
Application of the paste	Fill the chamber with the paste.	Leave enough space for sufficient sealing. Carefully remove any bleaching paste from enamel margins.
Sealing of the cavity	Seal with zinc-oxide cement and phosphate cement between appointments. If necessary, repeat the procedure 1-3 times at 1-week interval.	
Final seal	See A.	

PERIODONTAL DISEASE

EPIDEMIOLOGY

The predominant type of periodontal disease in children and adolescents is accompanied by few if any subjective symptoms. Consequently, there is great risk of neglect in the early stages. Data on prevalence and severity of gingivitis in childhood and adolescence are somewhat contradictory. This is partly due to differences in definitions and criteria used. In general, rural populations are more affected than urban. Children from low socio-economic groups have a higher prevalence of periodontal disease. Socio-economic factors appear to be more important than hereditary differences in population groups. Longitudinal and cross-sectional studies during childhood show that the prevalence and severity of gingivitis increase with age reaching maxima at 10-12 years of age. Approximately 4% of Scandinavian adolescents today exhibit periodontal disease characterized by minimal loss of connective tissue attachment and alveolar bone loss; this figure increases during adolescence.

Current prevalences of plaque, calculus and gingivitis of Scandinavian children and adolescents are presented in Table 13-1.

NORMAL CONDITIONS

Primary dentition

The gingiva starts to keratinize after the eruption of teeth, but the keratinized layer remains thin throughout the period of the deciduous dentition. Consequently, the vessels within the connective tissue are visible

TABLE 13-1

Individuals (%) exhibiting plaque, supra- and subgingival calculus and gingivitis at one or more teeth. From Scandinavian studies.

Age group	Visible plaque	Calculus		Gingivitis
		Supragingival	Subgingival	
5	80	5	-	64
10	98	20	4	97
15	97	30	4	74

through the epithelial layer, giving the gingiva, as well as the rest of the oral mucosa, a more reddish appearance and a more flaccid character than in adults. The typical stippling familiar in healthy gingiva develops slowly from the age of 2 or 3 years (Fig. 13-1).

The marginal edge of the gingiva has a more bulky and rounded appearance. This may be related to the pronounced cervical ridge of the crown in deciduous teeth. In areas with diastemata between primary teeth, the interdental tissues are comparable to saddle areas. When the molars have established proximal contacts the interproximal area is completely filled by an interdental papilla, with a marginal concavity, a col, corresponding to the contact area. The connective tissue has a comparatively less well-developed net of collagen fibres compared with the adult. Also later, when the primary teeth have erupted, the fiber bundles are fewer and appear less dense.

On x-rays, the alveolar bone surrounding the primary teeth has a distinct, but thin, lamina dura and a comparatively wide periodontal membrane. There are few trabeculae and large marrow spaces with a rich vascularization. The root cementum is also thin and mainly cellular.

Permanent dentition

During the period of slow passive eruption, i.e. the period of slow withdrawal of the marginal soft tissue, the length of the junctional epithelium is considerable in children. At an early age the junctional epithelium presumably originates from the reduced enamel epithelium. As a consequence of the character of its former stratum intermedium, a readiness to split up, a probe can easily be inserted deep into the marginal crevice area, intruding into the tissue proper and simulating an "eruption pocket".

Under normal conditions the gingival sulcus is a shallow groove with its bottom close to the gingival margin. Although instruments are easily inserted deeper along the tooth surface, there is no justification for unnecessary explorations interfering with the junctional epithelium. The gingival sulcus surrounding the permanent tooth is deeper than around primary teeth.

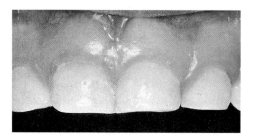 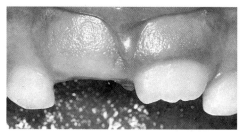

Fig. 13-1. Gingival stippling develops slowly in preschool children and is usually manifest by early school age.

PATHOGENESIS

One of the major problems in understanding the pathogenesis of periodontal disease is the difficulty in distinguishing clearly between normal and pathological conditions. When the gingival tissue is kept free from plaque, leukocytes will still be found migrating through the junctional epithelium towards the gingival sulcus. A few lymphocytes may also be present in the connective tissue.

The balance between the amount of irritation, and the individual phagocytic capacity and immunological competence, will be decisive for the severity of the disease. If plaque accumulation is minimal, and the defense mechanisms operate normally, there will be no clinical symptoms. More pronounced plaque accumulations, or defects in the defense reactions, result in clinical symptoms and the progression of periodontal disease.

Clinical picture

The clinically "normal" gingival crevice harbors inflammatory cells and produces exudate. But not until the vascular reactions have reached a certain level clinically noticeable signs of inflammation will occur. The free marginal gingiva becomes reddish, with a swollen appearance and papillae protruding from the interproximal spaces (Fig. 13-2). The surface is distended and shiny. Crevicular exudation is clinically obvious, especially when light pressure is applied to the free gingiva. There is also an increased tendency towards gingival bleeding on probing. The vascular and cellular reactions in the marginal gingiva should primarily be regarded as a natural defense against microorganisms. Since the causative factor is plaque accumulation, an efficient oral hygiene regimen will eliminate the clinical symptoms rapidly. However, a new period of poor oral hygiene will result in a

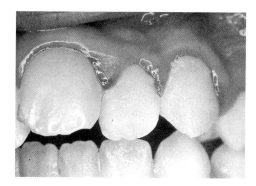

Fig. 13-2. Manifest gingivitis.

recurrence. Subclinical reactions and episodes of clinical gingivitis may alternate over long periods.

The tendency for gingival affections to remain superficial in healthy children is so pronounced that when a child of preschool or early school age, not known to have a disease which lowers the host defence, shows generalized periodontal disease with loss of bone, the dentist should regard it as mandatory to have the child's general health investigated.

Age-related differences

In an absolute majority of children the process of gingival inflammation remains superficial. Until the age of puberty, it appears to be a local resistance against involvement of the periodontal ligament and the alveolar bone. However, in adults the inflammatory reaction will advance, with continued loss of collagen and apical migration of the epithelium along the root surface leading to pocket formation.

The reason for these age-related differences in severity of periodontal disease are not fully understood. Lower amounts of spirochetes and black pigmented Bacteroides are present in microbial plaque in children. In addition, children do not develop calculus to the same extent as adults, a fact which may be related to the physiological proper-

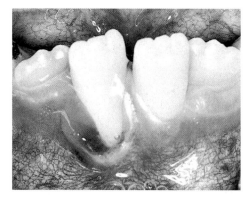

Fig. 13-3. Gingival recession at permanent lower central incisor.

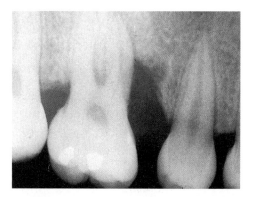

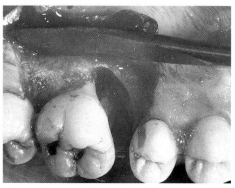

Fig. 13-4. Localized juvenile periodontitis. *Top*. X-ray. *Bottom*. Surgical exposure of the vertical bone destruction.

ties of their saliva and may be of importance.

Connective tissue has a greater vascularity, the increased cell-proliferation and turnover of collagen, compared with adults, may also be of importance. The number of plasma cells has also been found to be low in inflamed gingival tissue from children, indicating age-related differences in immunologic response.

Gingival recession

Localized gingival recession is found in approximately 10% of teenagers (Fig. 13-3). In young children the lesion occurs most frequently on the labial surfaces of the mandibular incisors while in older teenagers the buccal surfaces of upper molars and premolars are most affected. Such recession is often seen in association with a labial position of teeth, trauma from toothbrushing, a history of orthodontic therapy, or poor plaque control. Another predisposing factor to gingival recession is the high attachment of a frenum.

Slowly progressing periodontitis

This is the most prevalent form of periodontal disease in adolescence, characterized by minimal loss of connective tissue attachment and alveolar bone loss in the interdental areas of posterior teeth. These are the sites where plaque and gingivitis most frequently occur. Junctional epithelium begins to proliferate apically and a pathological periodontal pocket is formed. It has been observed that an increase of pocket depth and evidence of alveolar bone loss coincide with the shift in subgingival microflora, with *Porphyromonas gingivalis*, *Prevotella intermedia* and other anaerobic motile rods as the dominant cultured organisms. The conversion from a stable lesion, such as gingivitis, to a progressive lesion with alveolar bone loss may also involve a shift from a predominantly T-lymphocyte infiltrate in the tissue to a B-cell infiltrate.

Prepubertal periodontitis

Destructive periodontal disease in the primary dentition has been termed prepubertal periodontitis and is charaterized by a rapid destruction of the periodontal tissues. Prepubertal periodontitis has been classified into a localized and a generalized form. The localized form of the disease seems to affect appearantly healthy individuals. However, patients with the generalized form of prepubertal periodontitis are often suffering from systemic diseases.

Juvenile periodontitis

This is a rapidly progressive form of periodontitis, its onset is usually close to puberty, and the disease is associated with absence of pronounced clinical evidence of inflammation. Radiographically, the bone destruction has a vertical character localized mainly around molars and incisors (Fig. 13-4). It has been shown that the composition of the subgingival microflora in juvenile periodontitis is characterized by the presence of anaerobic microflora, i.e. *Actinobacillus actinomycetemcomitans*.

ETIOLOGY

There is unanimous agreement that chronic marginal gingivitis is caused by microbial plaque, nevertheless, gingivitis must be regarded as a multifactorial disease and a number of intrinsic and extrinsic factors influence the severity of its manifestation. The proportions of the predominant cultivable organisms from the normal dentogingival region in children with a deciduous dention, where gram-positive cocci are the major morphotype, appear in general to be much the same as in adults.

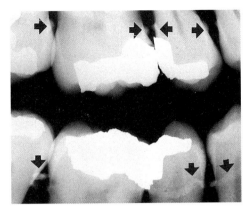

Fig. 13-5. Bite-wing x-rays showing subgingival calculus.

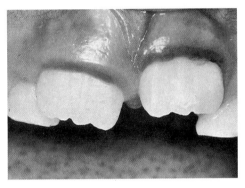

Fig. 13-6. So-called eruptive gingivitis.

Factors influencing plaque formation

If not removed from the tooth surface, microbial plaque may mineralize and form calculus. The surface of the calcified deposits is rough and enhances further bacterial colonization. The presence of supra- and subgingival calculus is, therefore, deleterious to periodontal health (Fig. 13-5).

Exfoliation of primary teeth and eruption of permanent teeth may enhance plaque accumulation mainly because discomfort during toothbrushing. So-called eruption gingivitis should not be regarded as a spe-

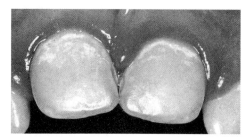

Fig. 13-7. Gingivitis at primary incisors with incipient carious lesions.

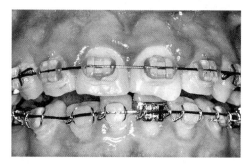

Fig. 13-8. Orthodontic treatment with appliances should be preceded and accompanied by training in adequate oral hygiene procedures to prevent development of gingivitis.

cific entity (Fig. 13-6). These lesions are also directly related to the amount of accumulated plaque.

Disturbances in enamel mineralization may cause a rough surface which accumulates plaque. The early stages of clinical eruption of hypoplastic teeth may be accompanied by pronounced gingivitis, which disappears later if the cervical part of the tooth has an unaffected enamel.

Malocclusions do not play a dominant role in the etiology of periodontal disease, but crowding of teeth may render oral hygiene measures difficult. There are indications that crowding may have greater implications for gingivitis in children than for periodontal disease in adults.

Caries. The manifest carious lesion increases plaque accumulation and gradually impairs oral hygiene. Cervical carious lesions are almost without exception accompanied by a local gingivitis (Fig. 13-7).

Restorations. The dentist who inserts the first proximal or cervical restoration has a great responsibility for the patient's future periodontal health. Defective margins, inadequate surface structure, and faulty contacts are all too often the cause of chronic gingivitis in children. Localized bone loss may also be seen adjacent to defective restorations.

Orthodontic appliances – Fixed appliances may impair normal oral hygiene procedures, bands and brackets accumulate plaque and removable plates can cause denture stomatitis (Fig. 13-8). Any possible harm to the supporting tissues caused by the appliances must be adequately treated and controlled.

Tobacco – Smoking appears to increase the susceptibility to periodontal disease.
Whether this is due to differences in amount and quality of plaque or to changes in defense mechanisms is still a matter of debate.

Factors modifying the defense system

Diabetes mellitus – It is generally held that adolescents and young adults with diabetes mellitus have an increased tendency to develop periodontitis. The reason for this is not completely understood, but impaired function of the polymorphonuclear leukocytes and vascular changes have been suggested. Children with diabetes also seem to be more susceptible to periodontal disease than healthy children. This tendency seems to be most pronounced in poorly controlled diabetic children (Fig. 13-9). Consequently, children with diabetes should be trained and motivated early to maintain efficient plaque control.

Leukemia – The most common form during childhood, acute lymphoblastic leukemia, is often accompanied by severe oral symptoms at the time of hospitalization and during the period of cytotoxic treatment. The low resistance of the tissues to infection is explained by drug interference with the replication of epithelial cells, in addition to a low number of circulating leukocytes. Therefore, plaque control is essential both before commencing cytotoxic treatment and during medical treatment.

Agranulocytosis – This malignant type of neutropenia is rarely seen in children but, as in cyclic neutropenia and chronic neutropenia, oral ulceration and periodontal manifestations are common. In chronic cases the gingiva will become hyperplastic, with granulomatous changes.

Sickle-cell anemia – A condition seen in American negroes, and thalassemia, which occurs in individuals of Mediterranean origin, are seldom seen in Scandinavia. Treatment is aimed at plaque control and palliative measures.

Heart conditions – Severity of oral manifestations is directly proportional to the general cyanosis. The gingiva has a bluish red hue. As the lowered tissue respiration impairs the defence against microorganisms, children with peripheral cyanosis exhibit a high gingivitis prevalence (Fig. 13-10). Indications for antibiotic prophylaxis are given in Chapter 18.

Mouth breathing – or deficient lip closure may cause frequent drying out of the gingiva in anterior areas. This is thought to result in vasoconstriction and a decreased host resistance. Clinical observations indicate an

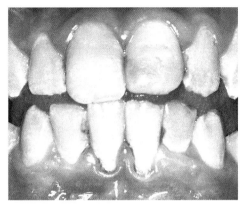

Fig. 13-9. Gingivitis in a patient with poorly controlled diabetes.

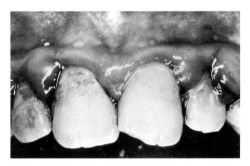

Fig. 13-10. Gingival condition in a child suffering from a heart condition with peripheral cyanosis.

association between gingival enlargement and mouth breathing, but epidemiological studies have been inconclusive.

Hormones – It is an established fact that hormonal changes contribute to the increased susceptibility to gingival affections during pregnancy. Correspondingly, a specific "puberty gingivitis" has been described, with pronounced edema in the marginal gingiva (Fig. 13-11). Epidemiologic studies have shown that the incidence of gingivitis reaches a peak 2 or 3 years earlier in girls than in boys, approximately coinciding with puberty. These findings suggest an influence of sex hormones on gingival status during puberty. Recent

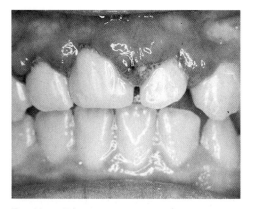

Fig. 13-11. Edematous gingivitis during puberty.

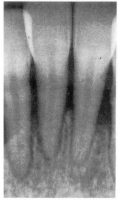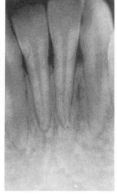

Fig. 13-12. Alveolar bone loss in children with Down's syndrome.
Left. A girl (18 years) suffering from heart condition with peripheral cyanosis. *Right*. A boy (18 years).

studies indicate an association between elevated hormone levels and an increase in certain species of black pigmented Bacteroides. However, puberty is also associated with a varying interest in personal oral hygiene.

Prepubertal periodontitis and juvenile periodontitis

The etiology of the severe types of early periodontitis is not fully understood. It has been reported that the microflora in the periodontal pockets is dominated by gram-negative species, e.g. *Actinobacillus actinomycetemcomitans*. This bacteria has been shown to be capable of invading the gingiva, as well as producing substances toxic to leukocytes, properties which make this bacteria a potential periodontitis pathogen. In addition, recent observations indicate that such host factors as reduced chemotactic and phagocytic response of polymorphonuclear leukocytes or monocytes are involved.

Syndromes involving early periodontitis

Down's syndrome – Children with Down's syndrome, mongolism, are exceptional in that they have a high prevalence of periodontal disease. Alveolar bone loss is more severe in the anterior segments, and especially in the mandible (Fig. 13-12). The reasons for the high susceptibility to periodontal disease in children with Down's syndrome are probably an impaired phagocytic function in neutrophiles and monocytes, combined with poor oral hygiene.

Hypophosphatasia – This is a hereditary metabolic syndrome resulting in low serum alkaline phosphatase activity, rickets-like skeletal changes and loss of alveolar-bone, mainly limited to the area of anterior primary teeth (Fig. 13-13). The result is a precocious exfoliation of these teeth. Microscopically, teeth from affected areas exhibit aplasia and hypoplasia of root cementum, large pulp chambers and interglobular dentin formation.

Acatalasemia – A deficiency of the enzyme catalase, which results in chronic ulcers of the oral mucosa and destruction of deeper tissues. The blood is not capable of decomposing the hydrogen peroxide produced by bacteria.

Chediak-Higashi syndrome – Defects in leukocytes and pigmentation, and mental retardation lead to an early onset of periodontal disease.

Histiocytosis-X (reticuloendotheliosis) – This may also cause alveolar bone destruction in connection with lesions in the jaws. Eosinophilic granuloma (histiocytosis in bone) is more frequent in the mandible than in the maxilla. Hand-Schuller-Christian disease (chronic disseminated histiocytosis) may lead to gross bone destruction extending around the roots and causing exfoliation. The treatment of the disease, with corticosteroids, irradiation and cytostatics, may produce secondary effects in the periodontium.

Papillon-Lefévre syndrome –This is a rare genetic disease affecting the hands and feet (*keratosis palmaris et plantaris*) and leading to fulminant types of periodontitis with rapid bone destruction. The oral symptoms start immediately upon eruption of the primary teeth and cease after the premature loss of the first dentition only to start again after eruption of the permanent teeth.

DIAGNOSIS

In clinical practice it appears sufficient to register whether the tooth surfaces harbor plaque or not. The Visible Plaque Index (VPI) is calculated as the number of positive findings as a percentage of the number of areas examined.

The early stages of gingival inflammation can be followed histologically or be measuring the gingival exudation. Symptoms visible to the eye, such as redness, swelling and bleeding tendency, may also give different implications in treatment planning.

Clinically, the tendency is now to sim-

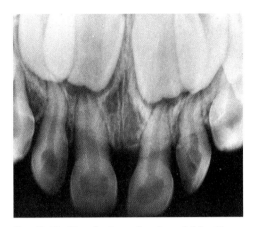

Fig. 13-13. Alveolar bone loss in a child with hypophosphatasia.

plify the diagnostic criteria for a marginal gingival lesion. The gingival bleeding tendency has been considered indicative of the condition of the gingiva. Such a system has been reintroduced by Ainamo & Bay, the Gingival Bleeding Index (GBI), based on one simple criterion: whether or not the marginal gingiva bleeds upon gentle probing. The index is calculated as the percentage of bleeding gingival units in relation to the number of units examined.

Owing to the specific morphology of children's gingiva, insertion of a probe into the crevice should be avoided. In general, there is no point in carrying out systematic measurements of pocket depth or probing attachment level until the age of 13-14 years, when pocket measurements may be indicated at incisors and molars. Together with the recording of clinical attachment loss, the diagnosis of periodontitis is based on X-rays taken. Microbial analysis of the subgingival samples of plaque is recommended in patients with marginal bone loss, but also in patients with early sign of clinical loss of attachment.

TREATMENT

Gingivitis

Edematous gingivitis involving marginal and papillary tissue is reversible with plaque control and heals without any permanent changes in the normal configuration of the tissue. However, parents must bear the responsibility for plaque control in their preschool children. A simplified Bass technique with a soft toothbrush is adequate in the cases of marginal gingivitis. The treatment of gingivitis should also include repeated education on etiology of the disease.

Gingival recession

The first step in the treatment of localized gingival recession is to identify the etiology and predisposing factors. If the gingival recession is associated with a high frenum attachment which retracts the marginal gingiva when the lip is stretched, frenectomy is recommended. Many cases of recession can be arrested by giving the patient instruction and motivation in adequate toothbrushing technique resulting in a good plaque control. The successful treatment of some cases of recession may require surgical intervention such as free gingival grafts. The main objective of the procedure is to increase of the width of the attached gingiva so that plaque control can be effectively practiced.

Slowly progressive periodontitis

The first sign of the disease may be detected in late puberty. Patients often have a number of pathologic periodontal pockets with an increased probing depth. Scaling and root planing are effective methods of pocket elimination and involve removal of calculus

and plaque both supra and subgingivally. Clinical treatment is always combined with a preventive program to reduce plaque accumulation. Scaling combined with oral hygiene instructions have been shown to maintain attachment levels and prevent further increases in pocket depth. Individualized plaque control programs must be instituted, for example every 3 months after initial treatment. At recall, patients' oral hygiene, gingival conditions, probing depth and attachment level must be re-examined as the risk of development of deeper periodontal lesions must be considered.

Prepubertal periodontitis and juvenile periodontitis

Data on the effects of treatment of early forms of periodontitis are sparse. Treatment is focused on eliminating such pathogenic bacteria as *A. actinomycetemcomitans*. It seems that this organism cannot be eradicated by such mechanical methods as scaling since bacteria occur not only in the periodontal pockets, but also in the gingival tissue. Thus, clinical studies suggest that subgingival curretage or flap surgery in combination with antibiotics is a good therapeutic approach. For juvenile periodontitis the antibiotic of choice is tetracyclin used systemically for a 3-week period. The effectiveness of such broad-spectrum antibiotics as tetracyclin is probably because *A. actinomycetemcomitans*, in particular is in most cases sensitive to it. For treatment of prepubertal periodontitis a careful selection of antibiotics is needed in order to avoid side effects on enamel formation. A specialized plaque control program must be carried out once every 3 months and the patients' oral hygiene, gingival condition, attachment level, alteration of bone defects, re-examined following therapy.

Bacteriological samples of the subgingival plaque should be taken on these occasions. Treatment of prepubertal periodontitis is essential as recent studies have indicated a strong correlation between prepubertal periodontitis and later development of juvenile periodontitis in the permanent dentition.

PREVENTION

Until recently it was assumed that virtually everybody was susceptible to serious, generalized periodontitis if oral hygiene was inadequate. The disease was thought to progress in a linear fashion throughout life from gingivitis to periodontitis. The current concept is that adult periodontitis progresses by acute bursts of activity, followed by period of quiescence. However, periodontitis has not yet been reported without preceeding gingivitis. So far, no predictors are available to identify patients at high risk for disease progression. Therefore, the prevention of gingivitis is clearly the most logical way of preventing periodontitis.

Mechanical plaque control

Mechanical removal of plaque by oral hygiene leads to remission of gingivitis. Plaque control is thus critical to the maintenance of gingival health. It has been shown that parents have to brush their children's teeth at least until school age to ensure optimal oral hygiene. Parents will also appreciate a simple, straightforward method, especially for use in small children. The simplified Bass technique, involving a horizontal movement of the toothbrush along the outside and the inside of the dental arches, is effective for both children and parents. A convenient method for a parent to brush a child's teeth is illustrated in Fig. 9-7. Systematic brushing of all toothsurfaces is important. The toothbrush recommended for children should be small, soft and have a large handel which is easy to hold. The quality of the oral hygiene is

more important than the frequency. Hastily performed and haphazard toothbrushing adds little to oral hygiene. It is vital to train parents and children in toothbrushing and to monitor the procedure with disclosing agents at regular intervals. Toothbrushing should be performed twice a day, in the morning and in the evening before bed. It is important that toothbrushing is kept simple.

Toothpicks – The use of toothpicks in children is recommended only in very specific cases and after careful instruction by a dentist or a dental hygienist. As the gingival tissues in children mostly fill out the interproximal spaces the use of toothpicks will result in gingival retraction and unnecessary exposure of the proximal surfaces.

Flossing – Interproximal areas are least accessible to toothbrushing, and dental floss is advocated as an aid to cleaning these regions. Studies have shown that flossing fails to improve situations where oral hygiene and gingival health are good, but if properly carried out it can benefit subjects whose gingival health is less satisfactory and also prevent the development of gingivitis.

Chemical plaque control

In recent years much attention has been focused upon the use of chemical agents which exhibit an effect on dental plaque, either as an inhibitor of plaque formation, or as an inhibitor of plaque metabolism. Both have potential for the prevention or reduction of periodontal disease. The most thoroughly investigated substance is chlorhexidine. Preparations are available as mouthrinses and dental gels in many countries. Regular or intermittent long-term use of chlorhexidine seems justified where no other effective means of oral hygiene are applicable. Considerable efforts are currently aimed at developing dentifrices which can improve and maintain gingival health.

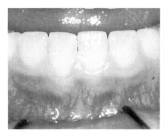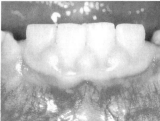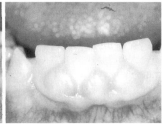

Fig. 13-14. Development of phenytoin-induced gingival overgrowth. The clinical appearance before the start and after 6 and 12 months of drug therapy.

GINGIVAL ENLARGEMENTS

Chronic marginal gingivitis in children is usually characterized by marked vascular reactions and tissue edema. In uncomplicated marginal gingivitis the edema is limited to the free marginal gingiva. Gingival enlargement dominated by edema is seen during puberty and in children with peripheral cyanosis. Enlargement of the gingival margin due to mouth breathing is also seen.

Drug-induced gingival overgrowth

Drugs such as calcium channel blockers (Nifedipine), immunosuppressives (Cyclosporin A) and anticonvulsants (Phenytoin) can induce gingival overgrowth (Fig. 13-14). Gingival overgrowth develops in 30% of cases using cyclosporin A. There is evidence that this side effect is dose related.

Phenytoin – The drug is used in children with grand mal but also in patients with psychomotor seizures. Connective tissue reactions are a common result of this antiepileptic treatment. Phenytoin-induced gingival overgrowth occurs more frequently in children than in adults. There have also been reports of the use of the antiepileptic agent sodium valproate resulting in development of gingival overgrowth.

Clinical appearance – The development starts as a lobulate enlargement of the interdental papillae. By introducing a plaque control programme before or at the start of PHT- therapy, gingival overgrowth can be minimized, but not totally prevented. In outpatients the thickness of the marginal gingiva is increased buccolingually, especially in the anterior region. Approximately 50% of children, where oral hygiene is not controlled, develop gingival overgrowth in the form of pseudopockets (probing depth > 4 mm). A few patients develop a severe form of gingival overgrowth where gingival tissue covers more than 60% of the anatomical crowns. In such cases surgical intervention is indicated, and an intensive preventive programme must be established to minimize the risk of recurrence of tissue enlargement. Gingival overgrowth represents tissue with an altered composition compared with normal gingiva, and contains an increased non-collagenous matrix with increased amounts of glycosaminoglycans (GAG).

Gingival fibromatosis

A specific type of diffuse, non-inflammatory gingival enlargement is idiopathic or hereditary gingival fibromatosis (Fig. 13-15). The fibrosis of the gingival tissue, generalized or localized to the molar areas, is usually symmetrical, and affects the entire gingiva up to the mucogingival junction. The extent can be so great that it changes the facial contour. Onset is early and the disease is often diagnosed in connection with retarded eruption. The enlargement is very firm and pale in color, and may be reduced by flap operations and wedge excisions.

ACUTE NECROTIZING ULCERATIVE GINGIVITIS (ANUG)

ANUG is a disease with rapid onset characterized by painful necrotic ulcerative gingival lesions and affected interdental papillae (Fig. 13-16). Occasionally, the necrotic ulcerative lesions may extend into the attached gingiva and oral mucosa, and are covered by greyish-white pseudomembranes.

ANUG is mostly seen in child populations suffering from malnutrition, but is today rare in developed countries. The principal bacteria associated with ANUG is *Bacteroides intermedius*. The pathogenic role of the microorganism is not fully understood, but ANUG cases are regarded as having reduced PMN chemotaxis and phagocytosis. In children, local treatment, i.e. plaque removal, is indicated combined with mouthrinsing with 0.5% hydrogen peroxide or with 0.1% chlorhexidine. Antibiotics are administered in cases with systemic effects, massive gingival necrosis, or a different spread of the infection.

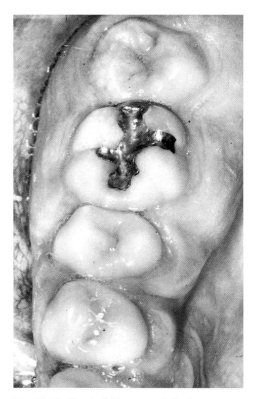

Fig. 13-15. Gingival fibromatosis in the posterior area.

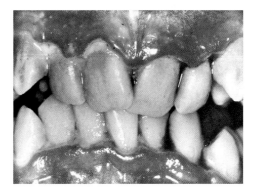

Fig. 13-16. Acute ulcerative gingivitis.

TRAUMATIC ULCERATIVE GINGIVAL LESION

These start in the marginal gingiva and are caused by bacterial superinfection of traumatized gingival tissue. Such trauma is predominantly the result of overintensive use of the toothbrush or by poor brushing technique. Bacterial infection is caused by the

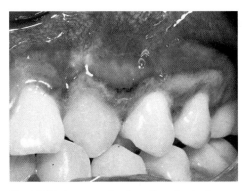

Fig. 13-17. A traumatic ulcerative gingival lesion.

normal mixed flora of the oral cavity. The ulcers are covered with a thin, yellowish or greyish, exudate and the patients often complain of pain in the affected area. The lesions are located in the buccal gingiva and there is no necrosis of the interdental papillae as in ANUG, or vesicles as in herpes simplex virus infections (Fig. 13-17). Initial professional cleaning of the teeth followed by cessation of toothbrushing for approximately 10 days is recommended. During this period the child should rinse its mouth twice daily with 0.1% chlorhexidine solution. Instruction in adequate toothbrushing technique should also be given.

Background literature

Aass AM, Albander J, Aasenden R, Tollefsen T, Gjermo P. Variation in prevalance of radiographic alveolar bone loss in subgroups of 14-year-old schoolchildren in Oslo. *J Clin Periodontol* 1988; **15**: 130-3.

Friis-Hansen B (ed). *Nordisk Lærebog i Pædiatri.* København: Munksgaard, 1985.

Hugoson A, Koch G, Rylander H. Prevalence and distribution of gingivitis-periodontitis in children and adolescents. *Swed Dent J* 1981; **5**: 91-103.

Lindhe J. *Textbook of clinical periodontology.* 2.ed, Copenhagen: Munksgaard, 1989.

Matsson L. *Development of experimental gingivitis at different ages in young individuals.* Thesis, Malmö 1979.

Modéer T, Dahllöf G. Development of phenytoin-induced gingival overgrowth in non-institutionalized epileptic children subjected to different plaque control programs. *Acta Odontol Scand* 1987; **45**: 81-5.

Sjödin B, Matsson L, Unell L, Egelberg J. Marginal bone loss in the primary dentition of patients with juvenile periodontitis. *J Clin Periodontol* 1993; **20**: 32-6.

Watanabe K. Prepubertal periodontitis: a review of diagnostic criteria, pathogenesis, and differential diagnosis. *J Periodont Res* 1990; **25**: 31-48.

TRAUMATIC INJURIES

EPIDEMIOLOGY

Dental trauma is seen by most dentists who deal with children. Thus, two prospective studies from Scandinavia showed that 30% of children had suffered traumatic dental injuries in the primary dentition and 22% in the permanent dentition.

The incidence of injuries to primary teeth is highest between 1 and 3 years of age. In the permanent dentition the most accident-prone time is between 8 and 11 years. Boys appear to sustain injuries to permanent teeth twice as often as girls. Even in pre-school children, boys are reported to outnumber girls.

Dental injuries usually affect one or two teeth, and the maxillary central incisors are the most frequently involved.

Distribution of various dental injuries in children is shown in Tables 14-1, 14-2.

ETIOLOGY

In a young child learning to walk and to run, coordination and judgement are incompletely developed and falling injuries frequently occur. It is pointed out that trauma to the orofacial area is often a component in child abuse. The abused child is generally very young and the symptoms include multiple bruises all over the body, as well as oral lacerations and injured teeth.

When the child reaches school age, accidents in the school yard are very common. Most of these injuries are caused by falls

TABLE 14-1

Distribution of dental injuries in the permanent dentition(3).

Type of injury	%
Crown infraction	8
Uncomplicated crown fracture	64
Complicated crown fracture	5
Root fracture	1
Concussion	7
Subluxation	10
Luxation	2
Exarticulation	2
Other injuries	1

TABLE 14-2

Distribution of dental injuries in the primary dentition(1).

Type of injury	%
Crown fracture	19
Root fracture	1
Concussion, subluxation and luxation	69
Exarticulation	7
Unknown	4

and collisions while playing and running. Injuries resulting from bicycle accidents are also prevalent in this age group. It is emphasized that children with maxillary protrusion are five times more susceptible to dental injuries than children with normal occlusion. Finally, injuries among teenagers, are often due to contact sports, such as ice hockey, soccer, football or basketball.

HISTORY

A history of the injury and a thorough examination should be completed in any situation. To ensure that all relevant data are recorded, a special injury form is recommended.

The patient is questioned about the following: time elapsed since injury, where injury occurred and how injury occurred.

General health – Did the trauma cause unconsciousness, amnesia, headache, vomiting, excitation or difficulties in focusing the eyes. With any of these symptoms, brain involvement is suspected and the patient is referred for medical care. The patient or its parents are questioned about the presence of medical problems such as bleeding disorders, epilepsy or allergic reactions.

Symptoms – Pain during mastication could indicate damage to the periodontium. Disturbed occlusion is indicative of tooth displacement or jaw fracture. Pulpal hyperemia is suspected when reactions to thermal changes are experienced.

Previous injury – to the tooth (teeth) in question. Repeated injuries are not uncommon. In these patients, prognosis may be less favorable.

CLINICAL EXAMINATION

In instances of associated severe injuries, a general examination is made with respect to signs of shock (pallor, cold skin, cold perspiration, irregular pulse), symptoms of brain concussion or jaw fractures.

Extra-oral examination

Limitation of mandibular movement or mandibular deviation on opening or closing of the mouth, indicate that the jaw may be fractured. Note is taken of lacerations to the face and lips. If a wound is located under the chin, the possibility of a jaw fracture should be considered. Crown-root fractures should also be suspected especially in the premolar and molar regions. If the patient has sustained a crown fracture, tooth fragments may penetrate and be retained in the lip. In this case, a swollen lip is suspect and should be examined both clinically and radiographically (Fig. 14-3).

Intra-oral examination

The examination must be systematic and include the recording of: laceration, hemorrhage and swelling of the oral mucosa and gingiva. Abnormalities in occlusion, displacement of teeth, fractured crown or cracks in the enamel.

Particular note is taken of the following factors:

Mobility – The degree of mobility is estimated in both a horizontal and a vertical direction, keeping in mind that immature permanent teeth and primary teeth undergoing root resorption have quite extensive physiologic mobility. When several teeth move together "en bloc", a fracture of the alveolar process is suspected.

Reaction to percussion – The handle of a mouth mirror is tapped gently against the tooth in both a horizontal and vertical direction. The contralateral uninjured tooth or another comparable tooth serves as a control.

Color of the tooth – Discoloration may appear almost immediately after the injury. In order to disclose the change in color as soon as possible, special attention is paid to the palatal (lingual) surface in the gingival third of the crown.

Reaction to sensitivity tests – In evaluating pulpal status, thermal tests carried out with heated gutta-percha or ethyl chloride are widely used. The electric test appears, however, to be a more reliable diagnostic aid, provided the operator is accurate and experienced in the technique and the patient is cooperative. It is important to explain the purpose of the test and explain the type of sensation to be expected. If the child is unfamiliar with the procedure, the dentist should demonstrate it using the child's thumb.

Neither negative nor positive sensitivity responses should be trusted immediately after an accident. It is claimed, that a positive response is the best prediction of continued pulp vitality. However, loss of vitality at a later stage should not be ruled out. Whereas an immediate negative response usually indicates pulpal damage, it does not necessarily indicate a necrotic pulp. The negative reaction is often due to damage to the apical nerve supply. In such cases the pulp may have a normal blood supply, but will not respond to stimuli.

X-ray examination

Details of examination, technique and analysis are given in Chapter 6.

CLASSIFICATION

A number of classifications of traumatic injuries have been presented. In this chapter the classification recommended by the World Health Organization and modified by Andreasen(2) will be used.

Injuries to the hard dental tissues and the pulp

Crown infraction – An incomplete fracture (crack) of the enamel without loss of tooth substance.

Uncomplicated crown fracture – A fracture confined to the enamel or involving enamel and dentin, but not exposing the pulp.

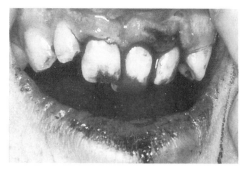

Fig. 14-1. A 13-year-old boy with severe displacement of three maxillary incisors after a bicycle accident.

Complicated crown fracture – A fracture involving enamel and dentin, and exposing the pulp.

Uncomplicated crown-root fracture – A fracture involving enamel, dentin and cementum, but not exposing the pulp.

Complicated crown-root fracture – A fracture involving enamel, dentin and cementum, and exposing the pulp.

Root fracture – A fracture involving dentin, cementum, and the pulp.

Injuries to the periodontal tissues

Concussion – An injury to the tooth-supporting structures without abnormal loosening or displacement of the tooth, but with marked reaction to percussion.

Subluxation – An injury to the tooth-supporting structures with abnormal loosening, but without displacement of the tooth.

Extrusive luxation – Partial displacement of the tooth out of its socket.

Lateral luxation – Displacement of the tooth other than axially.

Intrusive luxation – Displacement of the tooth into the alveolar bone.

Exarticulation – Complete displacement of the tooth out of its socket.

Traumatic injuries may involve injuries to the supporting bone such as comminution or fracture of the alveolar socket, fracture of the alveolar process, fracture of the mandible or fracture of the maxilla.

Injuries to the teeth are also often accompanied by the following injuries to the gingiva or the oral mucosa: laceration (a shallow or deep wound in the mucosa), contusion (a bruise usually causing submucosal hemorrhage), or abrasion (a superficial wound leaving a raw, bleeding surface).

PERMANENT TEETH: TREATMENT AND PROGNOSIS

Injuries involving permanent teeth can at first sight appear rather severe, particularly when associated with trauma to supporting tissues (Fig. 14-1). Fortunately, most traumatized teeth can be treated with success. However, it is emphasized that prompt and proper emergency treatment decreases the risk of complications.

The initial treatment phase is followed by a period of observation. It is pointed out that each injury has a specific prognosis (Table 14-3). Trauma cases should therefore be recalled often enough to disclose any complication as soon as possible in order to intervene at the right time. The intervals between re-examinations depend upon the severity of trauma and the expected type of complication, but the following time schedule may serve as a guide: examinations

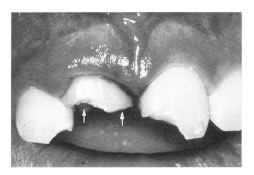

Fig. 14-2. Typical uncomplicated crown fractures involving either mesial corners or entire incisal edge. Intrusive luxation has also occurred in right central incisor (arrows).

Crown infraction

Infractions are incomplete fractures without loss of tooth substance. The fracture line stops before or at the dentino-enamel junction. Infractions may be seen as vertical, horizontal or diverging lines on the buccal surface of the crown. These lesions are frequent, but without the use of proper illumination, they are easily overlooked.

No active treatment is required. However, the energy of the blow may in these cases be transmitted to the periodontal tissues or to the pulp, resulting in pulp necrosis (Table 14-3). Periodic recalls are therefore necessary.

Uncomplicated crown fracture

Some typical examples are shown in Figs. 14-2, 14-3, 14-4. Uncomplicated crown fractures are also commonly associated with subluxation or luxation injuries (Fig. 14-2).

Enamel fracture – Minimal tooth substance is lost, and no restoration is needed. Most

after 1 week, 3 weeks, 6 weeks, 3, 6 and 12 months. Thereafter once a year for 4-5 years.

The follow-up examinations should include the testing of sensitivity, percussion and mobility and the inspection of the tooth color.

X-rays should be examined with respect to the periradicular condition and changes within the pulp cavity.

TABLE **14-3**

Type and frequency of complications in permanent incisors after various types of injuries. From Scandinavian follow-up studies in children and adolescents.

	Pulp necrosis	Pulp canal obliteration	Inflammatory resorption	Replacement resorption
Crown infraction	3%	-	-	-
Enamel fracture	1%	-	-	-
Enamel-dentin fracture	3%	-	-	-
Root fracture	20%	69%	2%	-
Concussion	3%	5%	-	-
Subluxation	6%	10%	1%	-
Extrusive luxation	26%	49%	6%	-
Lateral luxation	58%	31%	3%	1%
Intrusive luxation	68%	32%	47%	5%
Replantation	81%	15%	30%	41%

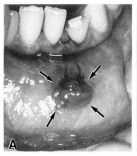
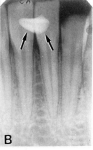

Fig. 14-3. A. Extensive crown fracture of mandibular lateral incisor and mandibular lip lesion (arrows). B. X-ray reveals fractured tooth fragment hidden in lip lesion (arrows).

often a slight contouring of a fractured angle will provide an esthetic result. The contralateral can be rounded off similarly to make the teeth symmetrical.

Enamel and dentin fracture – With the involvement of dentin, a number of dentinal tubules are exposed. These tubules constitute a pathway for bacterial products from plaque formed on the exposed surface.

In order to protect the pulp against external irritants, a calcium hydroxide liner should be placed on the exposed dentin as soon as possible. Restoration of fractured crowns with composite materials appears to be the treatment of choice in most cases. The acid etch composite restoration has been shown to be highly successful esthetically and functionally. With new improved composite systems, such restorations may even prove to be permanent treatment procedures. Details of the acid etch technique are discussed in Chapter 11.

If the fractured tooth fragment is found and brought to the clinic, considerations should always be given to attach the fragment to the fractured crown (Fig. 14-4). The coronal fragment has to be hollowed out with a diamond bur to allow optimal repositioning of the fragment over the dressing material. No other preparation is required, and care should be taken not to disturb the

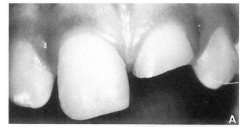
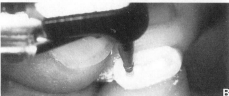
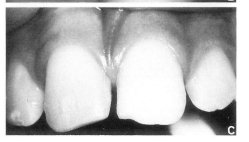

Fig. 14-4. Restoration of fractured incisor using the crown fragment. A. Enamel-dentin fracture of left central incisor. Exposed dentin is covered with calcium hydroxide liner. B. Part of dentin removed from tooth fragment with diamond bur, to provide space for dressing material. C. Fractured fragment bonded back in place.

enamel margins, since intact enamel is important to provide guidance for exact repositioning. After etching, rinsing and drying, light-curing resin is brushed onto the etched surfaces. The fragment is repositioned and held firmly while the material is cured with light.

A dry working field is a prerequisite for using the acid etch technique. Since extensive fractures can occur before the incisors are fully erupted, application of a rubber dam may be difficult. In such cases a preformed orthodontic band or the incisal end of a stainless steel crown should be adapted and cemented in place. These temporary restorations will serve adequately as retainers for the dressing material on the exposed dentin. As soon as further eruption has occurred, the tooth is restored with an esthetic bonded resin restoration.

Prognosis following infraction and uncomplicated crown fracture – Teeth without associated periodontal injuries are followed by remarkably few complications (Table 14-3). High-risk teeth with respect to pulp necrosis appear to be those with deep corner fractures.

A negative response to the electric pulp test must be accompanied by other clinical and/or radiographic signs before necrosis can be diagnosed. With infractions and uncomplicated crown fractures either a periapical inflammation, or a greyish discoloration should be expected as the definite sign of pulpal death. Most cases of necrosis are disclosed within 3 months after the accident.

Complicated crown fracture

The primary concern after pulpal exposures in immature teeth is preservation of pulp vitality in order to allow continued root development. The injured pulp must be sealed from bacteria so that it is not infected during the period of repair. In most cases partial pulpotomy (*ad modum Cvek*) is the treatment of choice.

Further information on the endodontic procedures is given in Chapter 12.

Crown-root fracture (uncomplicated and complicated)

These injuries involve enamel, dentin and cementum, and are often complicated by pulpal exposures. The fracture is sometimes vertical, that is with the fracture line in the same direction as the long axis of the root (Fig.14-5). A more typical finding is an ob-

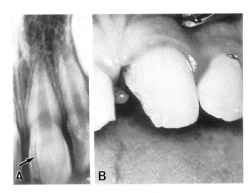

Fig. 14-5. A. Vertical uncomplicated crown-root fracture of left central incisor (arrow). B. Clinical condition after removal of mobile fragment.

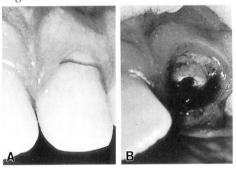

Fig. 14-6. Complicated crown-root fracture of left central incisor. A. Fracture line located about 2 mm incisally to gingival margin. B. Coronal fragment removed to allow inspection of fractured surface.

lique course as shown in Fig. 14-6. The fracture is then usually located a few millimeters incisally to the gingival margin on the buccal surface. Lingually the fracture is found to extend below the cementoenamel junction.

Treatment – In some cases fragments of crown-root fractured teeth can be splinted with composite materials using the acid etch technique, but the prognosis is rather doubtful. In fractures communicating with the oral cavity, periodontal breakdown and pulp necrosis are most likely to occur. Thus, with most crown-root fractures, the treat-

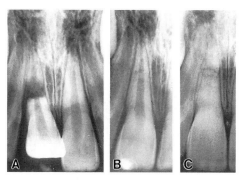

Fig. 14-7. A. Root fracture in right central incisor with severe dislocation of coronal fragment. B. Optimal repositioning performed within 1 h. C. Condition 2 years later with repair in fracture area and almost total pulp canal obliteration.

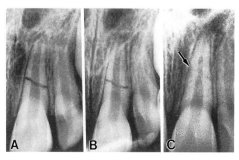

Fig. 14-8. Repair after rootfracture in left central incisor. A. At time of injury. B. During fixation period. C. 1 year later with a hardly discernible fracture line (arrow).

ment is to remove the loose fragment or fragments. Any pulpal involvement must be determined. If the pulp is exposed, treatment considerations are given in Chapter 12. Without pulpal exposures dentin covering procedures are carried out. Further treatment depends upon how deeply the fracture extends on the root surface. If the root portion is not too short, one of the following procedures is suggested: a) periodontal surgery to expose adequate amount of the root structure for a crown restoration; b) extrusion of the root portion (orthodontic or surgical) to a level where conventional crown treatment can be accomplished.

Prognosis following crown-root fracture – No studies have evaluated the long-term results of these treatment methods. It appears, though, that extrusion of the root fragment leads to stable periodontal conditions, whereas surgical exposure of the fracture surface has been found to lead to granulation tissue within the pocket. After some time this will result in migration of the restored tooth in a buccal direction.

Root fracture

Root fractures occur most often in the middle or apical third of the root and only rarely in the cervical third. The coronal fragment may be extruded or displaced in a palatal (lingual) direction.

Treatment – In case of displacement, every effort should be made to reposition the coronal fragment as soon as possible (Fig. 14-7). This is best accomplished by gentle digital manipulation. If the buccal socket wall is also fractured, it is necessary to reduce the fractured socket before attempting to reposition the coronal fragment. The position of the fragments should then be checked radiographically. Following reduction, the tooth must be stabilized for 8 to 12 weeks to allow repair (Fig. 14-9). Immediate, firm fixation should also be carried out in cases without dislocation, as close contact between the fragments is essential during the period of initial healing.

Splinting technique – An acceptable splint should be effective and easily constructed. It should neither add further trauma to the periodontal tissues nor interfere with occlusion. The splint should allow sensitivity testing and access to the root canal if endodontic treatment is required. A simple method based on the acid etch technique and fulfilling the above mentioned requirements is shown in Figs. 14-9, 14-12. The practical procedure is as follows: one or two uninjured teeth, on either side of the teeth, to be stabilized, are pumiced and rinsed with water. An orthodontic, twisted wire (dimension 0.032") is bent to conform to the buccal surfaces of the selected teeth. The surfaces are thereafter etched with phosphoric acid. The wire is attached to the uninjuried teeth first. Only a small amount of resin is necessary to hold the splint. The injured teeth are then attached to the wire. Care is taken to ensure that they are in proper position. The patients are instructed to rinse their mouths twice daily with a 0.1% solution of chlorhexidine.

Prognosis following root fracture – In about 80% of all rootfractured teeth the pulp remains viable and repair occurs in the fracture area.

Although the course of repair varies from one case to another, three main categories have been defined.

Repair with calcified tissue: invisible or hardly discernible fracture line (Fig. 14-8).

Repair with connective tissue: narrow, radiolucent fracture line and peripheral rounding of the fracture edges (Fig. 14-7).

Repair with bone and connective tissue: a bony bridge separates the two fragments.

In addition to changes in the fracture area, *pulp canal obliteration* is commonly seen (Table 14-3).

Fractures in the cervical third of the root are widely believed to be less advantageous as far as repair is concerned. However, as long as no communication exists between the fracture line and the gingival crevice, prognosis for repair is not reduced (Fig. 14-9).

Pulp necrosis – Necrosis is the main obstacle to repair and occurs with a frequency of about 20%. Severe dislocation of the coronal fragment significantly favours the development of pulpal death.

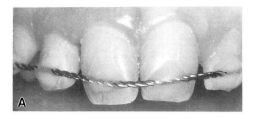
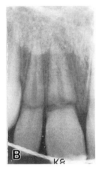
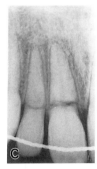

Fig. 14-9. Repair of fractures located in cervical third of roots. A. Fixation of fractured incisors using orthodontic, twisted wire, resin material and acid etch technique. B. During fixation period. C. 1 year later. Fracture lines still clearly visible. Note almost total obliteration of pulp cavities. (Palatal retainer bonded in place due to slightly increased mobility).

Most cases of necrosis are diagnosed within 3 months after a rootfracture injury. In teeth with persistent negative response to electric stimulation, necrosis is usually confirmed by radiolucencies adjacent to the fracture line (Fig. 14-10).

It is emphasized that the apical fragment almost always contains viable pulp tissue. In teeth with middle or apical third fractures, endodontic treatment is therefore usually confined to the coronal fragment. After completion of endodontic treatment, repair and union between the two fragments with connective tissue are consistent findings (Fig. 14-10).

When teeth with cervical third fractures develop necrosis, one of the following procedures is suggested: a) root canal filling of both fragments; b) extraction of the coronal

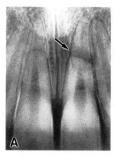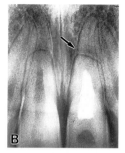

Fig. 14-10. Root fractures of both central incisors. A. Retained pulpal vitality and immediate repair in right incisor, whereas radiolucency corresponding to fracture line (arrow) indicates necrosis in left incisor. B. 2 years after completed root filling of left incisor. Union between segments is evident.

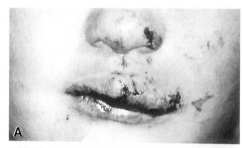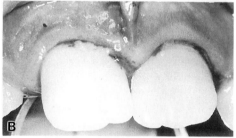

Fig. 14-11. A. External soft tissue damage. B. Bleeding from non-lacerated gingiva, indicating damage to periodontal tissue.

fragment with subsequent orthodontic extrusion of the apical fragment. The choice between the two treatment methods depends upon the root development, the level of the fracture, and the distance between the fragments.

Concussion

The involved tooth is tender to percussion and there may be a slight bleeding at the gingival margin indicative of damage to the periodontal tissues. In general the symptoms are few and moderate. Concussions are therefore easily overlooked, especially since they often occur in association with more conspicuous diagnosis.

No immediate treatment is required, but follow-up evaluation is important.

Subluxation

This type of injury is characterized by a varying degree of mobility without displacement. A marked bleeding from the gingival margin is nearly always present (Fig. 14-11).

Treatment – So far it has not been proven that splinting will improve the chance of pulp survival or periodontal repair. However, most dental schools still advocate splinting for 1-2 weeks in case of extreme loosening (mobility in both a horizontal and vertical direction). Should the tooth be only slightly loosened, it is sufficient to recommend a soft diet in the post-injury period. To achieve optimal plaque control, the patients are instructed to rinse their mouths twice daily with 0.1% chlorhexidine solution for 1 week.

Extrusive luxation

In this type of luxation a partial displacement out of the alveolar socket is observed.

Treatment – If the patient is seen shortly after the accident, the extruded tooth should as a rule be gently repositioned with finger pressure and a splint applied for 2-3 weeks.

Lateral luxation

Lateral luxation means displacement in either a palatal, buccal, mesial or distal direction accompanied by comminution or fracture of the alveolar socket. Most often a palatal luxation occurs (Fig. 14-12).

Treatment – If the patient is seen shortly after the accident, the displaced tooth should as a rule be gently repositioned with finger pressure. When bone fragments are also displaced, or when the apex is forced through the facial bone plate, pressure must be applied on the root apex to move it back through the fenestration, into the socket. Fractured cortical bone should also be molded back in place with finger pressure. Once reduction has been carried out, the involved tooth must be stabilized for 2-4 weeks using the acid etch splint.

If the repositioning procedure is delayed, the tooth is usually found to be quite firm in its new position due to formation of a blood clot in the socket. In these cases forceful manipulation may produce an additional injury to the periodontium. The tooth should either be allowed to realign spontaneously or it should be moved back orthodontically. Both methods appear to be less traumatic than a forceful manual repositioning.

Intrusive luxation

Intrusion is the most severe type of luxation. The tooth is forced axially resulting in comminution or fracture of the alveolar socket.

Treatment – There are three choices of treatment: await spontaneous re-eruption; perform an orthodontic repositioning, or bring the tooth down into position using forceps.

With immediate and total repositioning there is a tendency to lose a great deal of bone permanently. Surgical repositioning should therefore be avoided unless the

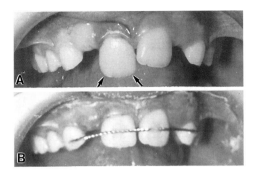

Fig. 14-12. A. Palatal luxation of right central incisor (arrows). B. Tooth repositioned and stabilized with an acid-etch resin and wire splint. Note that lateral incisors have not yet erupted. The orthodontic, twisted wire is bent to conform to buccal surfaces of central incisors and primary canines (courtesy of Dr. K. Størmer, Oslo).

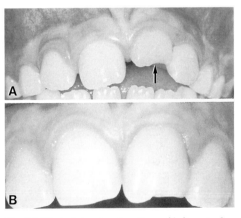

Fig. 14-13. A. Intrusive luxation of left central incisor in 8-year old girl (arrow). B. Spontaneous re-eruption 7 months later. Reactions to sensitivity and percussion are normal.

tooth is driven up into the floor of the nose or out into the soft tissue of the vestibulum.

Most intruded teeth should either be moved into position orthodontically or allowed to re-erupt spontaneously. The choice between the two treatment methods depends upon the degree of intrusion, since necrosis frequently develops and endodon-

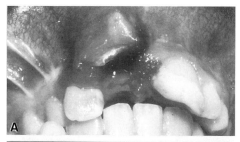

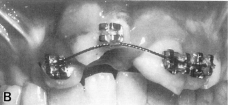

Fig. 14-14. A. Severe intrusive luxation of right central incisor in 8-year old girl. B. 4 weeks later. Tooth partially repositioned orthodontically. At this time endodontic treatment had to be started due to external inflammatory root resorption (courtesy of Dr. A. Stenvik, Oslo).

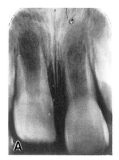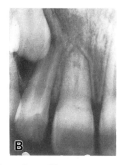

Fig. 14-15. A. Intrusive luxation of immature right central incisor. B. Spontaneous re-eruption, closure of apical foramen, and pulp canal obliteration have occurred.

tic treatment often has to be started within 3-4 weeks. If it is thought possible to gain access to the root canal with the tooth in its intruded position, spontaneous re-eruption is awaited (Fig. 14-13). Otherwise, the eruption is helped by orthodontic forces in order to make the endodontic treatment possible (Fig. 14-14).

Prognosis following concussion, subluxation and luxation injuries

Following the initial treatment it is hoped that pulpal and periodontal repair will take place uneventfully. However, as shown in Table 14-3 a number of complications may develop.

Pulp necrosis – Necrosis is the most common post-traumatic complication. It is diffi-

cult to establish the extent of pulpal damage shortly after the injury and to predict in which cases pulp necrosis will occur. However, as shown in Table 14-3 the survival or death of the pulp tissue is primarily related to the severity of the periodontal injury.

Several studies have also shown that necrosis occurs less frequently in immature teeth than in mature ones. With a large apical opening, slight movements of the apex can probably occur without disruption of the blood vessels. Furthermore, if circulatory disturbances do occur, the recovery capacity of a young pulp is extremely favorable (Fig. 14-15).

Diagnosis of necrosis – While most pulp necroses are diagnosed within the first 3 months after injury, up to 2 years may also pass before pulpal death is evident.

Sensitivity testing – More than half of all subluxated and luxated teeth do not respond to electric stimulation at the initial examination. It is, however, documented that a great number of teeth with subluxation later regain their sensitivity. Although less frequent, a change in reaction from negative to positive may also take place in luxated teeth. A return to normal sensitivity is commonly found within the first few months. However, it has also been observed as late as 2 years after the accident. A negative test alone should therefore not be regarded as proof of necrosis.

Endodontic treatment is always postponed until at least one other clinical and/or radiographic sign of necrosis appears.

Tooth discoloration – An almost immediate pinkish discoloration indicates intra-pulpal bleeding and not necessarily pulpal death. It is thought that injuries such as concussion and subluxation may sever or occlude the veins at the apical foramen. The arteries may not be disrupted, leading to continued blood flow into the pulp cavity and penetration of hemoglobin from ruptures in the subodontoblastic plexus into the dentinal tubules. The immediate observation is a pinkish discoloration. There is a fair chance that the vascular system will repair. In this event, discoloration slowly disappears, and the pulp will retain its vitality (Fig. 14-16). However, if the tooth crown turns progressively grey, necrosis should be suspected.

A greyish color that appears for the first time several weeks or months after trauma is regarded as a decisive sign of necrosis. In this case the grey color signifies decomposition of necrotic pulp tissue.

Periapical inflammation – Periapical involvement secondary to necrosis can be seen as early as 3 weeks after trauma. Frequently though, several months pass before an apical pathosis is evident.

Arrest of further root development – If necrosis involves the epithelial root sheath before root development is complete, no further root growth takes place. It should be borne in mind that necrosis may progress from the coronal to the apical part of the pulp. In this way vitality may apparently persist for a while apically, resulting in the formation of a calcified barrier across the wide apical foramen (Fig. 14-17).

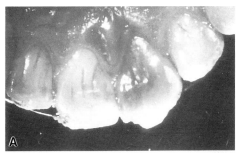

Fig. 14-16. A. Left central incisor in 10-year-old boy discolored within 1 week after subluxation injury. B. 3 months later. Discoloration has disappeared and tooth responds normally to electric pulp testing.

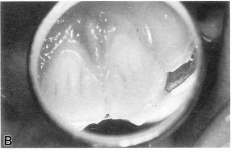

Fig. 14-17. Necrosis of right central incisor following intrusion. A. Re-eruption 3 months after injury. B. No further root development. Hard tissue formation (arrow) confused with continued vitality. C. Pulp necrosis diagnosed from periapical radiolucency (arrow), 1 year after injury.

Inflammatory root resorption (external) – This type of resorption is a decisive sign of necrosis, which calls for immediate endodontic treatment (Fig. 14-20). The resorptive

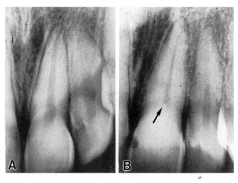

Fig. 14-18. Partial pulp canal obliteration in left central incisor. A. At time of injury. B. Condition 15 years later. Pulp chamber completely obliterated and root canal slightly reduced in size (arrow).

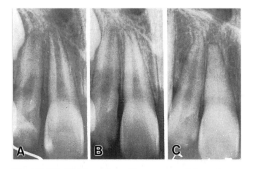

Fig. 14-19. Obliteration after successful replantation of right central incisor. Tooth replanted by the boy's mother within a few minutes. A. Normal findings 3 weeks later. B. X-ray 6 months later showing apical closure. C. 7 years after replantation. Total pulp canal obliteration and no sign of root resorption.

areas on the root surface are usually evident within 3 weeks to 4 months of the injury.

Pulp canal obliteration – Obliteration is the term used to describe the observation of progressive hard tissue formation within the pulp cavity. A gradual narrowing of the pulp chamber and root canal is observed on X-ray, leading to either partial or total obliteration (Figs. 14-18, 14-19). Because of the calcification, reduced electrometric response and even loss of sensitivity may be recorded. Another clinical observation is a slight yellowish color of the crown.

It is not understood what stimulates odontoblasts and possibly other cells to start the formation of hard tissue on the root canal walls. Obliteration appears however to be significantly related to teeth with incomplete root formation. Obliteration is also more frequent after extrusion, lateral luxation and intrusion than after concussion and subluxation (Table 14-3).

Although the X-ray gives the illusion of complete calcification, a minute strand of pulp tissue usually remains. In about 13% of these teeth the pulp becomes necrotic and periapical inflammation develops. This is a late complication usually seen 5-15 years after the injury. Endodontic treatment of these cases may be difficult on technical grounds. Therefore, prophylactic endodontic therapy of teeth showing progressive hard tissue formation has been recommended. Others do not support such measures mainly due to the rather low frequency of a complicating necrosis. Furthermore, in spite of the excessive calcification, the root canal is nearly always accessible for conventional endodontic treatment (Chapter 12).

Inflammatory root resorption (external) – Traumatic injuries with damage to the periodontal structure may cause progressive resorption of the root. Inflammatory resorption is the most common type of progressive root resorption and is most frequently seen after intrusive luxation and replantation (Table 14-3). The development seems to depend on cell damage of the periodontal ligament and the cementum induced by trauma, and the presence of infected necrotic pulp tissue. Bacterial products from the infected root canal will penetrate through the dentinal tubules into the periodontal ligament. Thus, an inflammatory response is provoked leading to further resorption of the root surface.

The diagnosis is made radiographically.

Bowl-shaped areas of resorptions are typical findings associated with radiolucencies in adjacent bone. Most frequently inflammatory resorptions are identified in the middle or coronal third of the root (Figs. 14-20, 14-21).

The first sign of resorption can be seen as early as 3 weeks after trauma. Most cases are disclosed within 4 months. If not present within the first year after injury, inflammatory resorption is unlikely to occur.

If allowed to progress, the resorptive process may destroy the tooth completely within a few months. The treatment of choice is therefore immediate removal of necrotic pulp tissue, canal debridement and long-term treatment with calcium hydroxide. In the majority of cases such treatment arrests the process, and cemental repair takes place (Fig. 14-21).

Root resorption (internal) – In addition to the post-traumatic complications listed in Table 14-3, internal root resorption is also a possible outcome. This type of resorption is an infrequent pulpal complication and is probably caused by a chronic pulpal inflammation.

Internal resorption is usually without clinical symptoms, and is first diagnosed on X-ray. The diagnosis is sometimes made soon after trauma and sometimes years later. The process may progress very rapidly, and endodontic treatment should be started as soon as the diagnosis is made. If the involved tooth is treated before resorption becomes extensive with perforation of the root surface, the treatment has a good chance of being successful.

Exarticulation

Replantation of avulsed incisors – Complete displacement of permanent incisors is a fairly uncommon injury, but when it occurs, replantation should nearly always be

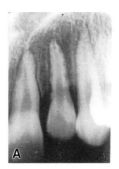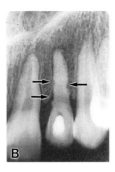

Fig. 14-20. External inflammatory root resorption along root surface of intruded lateral incisor. A. 6 weeks after injury. B. During endodontic treatment. Pulp cavity temporarily filled with calcium hydroxide. Persistent defects (arrows), but no further progression of resorptions.

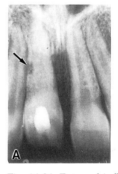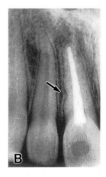

Fig. 14-21. External inflammatory root resorption following intrusive luxation of right central incisor. A. Area of resorption distally (arrow) 8 weeks after injury. Pulp canal temporarily filled with calcium hydroxide. B. 2 years later with persistent defect (arrow), but no further progression of resorption.

attempted. Replantation of avulsed teeth may offer only a temporary solution, due to a frequent occurrence of external root resorption (Table 14-3). However, even when resorption does occur, the replanted tooth can be maintained for years, serving as an ideal space maintainer.

A number of factors are associated with root resorption seen after replantation. Among these, the storage condition of the

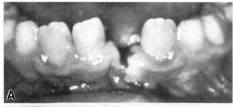
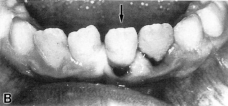

Fig. 14-22. Replantation of avulsed mandibular central incisor (arrow) performed 30 minutes after trauma. Tooth stored in the mouth of child's mother during trip to dental office. A and B. Situation before and immediately after replantation, respectively.

avulsed tooth before replantation seems to be most critical. It is of utmost importance that the periodontal ligament attached to the root is kept moist. Studies have demonstrated that the number of viable cells in the periodontal ligament declines very rapidly with an increase in the drying time. Twenty to thirty minutes seem to be the limit of drying of an avulsed tooth to avoid root resorption. Storage of the tooth in tap water is as damaging as dry storage, whereas saliva allows storage for about 2 hours. Milk is also well tolerated by the periodontal ligament. Teeth stored for as long as 6 hours in milk demonstrate the same low degree of resorption as in immediately replanted teeth.

Frequently the dentist is informed over the telephone that a tooth is "knocked out". The best advice is to replace the tooth immediately in the socket, and thereafter to seek dental aid. If the caller is unwilling or unable to carry out these instructions, he or she is advised to place the tooth in milk or in the child's mouth between the lower lip

and the teeth, and to seek a dentist immediately. If the child is too upset to cooperate, the tooth may also be stored in the mouth of a parent or another accompanying person.

Replantation procedure

– rinse the tooth in physiologic saline

– replace the tooth in the socket, using gentle finger pressure (Fig. 14-22)

– check the position by X-ray

– apply a splint

– administer antibiotic therapy in order to prevent inflammatory root resorption, and bacterial invasion of the pulp

– tetanus prophylaxis must be considered if the tooth or the wounds are contaminated with soil

– the patient is also advised to rinse the mouth twice daily with 0.1% chlorhexidine solution.

It is observed that rigid long-term splinting may increase the risk of ankylosis. It appears that a short splinting time favours both periodontal and pulpal healing. Removal of the splint after 1-2 weeks is therefore recommended.

Prognosis following replantation – The type and frequency of complications after replantation are shown in Table 14-3.

Pulp survival is not likely in the event of a closed apical foramen, and endodontic treatment must be started within 1-2 weeks to prevent the onset of inflammatory root resorption. The canal should be filled temporarily with a paste of calcium hydroxide for 6-12 months.

In teeth with a wide open apical foramen, revascularization of the pulp may occur (Figs. 14-19, 14-23). The pulp tissue of an avulsed tooth apparently has the potential to survive for up to 3 hours out of the socket. Therefore, in teeth replanted within

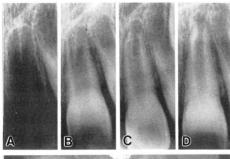

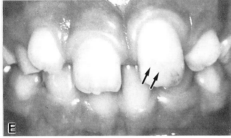

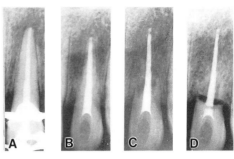

Fig. 14-24. Progression of replacement resorption after replantation of left lateral incisor. A, B and C. X-rays 6 months, 2 and 4 years after accident. D. Condition at time of removal of lateral incisor 7 years after replantation.

Fig. 14-23. Successful replantation of left central incisor. (arrows) Tooth stored in the mouth of child's mother for 45 minutes.
A, B and C. X-rays before, 12 days and 6 months after replantation, respectively.
D. 1 year after accident with continued root development and narrowing of pulp canal.
E. Clinical appearance 1 year after replantation.

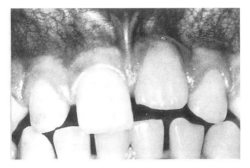

Fig. 14-25. Infraposition of left central incisor due to replacement resorption (ankylosis).

3 hours, endodontic treatment is postponed until pulp necrosis is evident. These teeth must be followed closely. With signs of necrosis such as inflammatory root resorption, endodontic treatment should be started immediately. It is recommended that a replanted tooth with incomplete root formation is examined radiographically every second week until pulp necrosis is confirmed or continued root formation is evident.

Replacement resorption (ankylosis) is the most severe type of external root resorption. This type of resorption is significantly related to replantation of avulsed incisors with an extended dry extraalveolar period (Table 14-3). Replacement resorption is caused by extensive cell damage to the periodontal ligament and to the cementum. A bony union (ankylosis) is established between the alveolar socket and the root surface, followed by continuous resorption of cementum and dentin. On X-ray, the normal periodontal space is found to disappear, and the tooth substance is gradually replaced by bone. Clinical examination may reveal this type of resorption before it can be seen on X-ray. A typical finding is a high, metallic percussion sound differing clearly from an uninjured tooth. It appears that most resorptions are evident within 2 months to 1 year after the accident.

Unfortunately, there is no effective treatment for an ankylosed tooth. The ultimate result is complete resorption of the root. However, the rate of progression is frequently slow, and the tooth can be maintained for several years. It may take from 5-8 years before the root is completely resorbed (Fig. 14-24).

A factor to consider is that ankylosis will disturb growth of the alveolar process in young patients due to infraposition of the tooth (Fig. 14-25). This occurrence may complicate further prosthetic solutions. For this reason extraction may be necessary. The procedure is to fracture the crown from the resorbed root at the bone level. The ankylosed root will then be transformed to bone during the remodelling process.

Alternative treatment methods following loss of permanent incisors

If it is decided not to replant a permanent incisor, or if extraction is required, an orthodontist should be consulted. Traditionally, further treatment consists of either orthodontic space closure or space maintenance by various prosthetic appliances. Finally, it should be mentioned that autotransplantation of premolars (see Chapter 17) or insertion of dental implants have also proved to be applicable in cases of avulsed and lost anterior teeth.

PRIMARY TEETH: TREATMENT AND PROGNOSIS

During its early development the permanent incisor is located palatally to and in close proximity with the apex of the primary incisor. Consequently, with injuries to primary teeth, the dentist must always be aware of a possible damage to the underlying permanent teeth.

The incidence of injuries to primary inci-

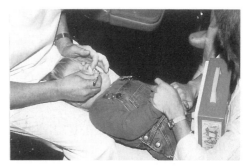

Fig. 14-26. Procedure for examination of a young child's mouth (see text).

sors is highest between 1 and 3 years of age. Since at this age the child is often unable to cooperate, the following procedure is suggested for clinical examination: The parent should be seated on an ordinary chair with the child on his or her lap, facing the parent. The dentist who is seated behind the child, receives and steadies the child's head in the lap, while the parent holds the child's arms and legs (Fig. 14-26). In this way a good examination of the oral structures can be done in a few minutes. However, active treatment such as splinting of loosened teeth may be extremely difficult. Therefore, in the majority of cases, the dentist has to decide whether the traumatized tooth is best treated by extraction, or whether it can be maintained without performing any extensive treatment. A primary incisor should always be removed if its maintenance will jeopardize the developing tooth bud.

If it is decided to preserve a traumatized primary tooth, it is carefully observed for clinical and X-ray signs of pulpal or periodontal complications. X-rays are also examined closely in order to disclose any damage to the permanent successor (Fig. 14-36). The intervals between re-examinations depend upon the type of injury and the extent of soft tissue damage. It may be necessary to see the child once a week until soft tissue has healed. Thereafter, re-examinations should take place at 3-6 monthly intervals

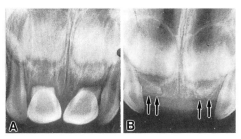

Fig. 14-27. A. Fractured roots of central incisors with dislocation of coronal fragments. B. 6 months after removal of coronal fragments. Resorption of apical fragments (arrows).

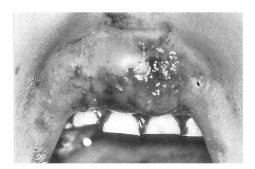

Fig. 14-28. Severe soft tissue lacerations with extensive hemorrhage. Central incisors and left lateral incisor extruded and extremely mobile. Right lateral incisor slightly subluxated.

for the first year, and then annually until the primary tooth is shed and the permanent successor is in place.

Uncomplicated crown fracture

If full cooperation of the child can be achieved, an enamel-dentin fracture can be capped with a calcium hydroxide compound and an acid etch restoration. In most instances, however, the treatment is limited to grinding of any sharp edges.

Complicated crown fracture

Normally, extraction is the treatment of choice. However, if the child is cooperative, the same procedure as outlined for permanent teeth can be followed.

Crown-root fracture

These cases involve fracture of enamel, dentin and cementum. Frequently the pulp is also exposed. Restorative treatment is extremely difficult, and the tooth is best extracted.

Root fracture

If the coronal fragment is severely dislocated, the primary tooth should be ex-

tracted. However, no effort is made to remove the apical fragment, as this might possibly damage the underlying permanent tooth. Without evident displacement, the coronal fragment may show little mobility, and no immediate extraction is required. The tooth should be kept under observation. Sometimes necrosis develops in the coronal fragment, whereas the apical portion nearly always remains vital. Following removal of the coronal fragment, uncomplicated resorption of the apical fragment should be expected (Fig. 14-27).

Concussion, subluxation and luxation injuries

These injuries dominate in the primary dentition. Most often the patients also have extensive soft tissue damage such as swollen lips, lacerations and hemorrhage of the oral mucosa and gingiva (Fig. 14-28). The parents are instructed to clean the traumatized area gently with 0.1% chlorhexidine solution, using cotton swabs (twice daily for 1 or 2 weeks). Normally the soft tissue heals quickly. Swelling will usually subside within 1 week.

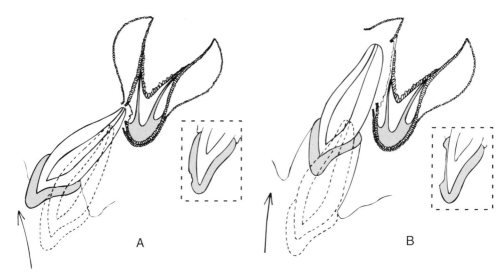

Fig. 14-29. Schematic drawings illustrating possible developmental disturbances of permanent tooth buds at the age of 2 years. A. Crown of primary incisor displaced buccally, forcing root into the crown of the developing permanent incisor. B. Severe intrusive luxation resulting in hypoplasia affecting enamel and dentin of permanent crown.

Concussion – Most concussions are not seen by the dentist at the time of the accident. The parents may see no need to seek dental treatment, or they may not be aware of the injury until tooth discoloration appears.

Subluxation – In case of extreme mobility, extraction is usually preferred. Should mobility be only slightly increased, the parents are advised to keep the traumatized area as clean as possible, and to give the child a soft diet for 1 or 2 weeks. Mobility should diminish within this period.

Extrusive luxation – An extruded tooth shows considerable mobility, and the tooth is best treated by immediate extraction (Fig. 14-28).

Lateral luxation – Palatal displacement of the crown is most commonly seen. In these cases the apex is forced in a buccal direction and thus away from the permanent tooth bud. There is nearly always an interference with the anterior occlusion. All the same spontaneous realignment should as a rule be awaited.

If the crown is displaced in a buccal direction, the root is displaced towards the permanent tooth bud (Fig. 14-29A) and extraction is the treatment of choice.

Intrusive luxation – Intrusion is the most common type of luxation. An intruded tooth often shows severe displacement (Fig. 14-29B). Sometimes it will be completely intruded into the alveolar process and mistakenly assumed to be lost, until an X-ray shows the intruded position (Fig. 14-30). With all intrusions the primary concern, is to clarify the direction of the displacement by a thorough X-ray examination (Chapter 6).

Treatment – If the primary root is displaced palatally i.e. towards the permanent successor, immediate extraction is recommended. Extraction is performed in order to minimize possible damage to the developing permanent tooth. With displacement of the root in a buccal direction, the intruded tooth is frequently allowed to re-erupt spontaneously. However, since there is a distinct risk of acute inflammation, the patient should be seen once a week, for the first 2-3 weeks. Re-eruption will generally take place within 1-6 months (Fig. 14-31). If re-eruption fails to occur, ankylosis should be suspected. An ankylosed tooth may interfere with eruption of the permanent successor and must be removed.

Exarticulation

Replantation of avulsed primary incisors is not recommended due to the risk of damage to developing tooth buds.

Space maintenance is not necessary following exarticulation or extraction of a primary incisor. When the loss occurs before eruption of the primary canine, minor drifting or migration of adjacent teeth may take place. With normal growth development, un-complicated eruption of the permanent incisors should be expected. However, early loss of a primary incisor may also result in a fibrous gingiva, which may prevent or delay eruption of the permanent tooth.

Pulpal and periodontal complications following trauma to primary teeth

Pulp necrosis – Necrosis is the most common complication. All traumatized teeth are therefore carefully observed for clinical or X-ray signs of pulpal death. In evaluating pulpal status, sensitivity testing is of limited value, due to the difficulty in obtaining adequate cooperation from the child. Most often diagnosis of necrosis is based upon inspection of tooth color and radiographic observation of the periapical condition.

Necrosis seems to be strongly related to discoloration of the tooth crown. It is ob-

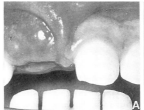
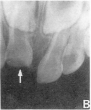

Fig. 14-30. A. Clinical examination shortly after trauma of an 18-month old child. Parents assumed that the right central incisor was lost. B. Conventional X-ray exposure reveals severe intrusive luxation. Primary tooth appears to be driven towards permanent tooth crown. Additional exposures (lateral projections) should be taken to disclose exact direction of the intrusion (Chapter 6).

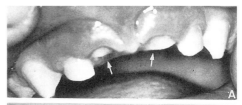
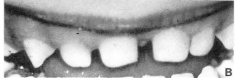

Fig. 14-31. A. Condition immediately after intrusion of both central incisors. B. Re-eruption is evident 6 months later.

served that traumatized teeth with a normal color only rarely develop periapical inflammation. A discolored tooth, on the other hand, is not necessarily necrotic. A greyish discoloration recorded shortly after a trauma, frequently reflects an intrapulpal bleeding. Upon further examination, the grey hue may gradually fade, and a return to normal or almost normal color is observed. In this case the pulp will retain its vitality. However, if the greyish color persists, necrosis is strongly suspected, and the tooth is examined radiographically at 3 monthly intervals

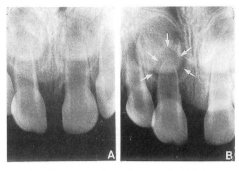

Fig. 14-32. A. X-ray 1 week after slight intrusive luxation of right central incisor.
B. 3 months after trauma with marked periapical inflammation (arrows).

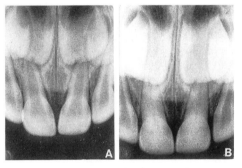

Fig. 14-33. Subluxation of both central incisors leading to pulp canal obliteration. A. At time of injury. B. 2 years later with almost total obliteration of pulp cavities.

in order to disclose any periapical inflammation as soon as possible.

Information on the pulpal condition can also be obtained by evaluation of the size of the pulp cavity. Normal physiologic reduction in size fails to take place if pulp death has occurred.

At the first sign of periapical inflammation (Fig. 14-32), extraction is the treatment of choice in order to prevent a possible sequela to the permanent successor.

Pulp canal obliteration – Obliteration of the pulp chamber and canal is a frequent reaction to trauma. The X-ray reveals either a partial or a total calcification of the pulp cavity (Fig. 14-33). Clinically, the tooth crown gradually assumes a yellowish hue. In the majority of cases, obliterated teeth remain unaffected up to the time of shedding. However, since a small percentage may develop periapical inflammation indicative of necrosis, radiographic examination should be performed once a year.

Root resorption – The etiology and pathogenesis are identical to root resorption in traumatized permanent incisors. External inflammatory root resorption is usually seen after intrusive luxation, whereas internal resorption may develp as a result of both subluxation and luxation injuries. Extraction is the treatment of choice with all types of root resorption.

INJURIES TO DEVELOPING PERMANENT TEETH

It is well documented that trauma to a primary tooth is easily transmitted to its permanent successor. Thus, developmental disturbances can be expected in about 50% of all cases. The highest and lowest frequencies of complications are found after intrusions and subluxations, respectively. In this connection, it is emphasized that exarticulation of a primary incisor may also disturb further growth and development of the underlying permanent successor (Fig. 14-35). The explanation for this is probably that a primary tooth is avulsed with a movement of the apex in the direction of the permanent tooth germ.

Most disturbances occur when the apex of the primary tooth directly traumatizes the permanent tooth bud (Fig. 14-29). However, it cannot be too strongly emphasized that harmful effects may also arise from periapical inflammation of the primary tooth. The type and severity of disturbances found among permanent incisors are also closely related to the age at the time of injury. A tooth germ is especially vulnerable during its early developmental stages. Thus, the most serious disturbances are seen when the damage occurs before the age of 3 years. Changes in morphology or mineralization of the crown of the permanent incisor are the most common types of complications. These lesions range from small enamel opacities to severe malformations (Figs. 14-34, 14-35, 14-36). A frequent finding is a yellow-brown discoloration, localized on the buccal surface, with or without hypoplasia of the enamel. Trauma may also interfere with root formation leading to bending of the root or partial arrest of the development.

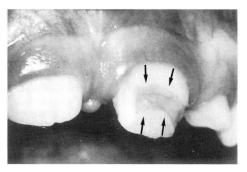

Fig. 14-34. External enamel hypoplasia of left central incisor (arrows) caused by intrusion of predecessor at the age of 15 months.

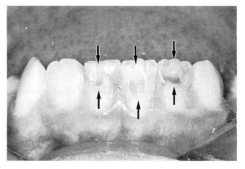

Fig. 14-35. Enamel defects in three lower incisors (arrows) resulting from exarticulation of corresponding primary incisors at the age of 2 years.

INJURIES TO THE SUPPORTING BONE

Treatment of comminution or fracture of the alveolar socket in the permanent dentition is described with root fractures and luxation injuries. Most fractures of the alveolar socket in the primary dentition do not require splinting due to a rapid bony healing in small children.

Fractures of the alveolar process are usually easy to diagnose, due to displacement and mobility of the fragment. Treatment always includes repositioning of the displaced fragment. In the permanent dentition splinting for 2-4 weeks is also carried out. Generally no measures are taken to stabilize a mobile fragment in the primary dentition, due to lack of sufficient teeth for the splinting procedure. After repositioning of the displaced fragment, the parents are advised to give the child a soft diet during the first weeks after the injury. The parents are also instructed to wash the traumatized

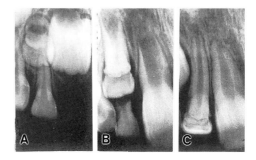

Fig. 14-36. Severe malformation of permanent lateral incisor following intrusive luxation of predecessor at the age of 2 years. A. Condition 1 year after trauma. B and C. Further development of deformed incisor and uncomplicated eruption, respectively.

area twice daily with 0.1% chlorhexidine solution.

Fractures of the mandible or the maxilla should be referred to an oral surgeon as soon as possible.

INJURIES TO THE GINGIVA AND THE ORAL MUCOSA

Soft tissue lesions must be adequately treated and recalled for evaluation. Minor lacerations of the mucosa, of the lip or the tongue should be sutured after careful debridement and cleansing of foreign bodies. With gingival lacerations it is necessary to achieve exact tissue positioning to ensure healing. Mouthrinsing or local treatment with 0.1% chlorhexidine solution is recommended to decrease the risk of infection during the wound healing.

It is emphasized that if the wound has been contaminated with soil, prophylactic vaccination against tetanus should be given as soon as possible.

Submucosal hematomas in the vestibular region or floor of the mouth may indicate a jaw fracture, and careful radiographic examination is indicated. Otherwise, no special treatment is needed.

PREVENTION OF DENTAL INJURIES

There is no easy way to prevent accidents leading to dental injuries in pre-school and school children. The dentist should, however, feel an obligation to visit schools and sports grounds in his or her neighborhood to point out any risk factors.

As pointed out in the beginning of this chapter, children with maxillary protrusion are particularly susceptible to dental injuries. In these children some traumas may be prevented by early corrective orthodontic treatment.

Although sports are the cause of relatively few dental injuries in children, these are often severe and involve a greater number of teeth than in other injuries. In the United States, football dental injuries have been reduced dramatically since the use of mouth protectors was made mandatory. The use of various types of mouth protectors should therefore be strongly encouraged for participants in all types of body-contact sports.

Background literature

Andersson L. *Dentoalveolar ankylosis and associated root resorption in replanted teeth.* Experimental and clinical studies in monkeys and man. Thesis. Stockholm, 1988.

Andreasen FM, Andreasen JO. Diagnosis of luxation injuries: the importance of standardized clinical, radiographic and photographic techniques in clinical investigations. *Endod Dent Traumatol* 1985; **1**: 160-9.

Andreasen FM, Vestergaard Pedersen B. Prognosis of luxated permanent teeth – the development of pulp necrosis. *Endod Dent Traumatol* 1985; **6**: 207-20.

Andreasen FM. Pulpal healing after luxation injuries and root fracture in the permanent dentition. *Endod Dent Traumatol* 1989; **5**: 111-31.

Andreasen JO. *Traumatic injuries of the teeth.* Copenhagen: Munksgaard, 1981.

Andreasen JO. Challenges in clinical dental traumatology. *Endod Dent Traumatol* 1985; **1**: 45-55.

Blomlöf L. Milk and saliva as possible storage media for traumatically exarticulated teeth prior to replantation. Thesis, *Swed Dent J* 1981, Suppl 8.

Cvek M. A clinical report on partial pulpotomy and capping with calcium hydroxide in permanent incisors with complicated crown fracture. *J Endod* 1978; **4**: 232-7.

Jacobsen I. *Traumatized teeth.* Clinical studies of root fractures and pulp complications. Thesis. Oslo 1981.

Schröder U, Wennberg E, Granath L-E. Traumatized primary incisors: follow up program based on frequency of periapical osteitis related to tooth color. *Swed Dent J* 1977; **1**: 95-8.

Tronstad L. Root resorption - etiology, terminology and clinical manifestations. *Endod Dent Traumatol* 1988; **4**: 241-52.

Literature cited

1. Andreasen JO, Ravn JJ. Epidemiology of traumatic dental injuries to primary and permanent teeth in a Danish population sample. *Int J Oral Surg* 1972; **1**: 235-9.

2. Andreasen JO. *Traumatic injuries of the teeth.* Copenhagen: Munksgaard, 1981.

3. Ravn JJ, Rossen I. Hyppighed og fordeling af traumatiske beskadigelser af tænderne hos københavnske skolebørn 1967/68. *Tandlægebladet* 1969; **73**: 1-9.

CHAPTER 15

DISTURBANCES IN TOOTH DEVELOPMENT AND ERUPTION

Dental anomalies

Variation in tooth size

Variation in tooth morphology

Numerical variations

Disturbances in hard tissue formation

Disturbances in tooth eruption

Disturbances in the eruption of primary teeth

Disturbances in the eruption of the permanent dentition

Symptoms associated with "teething"

DENTAL ANOMALIES

Variation in tooth size

The size of the teeth is mainly determined by genetic factors, however, it may also be influenced by external factors. Men have larger teeth than women. Racial differences are also seen. Tooth size is defined as abnormal when dimensions deviate 2 SD from the average. The deviation may be general or localized, and it may involve the whole tooth or only the root.

Microdontia is defined as teeth smaller than normal. General microdontia is a rare condition occurring in connection with congenital hypopituitarism, ectodermal dysplasia and Down's syndrome (Fig. 15-1).

Local microdontia, involving a single tooth, is more common and is often associated with hypodontia. Microdontia affects teeth which are congenitally missing and is regarded as a transitional form to agenesia: the upper laterals and the third molars are the most frequently affected teeth. The frequency of microdontia of the upper laterals is slightly less than 1%, unilateral in 65% of cases, with an autosomal dominant inheritance. Some environmental factors such as radiation to the jaws during tooth development may cause microdontia in the area involved.

Macrodontia is defined as teeth larger than normal. General macrodontia is extremely rare and is reported in connection with general gigantism. Bilateral enlargement of teeth with and without signs of fusion can

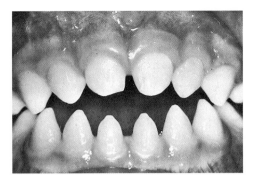

Fig. 15-1. Microdontia in lower anterior area.

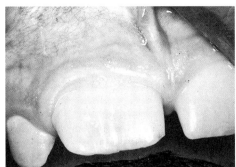

Fig. 15-2. Macrodontia due to fusion of teeth.

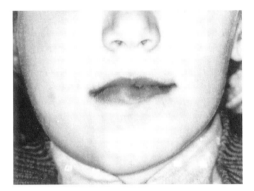

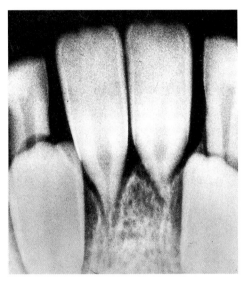

Fig. 15-4. Short roots in dentin dysplasia.

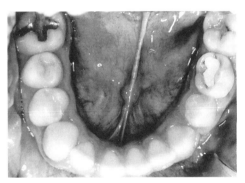

Fig. 15-3. *Top*. 12-year-old girl with hemifacial hypertrophy of the right side. *Bottom*. Clinical view. Observe the difference in size of the premolars and the canine between the left and right side.

be seen in the upper medial incisors (Fig. 15-2). In congenital hemifacial hypertrophy, macrodontia is seen unilaterally in the affected side (Fig. 15-3).

Root anomalies – The roots are considered shorter than normal when their lengths are equal to or less than the length of the crown. Short roots are supposed to be a constitutional anomaly of genetic origin (SR-anomaly). It is three times as common among girls than boys, predominantly affecting the upper central incisors. There is also a tendency of the affected teeth to root resorption. Short roots are seen in connection with osteopetrosis, hypoparathyroidism, and dentin dysplasia (Fig. 15-4). In single teeth short roots may be caused by trauma, pulpal complications or radiation to the teeth during their development.

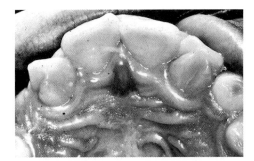

Fig. 15-5. Accentuated palatal tuberculum (left) and two palatal cusps (right) in permanent lateral incisors.

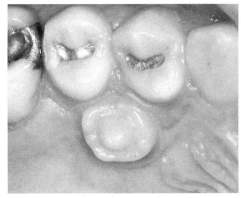

Fig. 15-6. Supernumerary premolar with evagination.

Abnormally large root length and root diameter is an unusual anomaly. This aberration is mainly found in the upper cuspids, where root lengths of up to 43 mm (17 mm normally) have been found. The enlargement can also partly be attributed to hypercementosis.

Variation in tooth morphology

The maxillary lateral incisors exhibit the most varied forms of the crowns. Peg-shaped types, T- and Y-forms, with an accentuated cingulum connected to the incisal edge are the most common forms (Fig. 15-5). The marked palatal cusp or ridge may interfere with the normal occlusion. A reduction by grinding has to be carried out gradually as there is usually a pulp horn in the cusp. The same anomaly may be seen in the center of the occlusal surface of a premolar and is then denoted dens evaginatus (Fig. 15-6). In the lateral incisors the evagination usally contains an extension of the pulp.

The maxillary first permanent molar and also the primary second molar may appear with an extra tuberculum, Carabelli's cusp, which is located on the palatal side of the mesiopalatal cusp. The second and third molars also display variations in number of cusps. However, the third molars exhibit the greatest variation of size and morphology of all teeth.

The shovel-shaped incisor appears to have a racial determination and is seen more frequently among Eskimos, Mongolians and American Indians.

Malformation, due to an invagination of enamel epithelium, consisting of a channel or lumen surrounded by hard tissues, in the tooth is called *dens invaginatus* (Fig. 15-7). The anomaly occurs most frequently in the permanent upper laterals, but can also be found in the upper centrals, the premolars, the canines and in the molars. The defect varies in severity from a hardly noticeable fossa to an invagination involving the major part of the crown pulp chamber. The prevalence of the *dens invaginatus* varies between different societies, possibly due to inconsistent classification. A Swedish population showed frequency of 3% for defects with a radiographically visible invagination. In 50% the invagination was bilateral.

Invagination can be suspected on clinical examination if the tooth has a marked cingulum or a palatal cusp. The entrance to the invagination can be extremely narrow, thus x-ray is necessary.

Defects of all hard tissues are commonly seen in the bottom of the invagination even with canals in to the pulp. Thus, the risk for

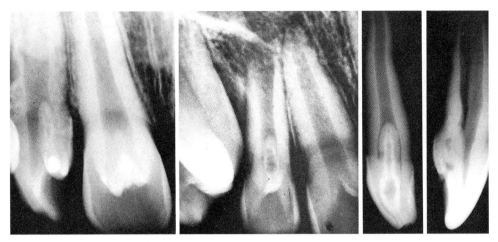

Fig. 15-7. Some examples of invaginations. Note enamel lining inside the lumen.

pulpal involvement is obvious after the eruption of the tooth. Due to packing of food in the fossa, caries may already attack the tooth before complete eruption. Small foramina may be restored with composite materials, while true invaginations should be treated as deep carious lesions. All softened or carious tissues should be removed. The risk for accidental pulpal exposure of the buccal side during excavation is obvious due to improper inclination of the burr. Extra long burs should thus be used to avoid guidance of the incisal edge of the tooth (Fig. 15-8). If the dentin at the bottom of the lumen is hard and the tooth is without any pulpal symptoms it is not necessary to extend the excavation into the frequently occurring canal seen as a small black spot in the bottom of the cavity. The bottom should be covered with a calcium hydroxide base and then filled with a composite resin material. If the pulp is exposed or if there are pulpal complications further treatment is dependent on root development, external morphology, etc.

Cynodontism (Greek kyon = dog) the reverse condition to taurodontism where the root-stem is practically absent. The roots

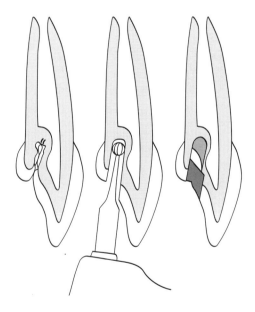

Fig. 15-8. The treatment of *dens invaginatus*. The lumen is reamed out with an elongated round bur. The bottom and buccal walls of the lumen are covered with calcium hydroxide compound.

appear to diverge directly from crown. This condition is characteristic for the primary molars (Fig. 15-9).

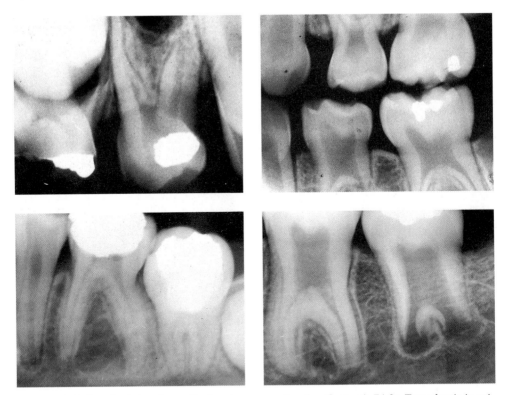

Fig. 15-9. *Left*. *Cynodontia* in primary (top) and permanent molars (bottom). *Right*. Taurodontia in primary (top) and permanent molars (bottom).

Taurodontism (Latin taurus = bull) is a rare anomaly found in multirooted teeth in both dentitions and is characterized by a prolonged root-stem with the furcation more apically than normally. The anomaly is genetically determined and the degree of taurodontism increases from the first to the third molar (Fig. 15-9).

Double-formation of teeth

Concrescence is defined as a condition where the roots of two or more teeth are fused only in the cementum. This anomaly may be caused by crowding or dislocation of tooth germs during root formation and is occasionally seen in the area of the second and third molars of the maxilla.

Fusion is defined as a union in dentin and/or enamel between two or more separately developed normal teeth. A fusion only in the enamel is very rare. Fusion may further be total or partial with complete or partially united pulp chambers. Fusion most often leads to a reduced number of teeth in the arch (Fig. 15-10). Occasionally, however, a normal and a supernumerary tooth may undergo fusion.

Gemination is attributed to an incomplete division of a tooth germ and thus there is no reduction of the number of teeth (Fig. 15-10). If the division is complete the condition is called twinning and it then involves a supernumerary tooth, which is a mirror image of its counterpart.

In contrast to other dental anomalies and anatomical variations, double-formations are more frequent in primary than in the permanent dentition. In both dentitions,

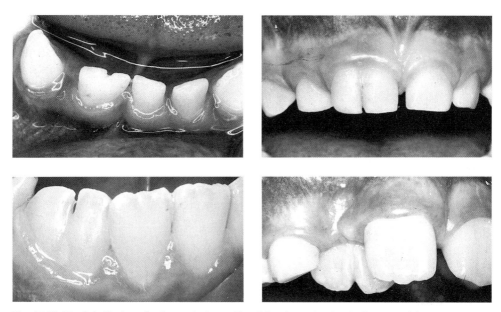

Fig. 15-10. *Top left*. Fusion of primary incisors. *Top right*. A gemination in the area of the primary central incisors. *Bottom left*. A fusion of a permanent lower incisor and canine. *Bottom right*. *Dens germinatus*, permanent lateral incisor.

double-formations occur most often in the front regions of the maxilla and the mandible. Double-formations, particularly fusions, in primary dentition are often followed by aplasia of the permanent successor. Double formation can frequently be observed in connection to congenital disorders, i.e. Down's syndrome and cleft palate.

The prevalence of double-formations in primary dentition is approximately 0.5%. The anomaly is very rare in permanent dentition. In general, fusions are more common than geminations.

In treatment of double-formations esthetic, skeletal and orthodontic consideration has to be given. As double-formations generally occur in the incisal regions, the cosmetic problems can be considerable. The teeth are enlarged and have a marked buccal fissure. Composite may improve the cosmetics and prevent caries in the fissure. The physiological resorption of these teeth is often retarded and may lead to delayed eruption of the permanent successor.

Numerical variations

Numerical variations of teeth appear to be a result of local disturbances in the induction and differentiation from the dental lamina. There is strong evidence that tooth number is genetically determined. Large differences in the incidences of numerical variations between ethnic groups are seen.

Congenital absence of teeth or agenesis of teeth may be of different severity: anodontia involves total absence of teeth, oligodontia describes agenesis of a number of teeth and hypodontia the absence of one or only a few teeth. The presence of supernumerary teeth is diagnosed as hyperdontia.

Early diagnosis of numerical variations is important to eliminate errors due to extractions and to give a proper treatment planning. X-ray examinations are important to verify diagnosis. It should be kept in mind that as second lower premolars exhibit large variations in onset of calcification, the diag-

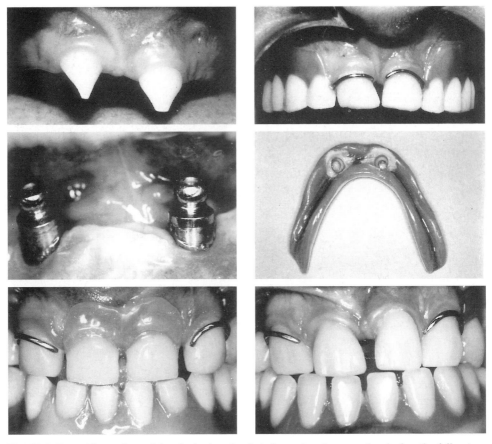

Fig. 15-11. Boy with ectodermal dysplasia. Anodontia in lower jaw. In upper jaw he has the following teeth: 53, 51, 61, 63, 16, 11, 21, 26. The incisors are malformed. *Top left*. At 2 years old only the conical primary incisors are erupted. *Top right*. At 3 years the incisors were morphologically rebuilt and a removable upper partial denture fitted. *Middle left*. At 6 years old, 2 osseointegrated implants were set in the lower jaw. *Middle right*. At the same time a specially designed lower denture was fitted. *Bottom left*. At 7 years old, the upper denture was modified due to exfoliation of 51 and 61. *Bottom right*. At 10 years old, his permanent incisors erupted and morphologically rebuilt with composite material.

nosis hypodontia cannot be established before the age of 7 or later.

Hypodontia in the primary dentition

Epidemiological investigations report a prevalence of hypodontia between 0.1 and 0.7%. The incisal areas are almost exclusively affected and then mainly the laterals. No sex difference in prevalence has been found. Anodontia or more extensive agenesis of primary teeth is rare, but may be found in connection with ectodermal dysplasia (Fig. 15-11). There is a rather strong correlation between hypodontia in primary and permanent dentition. Agenesis of a primary incisor is often followed by absence of its successor and even by an increased prevalence of hypodontia in other regions.

As hypodontia in primary dentition is relatively infrequent and generally affects

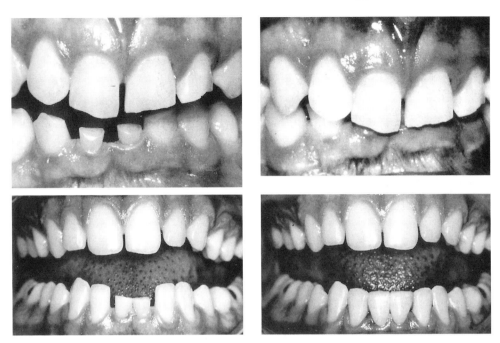

Fig. 15-12. Aplasia of permanent lower incisors. *Top*. Neglected case with collapse of the upper incisor region. *Bottom*. Treatment with composite retained onlay bridge to replace missing permanent lower incisors.

single teeth, there is normally no need for treatment.

Hypodontia in the permanent dentition

Hypodontia is more frequent in the permanent than in the primary dentition with a prevalence in a Scandinavian population between 6 and 10%, anodontia and oligodontia are extremely rare when the third molars are excluded. The most affected teeth are, in order, the lower second premolars, the upper lateral incisors, the upper second premolars and the lower central incisors (Fig. 15-12). Hypodontia is slightly more common among girls than boys. The prevalence of hypoplasia of the third molars varies between 10 and 35%.

Hypodontia in the permanent dentition usually affects two or more teeth in 50% of cases. (Symmetrical hypodontia often occurs for 12, 22; 35,45; 15,25 and 18, 28). There is a particular relation between hypodontia and microdontia in the upper laterals, and strong evidence that this form of hypodontia is inherited as an autosomal dominant trait.

A number of systemic disorders are connected with hypodontia in the permanent dentition. Congenital anhidrotic ectodermal dysplasia is a syndrome characterized by partial or complete absence of sweat glands, defects in lacrimal and salivary glands, sparse and thin hair, saddle nose, nail defects and extensive aplasia of teeth. Existing teeth are often peg-shaped. In Down's syndrome hypodontia is frequent. In patients with cleft lip and palate, hypodontia is also frequent outside the affected area and in the deciduous dentition.

Treatment planning in cases with aplasia of permanent teeth may be difficult. It is not only difficult to decide whether to close the

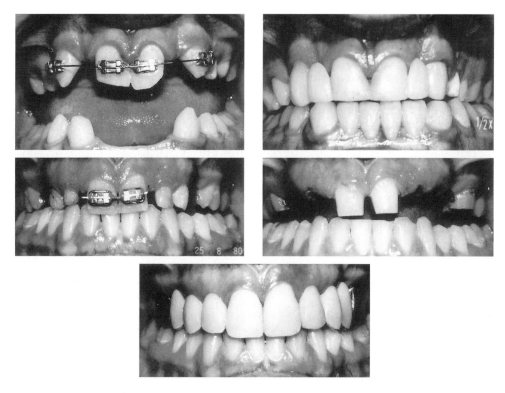

Fig. 15-13. Treatment of children with extensive aplasia. *Top left*. 12-year-old boy with aplasia of 12, 22, 42, 41, 31, 32. *Top right*. Treatment of the patient. After orthodontic correction and morphological rebuilding of 13, 11, 21 and 23 with composite material, onlay bridges replaced missing teeth. *Middle left*. 16-year-old girl with aplasia 15, 14, 12, 22, 23, 24, 25. Diastema between 11 and 21 has been closed. At 8 years old, 75 and 85 had been extracted to stimulate mesial drift of 16 and 26. *Middle right*. Treatment of the patient. Conventional preparation of 16, 11, 21, 26 for bridgeconstruction. Observe that the bite was raised about 5 mm. To adapt the patient to the new occlusion she was fitted with a temporary bridge for 6 months. *Bottom*. The final bridge was cemented when she was 17 years old.

space or not, but also to determine the time for intervention. Extraction of an existing primary tooth should be performed at a time when spontaneous closure of the space is most likely to occur. In the frontal area the morphology of the canines is important if it is expected to erupt in the place of a missing lateral incisor. Further, the esthetic problems of the canines in the region for the laterals are considerable, grinding or treatment with composites can to some extent improve the esthetics.

Orthodontic treatment of aplasias in the frontal region should always be considered before prosthetic therapy. Composite-retained onlay bridges are also commonly used today (Fig. 15-13). Aplasia of lower permanent incisors may result in a frontal collapse with a deep overbite. Early prosthetic treatment is therefore often indicated.

Extensive aplasia in the permanent dentition can be treated with partial dentures or different types of bridgework. It is important that all prosthetic treatment in young individuals is carefully planned and always seriously considers different aspects of growth, orthodontic treatment, etc.

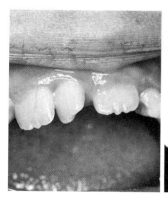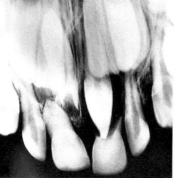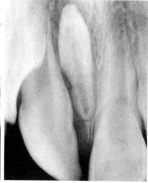

Fig. 15-14. *Left.* Erupting midline supernumerary incisor (mesiodens). *Middle.* Two midline supernumerary incisors. One of them inverted. *Right.* Inverted midline supernumerary incisor.

Hyperdontia in the primary dentition

The prevalence of supernumerary teeth in the primary dentition varies between 0.3 and 0.6%. Ninety per cent of all supernumerary teeth are located in the upper anterior region. Due to normal spacing in the deciduous dentition these teeth seldom create any clinical problems.

Hyperdontia in the permanent dentition

The prevalence of hyperdontia in the permanent dentition is 1-1.5%. Most supernumerary teeth are mesiodenses, located in the maxillary midline, followed by lower premolars and upper molars. There is a markedly higher prevalence among boys than girls. Para- and distomolars are almost always irregularly shaped. Multiple hyperdontia is generally symmetric.

Supernumerary teeth in the permanent dentition often cause disturbances in eruption, crowding and deviation of ordinary teeth. Thus, most supernumerary permanent teeth have to be extracted. Normally, the most deviant tooth in size, shape or position is chosen for extraction.

Mesiodenses (or midline supernumerary teeth) have a chronological development between the two dentitions. The prevalence is between 0.5 to 0.7% with higher pre-valence among boys than girls. About one-fifth of affected children have two or three mesiodenses. About 25% of mesiodenses erupt spontaneously and generally have a normal path of eruption, however, some may be inverted. Size and shape may vary, most being peg-shaped and smaller than normal maxillary incisors. Mesiodenses may cause delayed eruption or displacements of neighboring teeth (Fig. 15-14).

Disturbances in hard tissue formation

A disturbance of the enamel formation resulting in a macroscopically visible defect involving the surface with a reduced thickness of the enamel and with rounded borders is denoted *enamel hypoplasia* (Fig. 15-15). A defect without loss of enamel, but with changes in color and translucency of the enamel is called *enamel hypomineralisation* or *enamel opacity*. The surface of the opacity is normal.

Histology

Enamel hypoplasia is histologically characterized by the reduced enamel thickness and the rounded borders of the defect (Fig. 15-16). The bottom of the defect displays a

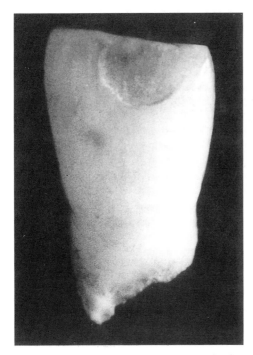

Fig. 15-15. Deciduous lower incisor with a half-moon shaped enamel hypoplasia at the incisal third.

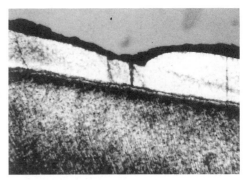

Fig. 15-16. Ground section of a deciduous incisor with an enamel hypoplasia. Note that the bottom of the defect corresponds to the neonatal line and the rounded cervical border.

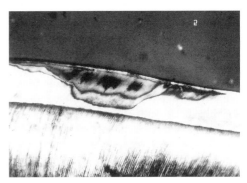

Fig. 15-17. Ground section of a deciduous incisor with an opacity. Note the porous area deep into the enamel.

more porous enamel than normal, the prism direction in the borders is perpendicular to the surface. The remaining enamel appears of normal thickness and morphology. The morphological appearence of the defect indicates that, whatever the cause of the disturbance, it is of short duration.

Enamel opacities are histologically characterized by a porous enamel under a well-mineralized surface (Fig. 15-17). The degree of hypomineralization and its extent into the enamel will determine the change of translucency, thus also the color of the opacity. In cases where the surface layer collapses, a macroscopical defect appears, which is then referred to as hypoplastic enamel.

Data on the chronology of dental development allow a rough estimation of the age at the time of disturbance when visible defects in the enamel are seen (Chapter 4). However, one must be aware that these data are based on normal gestational age. Therefore, data based on the start of the calcification of teeth and knowledge of the length of the pregnancy are more useful. Thus, timing of mineralization disturbances with macroscopical defects can be made with reasonable accuracy, in contrast to enamel opacities when timing is far more difficult.

Epidemiology

Enamel defects are the most frequently seen of the dental mineralization disturbances for obvious reasons, as dentin and cementum are hardly visible clinically. There are geographical and socio-economic variations

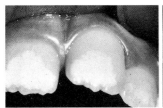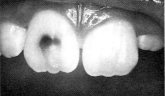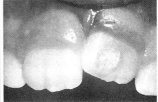

Fig. 15-18. Enamel lesions due to traumatic injuries of primary predessors. *Left*. Opacities. *Middle*. Opacity and discoloration. *Right*. Hypoplasia.

of enamel defects, even when the influence of fluoride in water supplies has been excluded. Good nutrition and health care play an important role, the developed countries thus have a lower prevalence. In Scandinavia, about 3% of children may be expected to have hypoplasias in their primary and 2-5% in their permanent teeth. Opacities are far more common with an estimated prevalence of 25-80% in the permanent dentition, depending on criteria used.

Etiology

In many cases of enamel defects there are no related factors to be found in the case histories. However, several etiology factors, local, as well as general, are known.

Etiology - local factors – A local factor can be suspected when an enamel defect affects a single tooth or has a local asymmetrical appearance. Acute mechanical trauma to the primary incisors may lead to a variety of disturbances in the developing permanent successor. If the root of the primary tooth penetrates the dental epithelium, the ameloblasts may be damaged and an enamel hypoplasia may result (Fig. 15-18). The disturbance may also be secondary to trauma, i.e. caused by tissue necrosis or pulpal complications induced by trauma. Depending on the stage of enamel development, an enamel hypoplasia or an enamel opacity may occur (Fig. 15-18).

The mineralization of premolars may be affected by periradicular osteitic processes of the primary teeth. The result of such a

local disturbance of infectious origin is called a Turner-tooth.

Therapeutic irradiation can severely disturb the dental development with loss of root formation, delayed or inhibited eruption.

Etiology - general factors – Symmetrical and chronological disturbances are caused by genetic factors, nutrititional disturbances, systemic diseases or intoxications. Different tooth groups and different parts of the teeth, corresponding to stage of development are affected.

In the primary dentition enamel hypoplasias show correlation to a number of different neonatal or perinatal disorders. Disturbances in the calcium homeostasis, such as neonatal tetany, severe rickets, vitamin-D-resistant rickets, respiratory distress syndromes, and gastro-intestinal conditions are associated with an increased frequency of enamel hypoplasias and enamel opacities. All these conditions have hypocalcemia as a common denominator. Vitamin-A-deficiency may also cause enamel defects.

In Scandinavia, severe hypocalcemic conditions rarely occur, however, a subclinical hypocalcemia may well predispose to increased sensitivity to other factors. Animal experiments and retrospective studies of children intubated at an early age, indicate that trauma to the dental arch is an etiological factor.

High fever and infectious diseases, especially in combination with diarrhea may lead to severe disturbances in calcium ho-

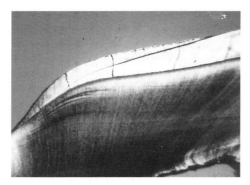

Fig. 15-19. Ground section of a deciduous incisor as seen in polarized light, with clearly visible neonatal line in the dentine.

meostasis and electrolyte balance, thus leading to enamel, defects.

In all primary teeth and in the lower first molars a neonatal line (birth line) can be seen histologically in the enamel as well as in the dentin (Fig. 15-19). The relationship between this incremental line and birth is well established. It is held to be an effect of neonatal hypocalcemia.

Fluorosis. – Long-term and high intake of fluoride during enamel formation results in changes of the enamel from thin white lines to chalky enamel, which breaks apart after eruption. There is a direct correlation between the amount of fluoride ingested during tooth formation and the degree of fluorotic changes. The first signs of fluorosis are found in the cuspal and incisal parts. After cleaning and drying the teeth, fine opaque

lines following the perikymata can be distinguished. The more affected the teeth are, the more pronounced and widened the lines will become, until the whole tooth surface exhibits irregular and opaque white areas (Fig 15-20). Even more affected tooth surfaces become entirely opaque and pitting of the enamel occurs, the most fluorotic teeth exhibit a total loss of surface enamel combined with brownish discoloration, due to uptake of different agents from the diet.

Primary teeth exhibit less dental fluorosis than permanent teeth. One explanation might be that most of the enamel is formed *in utero* with lower fetal serum-F.

The pathology of enamel fluorosis is not yet fully understood. Effects on calcium regulation, as well as toxic effects on the ameloblasts, have been proposed as possible factors. The treatment of fluorotic teeth varies with the degree of fluorosis. In slightly affected teeth, grinding and polishing of the enamel surface might be sufficient. More advanced defects can be treated with composites or crowns (Fig. 15-21). Dental fluorosis is basically a hypomineralization and should, therefore, be treated with topical application of fluorides, to attempt remineralization of the tooth surface.

Tetracyclins – Tetracyclins have a high affinity to mineralized hard tissues and may cause considerable discoloration of teeth. In many countries tetracyclins are for this reason not given to children below the age of 13, pregnant women or lactating mothers.

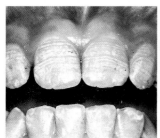
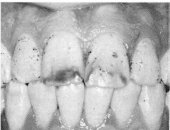
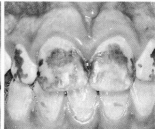

Fig. 15-20. Three cases of severe dental fluorosis.

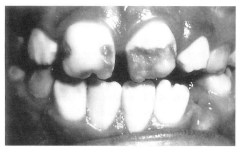

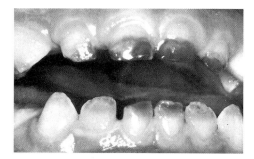

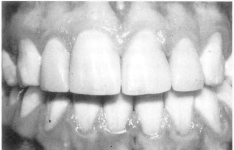

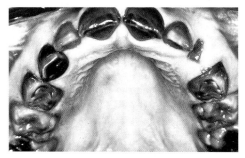

Fig. 15-21. Dental fluorosis. *Top*. Extensive hypo-mineralization caused by endogenous fluoride exposition, 10 ppm in drinking water.
Bottom. Upper incisors restored with composite materials.

Fig. 15-22. Tetracycline discoloration of primary (top) and permanent teeth (bottom).

Nevertheless, teeth stained by tetracyclins can occasionally be seen. The intensity and color of the teeth vary with different tetracyclins. In high doses tetracyclins may cause enamel hypoplasias (Fig. 15-22). As tetracyclins in hard tissues give a characteristic fluorescence in ultraviolet light they are easily identified in ground sections examined in a fluorescence microscope (Fig. 15-23).

Other toxic factors to be considered are the intake of cytostatic drugs, thalidomide and overdose of vitamin D (Fig. 15-24).

Several of the systemic disorders mentioned earlier have an hereditary character. However, there are a few specific disturbances of enamel and dentin formation with a genetic background.

Amelogenesis imperfecta is a hereditary anomaly exclusively affecting the enamel.

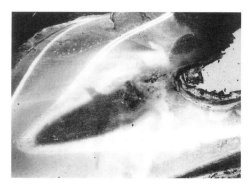

Fig. 15-23. Ground section of a deciduous incisor with characteristic tetracycline staining seen as 3 bands in the dentin in fluorescent light.

The prevalence in a Scandinavian population has been estimated to be 1 in 4,000 and 1 in 12,000-14,000 in a North American population. Both dentitions are generally affected. Several hereditary patterns have been observed, autosomal dominant inheritance being the most common.

Clinical classifications with up to 12 dif-

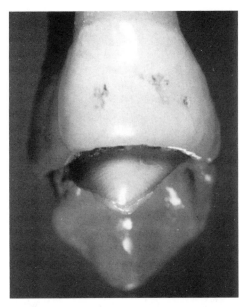

Fig. 15-24. Toxic effect on mineralization in a premolar of heavy doses of vitamin D given to a girl with vitamin D-resistant rickets at 3 years old.

ferent types have been described. However, many types appear to express variations of the same type (Fig. 15-25). The main classifications are the hypoplastic and hypomin-

eralization types. The hypoplastic types are mostly yellowish white to light brown with smooth, hard enamel, however, markedly reduced in thickness. The enamel is thin with a normal x-ray appearance. The hypomineralization types have yellow to dark brown crowns, a rough, uneven enamel with more or less normal thickness and morphology. The enamel is softer than normal and has a dentin contrast on x-rays and splits off easily.

Eruption may be delayed and some types are correlated to the development of anterior open bite. The susceptibility to periodontal diseases is greater than normal. The aberrant tooth morphology retains plaque and there are indications that the gingival epithelium may be defective. Patients with *amelogenesis imperfecta* generally show a low caries frequency, possibly due to loss of tooth substance and shallow fissures. An increased sensitivity of the teeth is sometimes found due to partial loss of enamel and/or porous enamel. There is no evidence that *amelogenesis imperfecta* is related to other ectodermal defects or other diseases. Similar dental defects may, however, appear in connection with, for example,

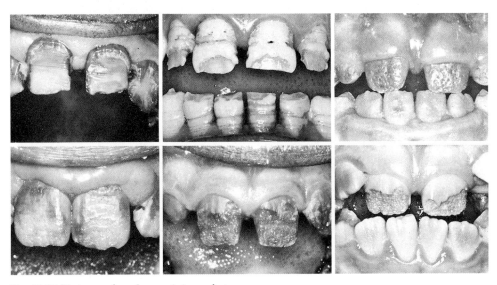

Fig. 15-25. Six types of amelogenesis imperfecta.

Fig. 15-26. *Top*. Amelogenesis imperfecta, hypomineralization type in a 14-year-old girl. Some
esthetic restorations have been placed, but with
an unsatisfactory result. *Bottom.* Same patient
(see top) with Dicor ceramic crowns (courtesy
by Dr B Torstensson).

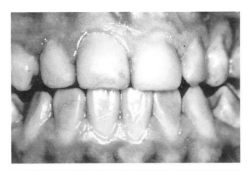

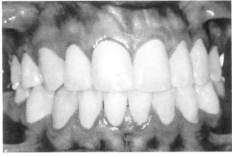

epidermolysis bullosa and pseudohypoparathyroidism.

Need for dental treatment is often very
high, for both esthetic and functional reasons. Esthetic problems can mainly be
solved by the use of composites or crowns
(Fig. 15-26). In cases with rapid attrition and
break down of the enamel, early placement
of gold crowns on the molars is recommended to stabilize the bite and avoid further destruction of the fragile teeth (Fig.
15-27).

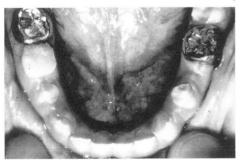

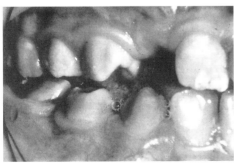

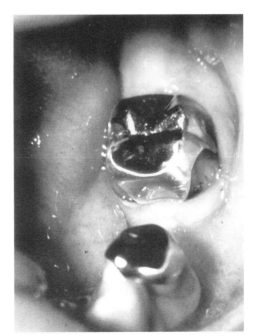

Fig. 15-27. Amelogenesis imperfecta. Risk for attrition and fractures due to chewing forces.
Top left. Nine-year-old girl with AI and very thin enamel (see incisors). To stabilize the bite and reduce the risk of enamel fractures, gold crowns are placed in all permanent first molars.
Bottom left and right. To reduce the risk of wearing down the soft enamel, gold inlays have been
placed in this 12-year-old girl with AI.

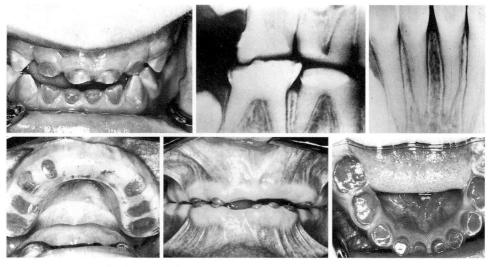

Fig. 15-28. Dentinogenesis imperfecta. Discoloration, attrition and pulpal obliteration (courtesy by Dr C Vincent).

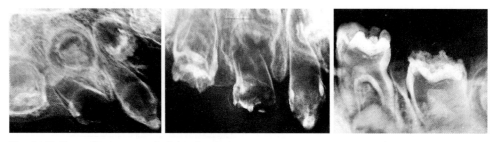

Fig. 15-29. X-rays from a case of odontodysplasia.

Dentinogenesis imperfecta. This autosomal inherited anomaly has an estimated prevalence in the North American population of 1 in 7-9,000. Both dentitions are affected. *Dentinogenesis imperfecta* appears both as an isolated trait and in association with *osteogenesis imperfecta*.

At eruption, the teeth have a normal shape and structure, however, with a yellowish color of the crowns, which is the reason the term "hereditary opalescent dentin" is also used for this condition. With time, and especially in the permanent dentition, the color changes to bluish grey shades. The teeth are subject to a rapid attrition, well marked in primary dentition, where the crowns can be worn down to the gingival margin. The enamel splits off easily and the exposed dentin gradually darkens (Fig. 15-28).

X-rays show the roots are short and underdeveloped, and the coronal pulp chambers and root canals often become totally obliterated shortly after eruption. In some cases abnormally large pulp chambers and practically no roots develop. This condition shows many similarities to the rare anomaly odontodysplasia.

Histologically, the enamel appears normal, but with an abnormal morphology of the dentino-enamel junction and the circumpulpal dentin. The body of the dentin has a laminar structure with undulating tubules.

Treatment of patients with *dentinogenesis imperfecta* creates considerable problems. Stainless steel crowns on the primary and permanent first molars may be of help. The cosmetic problems require appropriate attention and care.

Odontodysplasia is a very rare anomaly, where tooth development is arrested locally in one or several neighboring teeth, resulting in so-called shell-teeth with little or no root formation and huge pulp chambers. The affected teeth have a ghost-like appearance in x-rays (Fig. 15-29). Odontodysplasia is most often localized to one or two regions of the jaws. The etiology is unknown, however, local trauma appears to be one factor to be considered.

Dentin dysplasias are extremely rare hereditary anomalies of two types. The pulpal dentinal dysplasias result in voluminous coronal pulp chambers, but relatively normal roots. In radicular dentinal dysplasia, the crowns have a marked cervical constriction and the roots can be extremely small and thin. In this type, the cervical enamel and the root dentin show abnormal histological features. As in odontodysplasia, pulpal complications and early exfoliation are the dominant clinical problems.

Root cementum anomalies. Hypolasia or even aplasia of root cementum is seen in hypophosphatasia, a condition leading to severe periodontal disease. In cleidocranial dysostosis there is no deposition of cellular cementum.

DISTURBANCES IN TOOTH ERUPTION

The chronology of the clinical eruption of teeth is presented in Chapter 4, Table 4-2 (primary teeth) and Table 4-3 (permanent teeth). The total time span for the eruption

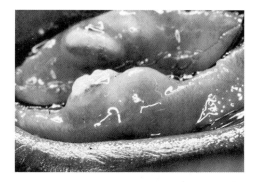

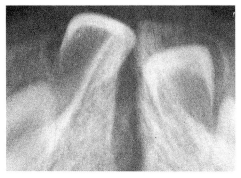

Fig. 15-30. *Top*. Natal tooth and bulge of a neonatal tooth erupting 2 days later. *Bottom*. X-ray showing the superficial position of a natal tooth.

of the primary dentition is only 20 months, with minor deviations from average figures, and with no significant sex differences. The total time span for the eruption of the permanent dentition, however, is about 14 years, sex differences are significant, and the deviations from average figures are large, especially for the last teeth to erupt.

Disturbances in tooth eruption involve premature and retarded eruption, ectopic eruption and impaction of teeth. In addition soft tissue problems may arise during eruption in both dentitions.

Disturbances in the eruption of primary teeth

Normally the eruption of primary dentition is uneventful because they have no prede-

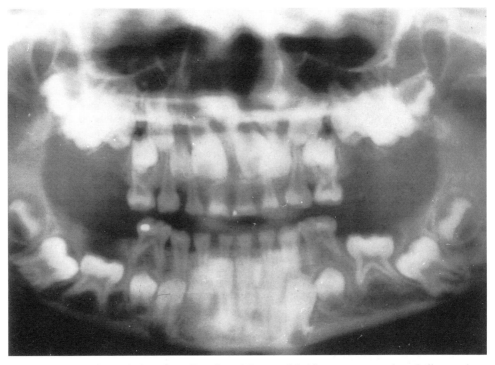

Fig. 15-31. Inherited retarded eruption. Female at 8.5 years old. All permanent teeth and all second primary molars are still unerupted.

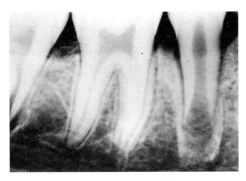

Fig. 15-32. After the extraction of the predecessor, the lower second premolar has erupted rapidly "leaving the alveolar bone behind".

cessor to be resorbed, a short distance to move, and are seldom short of space. However, certain general symptoms are said to be associated with "teething" (see p.272).

The normal span of eruption for the first tooth should be from the 4th to 10th month (Mean ± 2SD) and for the last from the 20th to 36th month. However, even eruptions beyond these limits will often be within normal genetic/familiar variation. Tooth eruption before that time may be defined as premature, and beyond that time as retarded, and the cause for the abnormality should be investigated.

Premature eruption in the primary dentition is rare. The most extreme manifestations are the natal and neonatal teeth (*dentitio connatalis* and *neonatalis*). The frequency is estimated at 1 case per 2,000-3,000 births, and there are no sex differences. Most of the teeth belong to the normal primary dentition and have a normal shape. The most prevalent tooth is the lower central incisor(s). The root has not yet developed, and the tooth is loosely attached to the gingiva (Fig. 15-30). The etiology is poorly understood, but there seems to be an heriditary

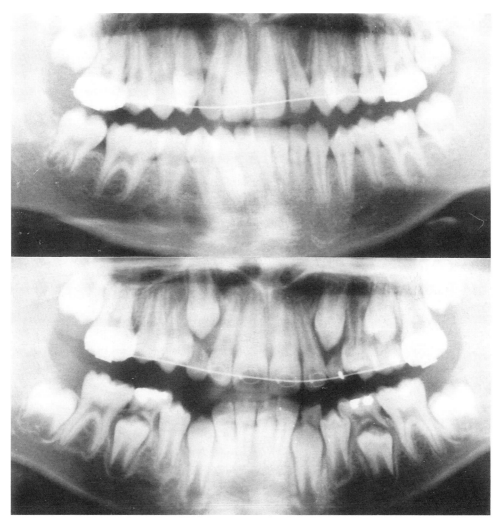

Fig. 15-33. OPG of monozygous twins at 10 years. *Top*. A twin with *pubertas praecox* (early production of sex hormones). *Bottom*. His normal twin brother. Differences in eruptional stages amount to 2.5 years.

background. Natal teeth may also be part of certain syndromes (e.g. chondro-ectodermal dysplasia, *Pachyonychia congenita*).

The symptoms related to natal/neonatal teeth include gingivitis and extreme tooth mobility, which may cause discomfort to the child during feeding, ulceration of the tongue, possibilities for exfoliation and aspiration, and also trauma to the mother's breast. Natal and neonatal teeth should be

extracted only if they are loose enough to involve risk of exfoliation or if feeding is severely disturbed.

Retarded eruption in the primary dentition may be caused by the same factors as those of the permanent teeth (Tables 15-1, 15-2), but most of the local factors will naturally be lacking. Premature children show retarded eruption of their first primary teeth, but the delay will usually be

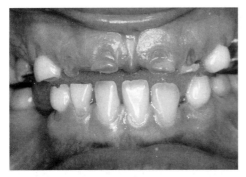

Fig. 15-34. Intra-oral photograph of a 17-year-old girl with inherited retarded eruption. Only the first permanent molars and 3 lower incisors have erupted.

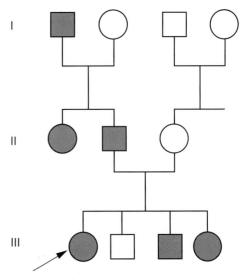

Fig. 15-35. Pedigree through 3 generations of a family with inherited retarded eruption. In the first generation there is one affected man, in the second generation 2 affected siblings (male and female), and in the third generation 3 affected siblings (1 male, 2 females).

caught up. Primary dentition is also less vulnerable to most of the systemic factors (e.g. hypovitaminosis, endocrine deficiencies), and in cases of inherited retarded eruption often only the second primary molars may be affected (Fig. 15-31).

Disturbances in the eruption of the permanent dentition

Premature eruption beyond the normal variation is rare. The main local cause is early loss of the predeceding tooth (Fig. 15-32). Systemic factors may be hyperproduction of thyroid, pituitary and sex hormones (Fig. 15-33), but the effects of these hormones on tooth maturation and eruption are considerably less than on skeletal parameters. Other factors which increase the metabolism have also been suggested to stimulate eruption (e.g., fever and high blood pressure).

Retarded eruption in the permanent dentition is quite common and may either be local, affecting one or few teeth, or systemic, affecting the whole dentition. Before considering systemic retarded eruption, allowance should be given for the normal variation (2SD) and for sex differences. Systemic

causes of retarded eruption are listed in Table 15-1. In most of them (hypovitaminoses, endocrine hypofunction, syndromes and single gene disorders), the other somatic aberrant features are quite obvious and offer no difficulties in diagnosis. With

TABLE **15-1**

Disease and some syndromes associated with retarded eruption of teeth

Hypopituitarism
Hypothyroidism
Hypovitaminosis D
Down's syndrome
Cleidocranial and cleidofacial dysostosis
Osteopetrosis
Ectodermal dysplasia
Achondroplasia
Amelogenesis imperfecta
Inherited retarded eruption

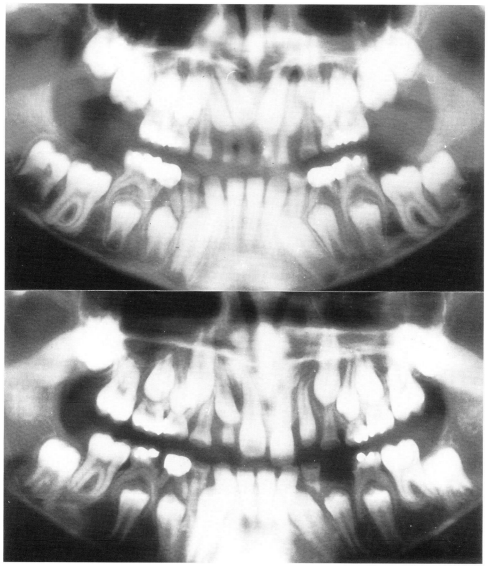

Fig. 15-36. *Top*. OPG at 12 years of a boy with inherited retarded eruption. In the permanent dentition, only the lower incisors are erupted. *Bottom.* OPG at 14 years. All first molars and 3 of the upper incisors have erupted meanwhile, despite being deeply seated in the jaws and had completed roots with hooking or bending.

the exception of Down's syndrome all the listed disorders are rather rare.

In inherited retarded eruption, late eruption is the only aberrant feature in an otherwise completely healthy child. The tooth formation/maturation schedule is close to normal, while the eruption may be 10-15 years delayed (Fig. 15-34). Thus, the root formation will proceed in an inward direction, often creating severe deviation and hooking of the roots.

Transmission seems to be autosomally

dominant (Fig. 15-35), but the pathogenic mechanism is unknown (as is the mechanism for normal eruption), but some genetically programmed factors may, in some way, prevent the start of eruption. When the eruption is "released", it may be rapid despite the tooth often having a long eruption path or hooked roots (Fig. 15-36). In inherited retarded eruption, teeth both with and without predecessors are affected. Extraction of the predecessor will normally not provoke eruption. When teeth erupt they will usually follow the normal sequence (lower first incisors, 6-year molars, etc.).

Local factors delaying eruption are presented in Table 15-2. The most prevalent cause is lack of space, caused by caries or ectopic eruption of the 6-year molars. Unerupted teeth should be searched for if their eruption is 2-3 SD beyond normal eruption time, or if their contralateral tooth has been erupted for some time. However, it should be kept in mind that SD is only half a year for incisors and first molars, while it is about one and a half years for canines, premolars and second molars.

Symptoms associated with "teething"

Often the primary teeth pierce the gum without causing any symptoms. However, in at least two-thirds of all infants local symptoms of varying severity may be noted at the area of breakthrough. Examination reveals redness and swelling in the oral mucosa overlying the tooth. These symptoms appear a few days before clinical eruption. During this period the child may show signs of local irritation and has a tendency to rub the gum with his fingers or with some object. This will result in drooling. Shortly before the tooth pierces the oral mucosa, a whitish area is seen exactly at the future point of breakthrough, correspond-

TABLE 15-2
Local disturbances leading to retarded eruption
Lack of arch space Ectopy Sequelae to trauma Persisting root remnants Anchylosis of predecessor Premature loss of predecessor Cysts Supernumerary teeth Double formations

ing to the keratinization of the fused dental and oral epithelia. The actual exposure of the tooth will take place a few days later. This is not normally accompanied by any ulceration of the soft tissue.

The eruption of permanent teeth may be accompanied by similar local manifestations, but the subjective symptoms are far less pronounced. The exposure of hard tissue in the oral cavity undoubtedly represents altered bacteriological conditions and a new relationship between the soft tissue and the microbial flora of the oral cavity. As the confluence between oral and dental epithelium is permeable, an accumulation of inflammatory cells occurs in the adjacent tissue. The initial phase is acute and dominated by polymorphonuclear leukocytes. This acute reaction may be a possible cause of the local reactions noted in the days around the actual eruption into the oral cavity. The chronic inflammation noted a couple of days after eruption then represents an unspecific marginal gingivitis.

After eruption, soft tissue often remains for a relatively long time in the distal part of the occlusal surface (Fig. 15-37). This lobe is known as an *operculum gingivae*. The tendency to a persisting operculum is greater when eruption takes place early in relation to the growth of the jaw. In such cases the tooth erupts partly into the retromolar mu-

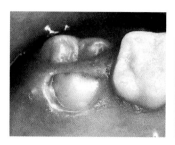 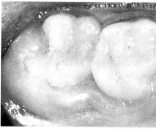

Fig. 15-37. *Left*. A string of tissue still covers the central part of an erupting molar. *Right*. *Operculum gingivae*.

cosa, a tissue which is more resistant to resorption than the future gingiva.

Mechanical trauma or plaque accumulation at the operculum may cause inflammation and considerable swelling of a type most often seen around lower third molars.

Even if it is accepted that an accumulation of leukocytes in the mucosa at the onset of clinical eruption may be the cause of local symptoms, the question still remains whether tooth eruption has any influence on the general condition of the child. In modern dentistry the term *dentitio difficilis,* difficult teething, refers primarily to the eruption of third molars. Formerly the term was mainly associated with the eruption of primary teeth.

Hippocrates maintained that tooth eruption may cause severe illness. This opinion remained deep-rooted in ancient medicine and is also reflected in death statistics. During the 18th century almost half of all deaths in infancy in France were ascribed to "teething troubles".

The general symptoms most often mentioned in the literature are irritability, fever, infections in the respiratory tract, anorexia, constipation, diarrhea, hypersalivation and skin rashes.

The question arises whether teething can cause any of these symptoms, or the symptoms can hasten tooth eruption, or whether they can occur simultaneously, but independently.

A general irritability of the child in connection with the eruption of teeth may induce agitation, restlessness and insomnia. The presence of an acute local inflammation

in the gingiva is sufficient explanation for such symptoms.

In contrast to earlier opinions, there is no evidence that convulsions or seizures may be due to tooth eruption. In most instances hysterical convulsions or temper tantrums are assumed by laymen to be teething convulsions. In this context it is interesting, if only from a historical standpoint, to read about the feared teething convulsions which once dominated death statistics. The few case histories preserved show very clearly that the dominating cause was hypocalcemic seizures due to severe rickets, so-called spasmophilia.

The relationship between fever and tooth eruption has been considered two-fold. Firstly, fever from other causes may increase the basal metabolism and, thereby, hasten eruption. Secondly, there is a possibility that the local oral inflammation at the eruption site may affect body temperature. However, observations have been contradictory and have failed to show a general tendency. It cannot be excluded that some children may have small peaks in body temperature during the eruption of primary teeth.

The often described hypersalivation is rather a drooling due to the child's manipulations in the oral cavity. This may in turn give rise to irritation and reddening of the skin, described as skin rashes.

The conclusion must be that there is no absolute association between tooth eruption and disturbances in the general condition of the child. However, local inflammation at the site of eruption may make the child irritable and, occasionally, even cause a rise in body temperature or mild change in peristalsis.

Therapy for "difficult teething"

Treatment for teething troubles was formerly directed at both local and supposed general symptoms. Since local massage of the gum pads obviously relieves the discomfort, various remedies with which to rub the gum have been prescribed. Some of these "teething powders" contained mercury and caused severe illness, other preparations contained ethanol and gained wide popularity because of their sedative effects.

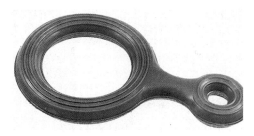

Fig. 15-38. Bite-ring of rubber.

Today, a bite ring of rubber may possibly be recommended because it is easy to clean, cannot be swallowed and does not injure the gums (Fig. 15-38).

Background literature

Norén JG. *Human deciduous enamel in perinatal disorders*. Morphological and chemical aspects. Thesis. Göteborg, Sweden 1983.

Pindborg JJ. *Pathology of the dental hard tissues*. Copenhagen: Munksgaard 1982.

Pindborg JJ. Aetiology of developmental enamel defects not related to fluorosis. *Int dent J* 1982; **32**: 123-34.

Rasmussen P, Hansen AS, Berg E. Inherited retarded eruption. *J Dent Child* 1983; **50**: 268-73.

Roberts MW, Li SH, Comite F, et al. Dental development in precocious puberty. *J Dent Res* 1985; **64**: 1084-6.

Sundell S. *Hereditary amelogenesis imperfecta*. An epidemiological, genetic and clinical study in a Swedish child population. Thesis. Göteborg, Sweden 1986.

CHAPTER 16

DISTURBANCES OF OCCLUSAL DEVELOPMENT AND FUNCTION

Morphologic malocclusion
Functional malocclusion
Craniomandibular disorders

MORPHOLOGIC MALOCCLUSION

Classification

The term "malocclusion" covers a number of different morphologic deviations which may occur as single traits or in various combinations. To specify the concept, methods have been developed to systematically describe morphologic malocclusions based on groupings of single traits of malocclusion in three main categories, subdivided as shown in Table 16-1.

A relatively simple, but very useful, classification to be employed in connection with diagnosis and treatment planning is to divide the malocclusions into two major groups:

– dento-alveolar malocclusions
– skeletal (basal) malocclusions

Dento-alveolar malocclusions are primarily related to deviations within the dental arches and alveolar processes. Skeletal malocclusions are primarily caused by deviation in jaw relationships. Definitions of single malocclusion traits according to Björk et al(2) will be given in the following.

Sagittal malocclusion – Extreme maxillary overjet is defined as ≥ 4 mm in primary and ≥ 6 mm in permanent dentition (Fig. 16-1); mandibular overjet > 0 mm. In the latter, the presence of anteriorly forced bite should be recorded.

Distal or mesial occlusion is defined as a 1/2 cusp or more deviation from normal occlusion (Figs. 16-2, 16-3).

Vertical malocclusion – Deep bite is defined as ≥ 3 mm in primary and ≥ 5 mm in permanent dentition (Fig. 16-4). Open bite measured at the central incisors > 0 mm. Open bite in the lateral region is recorded for the canine, premolar and molar section on each side.

Transverse malocclusion – Crossbite is recorded on each side for the canines, premolars and molars if the buccal cusp of the upper teeth occludes lingually to the cusp of the corresponding lower tooth (Fig. 16-5A).

Scissors bite is recorded if the lingual

cusp of the upper tooth occludes buccally to the buccal cusp of the corresponding lower tooth (Fig. 16-5B). Crossbite and scissors bite are registered only when the cusps have passed each other.

Transverse forced bite is registered if the lower jaw from first tooth contact to full occlusion is displaced laterally by at least 2 mm measured at the incisors.

Space anomalies – Crowding and spacing may be recorded after the primary dentition is fully erupted. The registration is made separately for the incisor section and for the lateral sections (canines and premolars). The incisor segment is demarcated by the distal contact points of the two lateral incisors when these teeth do not deviate labially or lingually in relation to the midline of the alveolar process. The lateral segments are limited by these points and the mesial contact points of the first permanent molars. When a lateral incisor deviates, the demarcation point is taken at the mesial contact point of the canine. When both lateral incisor and canine deviate, a point is used on the midline of the alveolar process between the two contact points. Crowding or spacing is registered when there is a deviation from normal of at least 2 mm in a section. Before shedding of primary teeth, crowding and spacing is judged from the size of the primary teeth, after shedding from that of the permanent teeth. The maxillary medial diastema should be recorded separately.

Prevalence

Dentitional anomalies were dealt with in Chapter 15, and only the prevalence of occlusal and spatial anomalies will be discussed here.

The prevalence of morphologic malocclusions in Scandinavia has been studied by several authors(5,9,11). Prevalence of malocclusions in Danish children classified according to(2) is given in Tables 16-2 to 16-5.

TABLE 16-1

Classification of morphologic malocclusion according to Björk et al(2).

Malocclusion

Dentitional anomalies
    Formation
        Hyperdontia
        Hypodontia
        Malformation
    Eruption
        Ectopic eruption
        Transposition
        Delayed eruption
        Arrested eruption
        Persistent primary teeth
    Position
        Rotation
        Tipping
        Inversion
Occlusal anomalies
    Sagittal anomalies
        Extreme maxillary overjet
        Mandibular overjet
        Distal molar occlusion
        Mesial molar occlusion
    Vertical anomalies
        Deep bite
        Open bite, frontal
        Open bite, lateral
    Transversal anomalies
        Crossbite
        Scissors bite
        Midline displacement
Space anomalies
    Upper jaw
        Crowding
        Spacing
    Lower jaw
        Crowding
        Spacing

Some of the occlusal anomalies show marked changes in prevalence from primary to permanent dentition, for example, distal molar occlusion which is a common

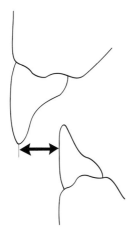

Fig. 16-1. Measurement of overjet.

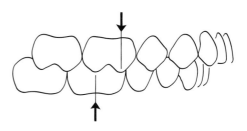

Fig. 16-2. Distal molar occlusion.

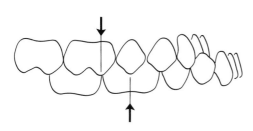

Fig. 16-3. Mesial molar occlusion.

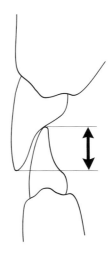

Fig. 16-4. Measurement of overbite.

physiologic malocclusion before eruption of the permanent first molar, and frontal open bite, which in most cases disappears spontaneously following discontinuation of sucking habits.

Prevalence of spatial anomalies in primary and permanent dentition also shows marked differences. Thus, crowding is practically non-existent in primary dentition, whereas it is present in the permanent dentition of at least one third of children. In contrast, spacing is very common in primary dentition and rare in the permanent.

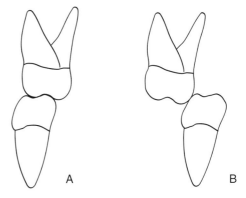

Fig. 16-5. A. Crossbite. B. Scissors bite.

TABLE **16-2**

Frequencies of sagittal malocclusion, %. From(5,10).

	Full primary dentition		Full permanent dentition	
	Boys	Girls	Boys	Girls
Increased maxillary overjet ≥ 4mm	35.8	41.8	-	-
Increased maxillary overjet ≥ 6mm	11.9	11.9	15.9	12.5
Distal molar occlusion ≥ 1/2 cusp width	49.5	49.0	23.2	25.8
Mandibular overjet > 0 mm	0	0	0.7	0.2
Mesial molar occlusion ≥ 1/2 cusp width	1.0	2.4	4.1	4.5

TABLE **16-3**

Frequencies of vertical malocclusion, %. From(5,10).

	Full primary dentition		Full permanent dentition	
	Boys	Girls	Boys	Girls
Frontal open bite > 0 mm	21.8	23.9	2.3	1.8
Frontal deep bite ≥ 3 mm	18.1	18.9	-	-
Frontal deep bite ≥ 5 mm	3.6	2.0	22.7	14.5

Etiology

Several factors are of significance in the etiology of malocclusions. A malocclusion may develop as a result of genetic and/or environmental factors. The genetic mechanisms may be simple, for example, autosomal dominant transmission, or more complicatedly, polygenic, where several different genes are acting. Such environmental factors as oral habits, hypertrophic tonsils and adenoids, dental trauma, early loss of primary teeth and severe, chronic diseases in childhood (juvenile rheumatoid arthritis of the temporomandibular joint), may be of importance in the development of malocclusion.

As discussed in Chapter 4, the dento-alveolar compensatory mechanism may reduce the effects of aberrant jaw relations. In less extreme cases the dento-alveolar compensatory mechanism may be successful in maintaining normal occlusal relations in spite of changing jaw relationships, however, often at the expense of the deterioration of the space condition. In children with extreme deviations in jaw relationships, the dento-alveolar compensatory mechanism may become insufficient leading to a so-called "skeletal" malocclusion. The presence of primary crowding, abnormalities in eruption, tooth migration, oral habits, mouthbreathing and abnormal tongue posture may impair the dento-alveolar compensatory mechanism and thus lead to malocclusion.

In conclusion, the developement of malocclusion is most often caused by a non-functioning, incomplete or impaired dento-alveolar compensatory mechanism rather than by the actual discrepancy in jaw relationships.

Sagittal malocclusion – An increased maxillary overjet may be the result of (Fig. 16-6):

Frequencies of transversal malocclusion, %
From(5,10).

	Full primary dentition		Full permanent dentition	
	Boys	Girls	Boys	Girls
Crossbite	10.6	17.3	9.4	14.1
Scissors bite	0	0.5	7.1	7.9
Midline displacement	4.6	5.8	14.0	13.9

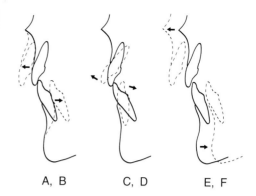

A, B   C, D   E, F

Fig. 16-6. Development of increased maxillary overjet. Adapted from(1).

TABLE 16-5

Frequencies of crowding and spacing, %.
From(5,10).

	Full primary dentition		Full permanent dentition	
	Boys	Girls	Boys	Girls
Crowding, upper jaw	1.5	2.9	20.6	26.3
Crowding, lower jaw	0.5	1.9	33.0	31.7
Spacing, upper jaw	51.0	43.3	8.1	4.3
Spacing, lower jaw	41.9	39.9	5.1	2.5
Medial diastema	8.6	9.6	0.8	1.0

A, B   C, D   E, F

Fig. 16-7. Development of mandibular overjet. Adapted from(1).

A mandibular overjet may develop as a result of (Fig. 16-7):

A protrusion of the maxillary alveolar process. B retrusion of the mandibular alveolar process. C increased labial inclination of the upper incisors. D lingual inclination of the lower incisors. E protrusion of the maxilla. F retrusion of the mandible.

A retrusion of the maxillary alveolar process. B protrusion of the mandibular alveolar process. C increased labial inclination of the lower incisors. D lingual inclination of the upper incisors. E protrusion of the mandible. F retrusion of the maxilla.

Oral habits, especially finger sucking, may have an adverse effect on incisor inclination (Fig. 16-8). Incompentent lip closure with the lower lip resting behind the upper incisors may be the result.

Mandibular prognathism is often genetically determined. Retrusion of the maxilla can be seen in pathological conditions with synostosis of maxillary sutures as seen in Crouzon syndrome.

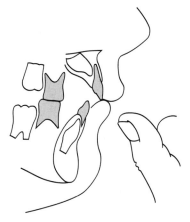

Fig. 16-8. Development of dento-alveolar open bite due to finger sucking.

Distal molar occlusion (Fig. 16-2) may arise because of:

– mesial migration of the permanent upper molars due to ectopic eruption or early loss of primary molars because of caries

– inappropriate adjustment of the first permanent molars during the mixed dentition

– retrusion of the mandible

– protrusion of the maxilla

Mandibular retrusion is most often caused by genetic factors in otherwise healthy children, but may also be observed in children with congenital or acquired anomalies of the mandibular condyles, e.g. Treacher-Collins syndrome and juvenile rheumatoid arthritis.

Mesial molar occlusion most often occurs as a result of skeletal mandibular prognathism.

Vertical malocclusion – Frontal open bite of dento-alveolar origin may be due to:

– incomplete eruption (infraposition) of the upper or lower incisors

– reduced vertical development of the alveolar process in the incisor region

Dento-alveolar open bite most often develop as a result of oral habits (dummy/finger sucking or tongue thrust). Depending on the type and duration of the habits, there is a tendency for spontaneous correction of frontal open bite especially if the habit is broken before eruption of the permanent incisors.

Skeletal open bite may develop if the mandible during the adolescent growth period rotates in a backward direction (Fig. 16-9) to such a degree that the compensatory dento-alveolar mechanism becomes insufficient. The compensatory mechanism may also be hampered by the development of a tongue thrust or by interposition of the tongue between the dental arches, as often seen in children with hypertrophic tonsils. Children with hyperthrophy of the adenoids with constriction of the airways also often exhibit a backward rotation of the mandible and frontal open bite. Children with this type of growth pattern are characterized by an increased anterior facial height (Fig. 16-10).

Dento-alveolar deep bite may develop in cases with increased overjet. Excessive eruption of the incisors may occur when normal contact between upper and lower incisors is absent. In this type of occlusal development the vertical jaw relationship is usually normal.

Skeletal deep bite may develop if the mandible during growth rotates in a forward direction (Fig. 16-11). In children with an unstable incisor occlusion and extreme vertical growth direction of the mandibular condyles, a deep bite and reduced anterior lower face height may develop as a result of forward rotation of the mandible (Fig. 16-12). Also, extreme force in the masseter and temporalis muscles or extensive tooth wear or tooth loss may cause deep bite and reduced anterior lower face height.

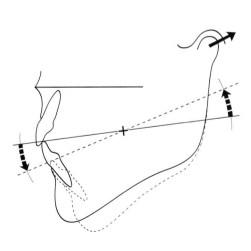

Fig. 16-9. Backward growth rotation of the mandible. From(3).

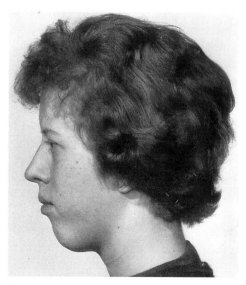

Fig. 16-10. Girl with increased anterior facial height and open bite secondary to backward mandibular growth rotation. From(3).

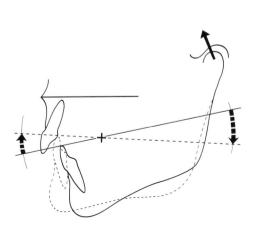

Fig. 16-11. Forward growth rotation of the mandible. From(3).

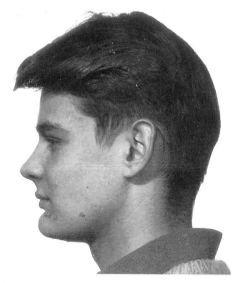

Fig. 16-12. Boy with reduced anterior facial height and deep bite secondary to forward mandibular growth rotation. From(3).

Transverse malocclusion – Dento-alveolar crossbite or scissors bite of single teeth are often the result of crowding. A total unilateral crossbite is most often associated with a midline deviation of the mandible to the side of the crossbite. This situation is often seen in cases with a narrow maxillary arch. A lateral shift of the mandible may then

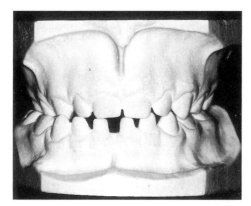

Fig. 16-13. Functional crossbite on the right side. Note the marked midline deviation towards the side of the crossbite. From(11).

occur due to intercuspal guidance, most often in the canine region, into so-called "functional crossbite" (Fig. 16-13).

A total unilateral scissors bite may be caused by a narrow mandibular arch, a wide maxillary arch or a combination.

Skeletal unilateral crossbite or scissors bite may be caused by asymmetry in the cranial base, the maxilla or the mandible. Asymmetry of the cranial base is common in the newborn as a result of prenatal factors or birth trauma. This anomaly is usually self-corrected, but if not a compensatory asymmetrical growth of the jaws may be observed. Primary asymmetry of the cranial base and the mandible may be caused by congenital or acquired growth disturbances in specific growth zones e.g. plagiocephaly of hemifacial microsomia. Likewise, primary asymmetry of the maxillary complex may be caused by congenital or acquired growth disturbances (e.g. unilateral maxillary synostosis or unilateral cleft lip and palate).

Bilateral crossbite or scissors bite are rare types of malocclusion. They are most often of a skeletal nature and in many cases they are combined with deviations in the sagittal and vertical dimensions.

Spacing anomalies – Crowding and spacing in the dentition depend upon the available space in the dental arches and the mesio-distal diameter of the teeth.

Both tooth size and jaw size are strongly genetically influenced. However, crowding has become very common in modern man, probably due to minimal wear of teeth.It is suggested that lack of occlusal and interproximal dental wear in modern man partly explains the marked increase in occlusal anomalies, since the consequent crowding impairs the compensatory dento-alveolar mechanism.

Early loss of primary teeth is also a cause of dento-alveolar crowding in the permanent dentition and depends on several factors:

– the region involved; mesial migration is most pronounced following premature loss of the upper second primary molar

– developmental stage; loss of primary molars before the age of 7 years seems to cause crowding in the permanent dentition

– the general space conditions in the dental arches; i.e. the more initial crowding, the more space loss

– intercuspal locking; a stable occlusal locking of the first permanent molars reduces the amount of migration following early loss of primary teeth

Basal crowding or spacing may develop in cases with congenital or acquired anomalies of tooth development (microdontia, aplasia, macrodontia, supernumerary teeth) or jaw development (maxillary or mandibular hypo- or hyperplasia).

Prevention

Caries prevention and therapy – Caries prevention serves to keep primary teeth functional until natural exfoliation and is, thus, a significant tool in prevention of malocclusion. In restorative therapy it is important to maintain the mesio-distal dimensions of the primary teeth to avoid mesial migration of teeth with subsequent loss of space in the dental arch.

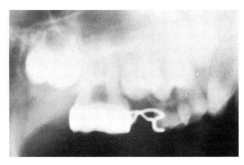

Fig. 16-14. Space maintainer welded on to orthodontic band.

Space maintainers – Space maintainers may be needed if a primary molar is lost prematurely, especially if the occlusion of the first permanent molar is not fully established, and if there is no excess space in the dental arches. A variety of simple appliances are used: removable plates, headgear, lip bumper, lingual arch, orthodontic band with a welded piece of archwire, band-tube-loop space maintainer or Sannerud's model (Fig. 16-14).

The following factors should be considered when a space maintainer is planned:

- it should keep the space for the permanent successor
- it should allow normal development of the teeth and alveolar process
- it should stop elongation of antagonists
- it should not impair function
- it should be constructed with minimal damage to the tissues
- it should meet both hygienic and cosmetic demands

Habit breaking – Habit breaking may be needed to prevent or stop the development of anterior open bite in the primary dentition. Anterior open bite is usually corrected spontaneously if the sucking habit is broken before emergence of the permanent incisors. After eruption of the permanent incisors sucking habits, especially finger-sucking, may cause labial tipping of the upper incisors and lingual tipping of the lower incisors, which again may lead to dysfunction of the lower lip and also of the tongue. An abnormal lip or tongue function may impede self-correction of the malocclusion after the sucking habit has ceased. Thus, parents and child should be informed about the unfavourable effects of prolonged sucking habits.

Tonsils and adenoids – Removal of adenoid tissue from the nasal airway and medical care of allergies to secure nasal breathing also play an important role in the prevention of malocclusion. Hypertrophic tonsils may interfere with the function of the tongue leading to a low and protruded tongue posture which again may exert an adverse effect on the occlusion leading to crossbite, mandibular overjet and anterior open bite. Thus, tonsillectomy may be indicated to prevent the development of malocclusion. Consequently, the parents and the family doctor should, when necessary, be informed about these factors.

Extraction of primary teeth – Crowding may cause ectopic eruption of permanent incisors with premature unilateral exfoliation of a primary lateral incisor or canine. To prevent midline deviation, extraction of the contralateral primary tooth may be con-

TABLE 16-6

The associations between the potential risks and single malocclusion traits. From(6) with modifications. +: association exist; (+): association uncertain.

	Extreme overjet	Mandibular overjet/ inversion	Extreme deep bite	Extreme open bite	Crossbite	Scissors bite	Crowding	Spacing	Ectopic eruption
Caries	-	-	-	-	-	-	-	-	-
Periodontal disease	(+)	(+)	(+)	-	(+)	-	(+)	-	-
Attrition	-	(+)	(+)	-	(+)	-	-	-	-
Trauma	+	-	-	-	-	-	-	-	-
Root resorption/ cyst formation	-	-	-	-	-	-	-	-	+
CMD	-	(+)	(+)	-	(+)	-	-	-	-
Chewing problems	-	-	-	+	(+)	(+)	-	-	-
Speech problems	(+)	-	-	+	-	-	-	(+)	-
Psycho-social problems	+	+	-	-	-	-	+	+	(+)

sidered. Primary crowding problems cannot, however, be solved by this treatment and such children will most often end up requiring corrective orthodontic treatment. To avoid malposition of individual permanent teeth, a primary tooth should, generally, be extracted if it persists after its successor has pierced the gum.

Indications for treatment

Investigations dealing with the causal associations between morphologic malocclusion and potential adverse effects on oral health have given somewhat conflicting results.

Potential risks can be divided into four categories:

- risk of adverse effects on teeth and surrounding structures

- risk of development of craniomandibular disorders (CMD)

- risk of psychosocial problems

- risk of late developing dento-facial disturbances (e.g. mandibular prognathism or facial asymmetry)

In Table 16-6 the associations between the potential risks and single malocclusion traits, as suggested by Helm(6) are given with a few modifications. In general, it would seem that currently orthodontic treatment is indicated in 25-30% of Scandinavian children, taking general oral health and current social norms into consideration.

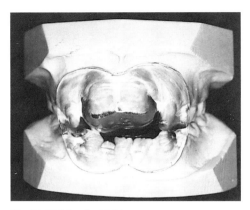

Fig. 16-15. Mouth shield.

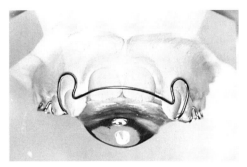

Fig. 16-16. Removable plate with tongue shield.

Treatment

Orthodontic treatment of malocclusion is a vast area and extensive postgraduate education is needed for its performance. Since this chapter is intended for education in pedodontics, only a few interceptive treatment methods will be mentioned. For further information the reader is referred to orthodontic textbooks.

Dividing orthodontic therapy into *interceptive* and *corrective* treatment is somewhat artificial. However, interceptive treatment is usually thought to be of short duration and to take place in the primary or early mixed dentition. The treatment consists of relatively simple procedures which aim to eliminate factors having a further harmful effect on the future development of the occlusion and the surrounding structures.

Interceptive treatment

Sagittal malocclusion – Maxillary overjet caused by sucking habits, in primary or early mixed dentition, may be treated effectively by a mouth shield (Fig. 16-15). The shield is worn in the vestibulum, where pressure from the musculature will exert a retruding force on the shield and thereby on the incisors. It should be used every night

and for about 4 hours during the day. If the overjet is combined with distal occlusion on the first permanent molars, the child should be referred to an orthodontist.

Mandibular overjet should generally be treated by an orthodontist, but single inverted incisors may be treated by the pedodontist if:

– there is sufficient space in the region

– the inclination of the inverted tooth is favourable

– the tooth has not erupted into a deep bite

Treatment can be carried out with a tongue blade (a wooden spatula) which is reduced to the width of the incisor. The tongue blade is placed behind the inverted tooth as vertically as possible. When the child bites on the blade it acts as a lever. This biting exercise should be carried out at least three times a day for periods of 10 minutes (2 minutes' biting, 1 minute's rest and so on). The exercise should be done with parental control. If the condition is not corrected within 2-3 weeks, appliance therapy is needed.

Vertical malocclusion – Open bite persisting after a sucking habit has ceased, may be due to tongue thrust or dysfunction of the lower lip.

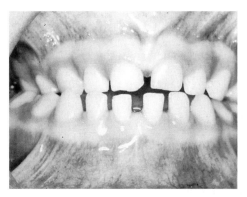
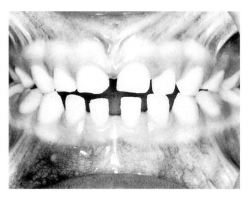

Fig. 16-17. Functional crossbite corrected by grinding of occlusal interferences (11).

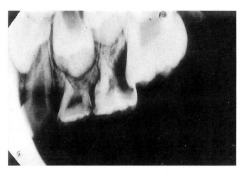

Fig. 16-18. Ectopic eruption of first upper permanent molar with resorption of the disto-buccal root of the second primary molar.

A tongue thrust may be eliminated by a removable upper plate with a shield which inhibits protrusion of the tongue between the upper and lower incisors (Fig. 16-16). The appliance should be used day and night except during meals. Lip dysfunction may be treated with a mouth shield. The child exercises the correct lip posture and at the same time the shield will retrude the upper incisors. In general, if these types of treatment have not improved the situation during a 3 or 4-month period, the child should be referred to an orthodontist. Cases of deep bite where the lower incisors occlude on the palatal mucosa should also be referred to an orthodontist.

Transverse malocclusion – Functional crossbite is relatively simple to correct, and treatment should be carried out in the primary or early mixed dentition. Functional crossbites can be treated either by grinding of primary teeth (Fig. 16-17) or with orthodontic appliances.

If the width of the upper dental arch measured at the canines and the molars, is greater than the width of the lower arch, grinding of the occlusal interferences may lead to spontaneous correction of the crossbite. It is important that the facets created by the grinding are steep, to secure stability and proper guidance into the correct intercuspation. If the width of the upper dental arch is smaller than that of the lower dental arch an orthodontic appliance, either an expansion plate or a fixed lingual arch, is needed to correct the malocclusion (see below).

Dentitional anomalies – Ectopic eruption of the first upper permanent molars is seen in 2-3% of children (Fig. 16-18) and causes premature and atypical resorption of the distal root of the second primary molar. Clinically, the problem is recognized by delayed eruption of the first permanent molar. However, about 50% of cases show self-correction and an observation period of 4-6 months is therefore recommended before treatment is commenced.

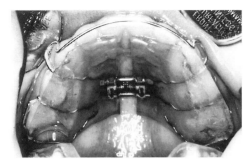

Fig. 16-19. Expansion plate. Note the covering of the occlusal surfaces.

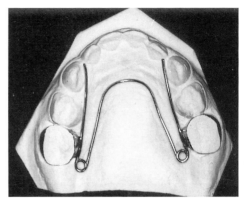

Fig. 16-20. Lingual arch of the Quad Helix type.

The choice of treatment depends upon the status of the primary molar. If root resorption is not too advanced the permanent molar can be moved distally by means of separating elastics or brass wire ligation. If root resorption is severe, the tooth is extracted to allow the first permanent molar to erupt. This will always lead to loss of space in the dental arch. Regaining of the space may be achieved by corrective orthodontic treatment (see below). Ectopic eruption of the upper canines may also occur. If the eruption path is too mesially inclined, the roots of the lateral and even the central incisors can be resorbed. In some cases extraction of the primary canine may normalize the eruption path for the permanent canine.

Treatment

Corrective therapy involves the use of removable or fixed orthodontic appliances to correct tooth or jaw position. In this context only the most simple appliances and treatments will be discussed.

Primary dentition – Functional or dento-alveolar crossbites may be treated with an expansion plate (Fig. 16-19) or a lingual arch attached to the second primary molars (Fig. 16-20). The expansion plate may have acrylic covering of the upper occlusal surfaces

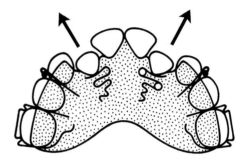

Fig. 16-21. Plate with protruding springs to correct inverted incisors.

to unlock the occlusion and thereby facilitate lateral tooth movement. The lingual arch has the advantage of being fixed, thereby eliminating possible cooperation problems.

Early mixed dentition – Inverted permanent incisors that have erupted into deep bite may be corrected using a plate with protruding springs combined with covering of the occlusal surfaces to open the bite allowing the incisors to move labially (Fig. 16-21). If good incisal overlap is achieved no retention is required after the inverted tooth has been brought into correct position.

Distal molar occlusion and crowding caused by mesial migration of the upper

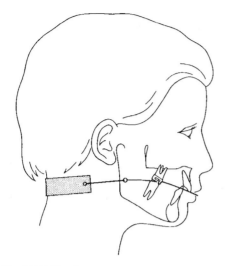

Fig. 16-22. Headgear.

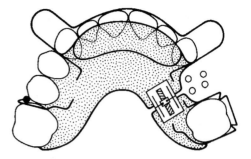

Fig. 16-23. Plate with expansion screw to distalize molar.

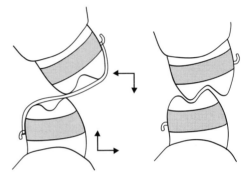

Fig. 16-24. Cross-elastic used to correct scissors bite.

first permanent molar following premature loss of the upper second primary molar may be corrected by using a headgear (Fig. 16-22), a removable plate with a spring, or an expansion screw, (Fig. 16-23) to distalize the permanent molar.

A dento-alveolar crossbite localized to a single lateral tooth pair can often be successfully treated with cross-elastics. Orthodontic buttons are bonded on the palatal surface of the upper tooth and on the buccal surface of the lower tooth. An elastic band (3/16", 3.5 oz.) is used between the buttons day and night except during meals.

Scissors bite of a tooth pair is treated similarly, but the buttons are placed on the buccal surface of the upper tooth and on the lingual surface of the lower tooth (Fig. 16-24). Bite opening may be needed if the teeth are in deep bite.

Dento-alveolar crossbite on several teeth can be corrected with an expansion plate or a fixed lingual arch in the upper jaw (e.g. Quad Helix; Fig. 16-20).

Treatment of skeletal deviations with functional appliances could be initiated in this period but such treatments should, in general, be carried out by an orthodontist.

Late mixed dentition – This stage is most often close to the onset of the pubertal growth spurt and treatment of skeletal distal occlusion and increased overjet may sucessfully be performed with functional appliances or headgear at this stage. These treatments should generally be carried out by, or in collaboration with, an orthodontist.

Distalization of upper first molars which have drifted mesially becomes increasingly difficult with development and eruption of the second permanent molar.

Permanent dentition – In the full permanent dentition corrective orthodontic treatment with or without extractions is carried out. Most often fixed appliances are needed, and planning and treatment should be carried out by an orthodontist.

In conclusion, the role of the pedodontist with regard to corrective orthodontic therapy is limited to relatively simple treatments with simple removable or fixed appliances. Such treatment should show improvement in the condition within 3-4 months. If this is not the case, the child should be referred to an orthodontist.

FUNCTIONAL MALOCCLUSION

Classification

Functional malocclusion is synonymous with occlusal interferences and can be defined as: occlusal contacts hampering or hindering harmonious jaw movements with the teeth maintaining contact.

The most common functional malocclusions are:

– interferences between retruded contact position (RCP) and intercuspal mandibular position (ICP) as a: a) lateral slide between RCP and ICP or lateral forced bite; b) sagittal slide (>2 mm) between RCP and ICP; c) Unilateral contact in RCP

– non-working side interferences with contact only on the non-working side. Functional non-working side interference occurs on lateral movement (≤ 3 mm)

Prevalence

The occlusion is continuously changing during childhood and so is the prevalence of occlusal interferences, e.g. non-working side interferences occur twice as often in children at 7 years as at 10 years or older. Interferences between RCP and ICP laterally and/or antero-posteriorly and/or functional interferences, may be found in about 20% of children of 10 years of age or older.

Diagnosis

The retruded contact position (RCP) is a reference position, for registration of the functional occlusion, whereas morphologic malocclusion is assessed in intercuspal mandibular position (ICP). In ICP the condyles should be centered in the glenoid fossae whereas in RCP the condyles are in a posterior position in the fossae. During childhood it is therefore important to examine the relation between RCP and ICP and even interferences during function, as non-working side interferences.

An individual with excellent morphologic occlusion may show severe functional malocclusion and vice versa. Nevertheless, some morphologic malocclusions e.g. crossbite, frontal open bite, and distal and mesial occlusion, may often be connected with occlusal interferences as lateral forced bite and non-working side interferences.

Indication for treatment

Functional malocclusion has been considered more important than morphologic malocclusion in explaining mandibular dysfunction. The literature contains, however, insufficient information as to the specific effect of occlusal disturbances in this connection. An explanation might be that the influence of occlusal interferences depends on how the individual adapts to them. The adaptive capability is much greater in young children than in adolescents and adults.

Treatment

Treatment of morphologic malocclusions with occlusal interferences and forced bite has been described above. This type of treatment serves to establish a correct condyle-fossa-relationship as early as possible and to normalize the function of the TMJ allowing for normal growth. Treatment of craniomandibular disorders are discussed below.

CRANIOMANDIBULAR DISORDERS

The functions of the masticatory system include normal functions such as chewing, swallowing, speech, etc., but also such parafunctions as sucking habits, grinding or clenching of teeth. These functional disturbances have been given many names in the literature, for example, "Costen syndrome", "TMJ dysfunction syndrome", "myofascial pain dysfunction syndrome", "mandibular dysfunction" and "craniomandibular disorders (CMD)". Although a disparity of opinions about the etiology of functional disturbances still exists, it is largely agreed that the symptoms included are: pain or tenderness in the TMJ and the masticatory muscles and/or limited or irregular movements of the mandible and/or TMJ sounds.

Disturbances of musculature

There is evidence that many symptoms of pain, headache and dysfunction arise from the jaw muscles, most probably due to inflammatory responses (myosis) caused by hyperactivity. Muscle affection is usually assessed by palpation and by information from the patient about pain. Sometimes muscle hypertrophy may be so dramatic that it can be observed clinically.

Hypofunction of masticatory muscles may be due to hypoplasia or atrophy. This is a rare condition but can be seen in a number of congenital or acquired diseases, e.g. hemifacial microsomia, muscular dystrophy and juvenile rheumatoid arthritis.

Disturbances of TMJ

The TMJ may be affected by congenital aplasia of the condyle as in hemifacial microsomia and Treacher-Collins syndrome, causing abnormal growth and function. The TMJ can be affected by many diseases, which might influence mandibular growth, but even if there is primary affection of the TMJ it will not always trouble the patient.

Acquired disturbances of different parts of the TMJ may be:

TMJ sounds, i.e. clicking and crepitation. The clicking sound may be ascribed to disc displacement, to structural changes of disc and joint surfaces, to muscular incoordination or to subluxation. Clicking may start without any obvious cause, but is also reported to start in connection with chewing, trauma, or during dental visits.

Osteo-arthrosis is defined as a non-inflammatory disease characterized by deterioration and erosion of the articular surfaces. The condition is rare in young children, but in some cases the resistance of joint structures is so low that even normal function may be sufficient to cause overloading leading to arthrosis (juvenile arthropathy). In most of these patients the clinical problems will gradually cease and function will often normalize.

Juvenile rheumatoid arthritis (JRA) – More than 50% of children with JRA get involvement of the TMJ during childhood. The arthritis causes destruction of the condyles and other joint structures. Some of these children may develop mandibular micrognathia, mandibular asymmetry, open bite and abnormal oral function with reduced opening capacity, and loss of muscle strength.

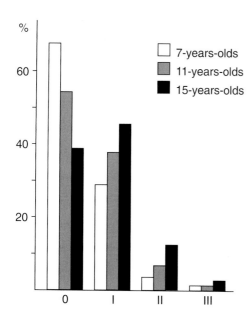

Fig. 16-25. Clinical dysfunction index at different ages. Slight dysfunction (I) is common whereas moderate (II) and severe (III) dysfunction are less prevalent but increasing with age.

Traumatic injuries to the jaws may cause reactions in the joints. In cases with severe trauma, fracture of the condylar process may occur. At opening of the mandible there is a shift towards the affected side if the fracture is unilateral and mandibular growth may become asymmetrical. However, subjective symptoms are usually not persistent in children but further development should be followed carefully.

Unilateral hyperplasia of the condyle is rare but may occur around the time of puberty leading to skeletal crossbite and midline deviation and sometimes to functional problems such as asymmetric jaw movements and tenderness and pain from muscles and joints.

TABLE 16-7

Distribution of TMJ clicking at different ages.

TMJ clicking	7 years	11 years	15 years	20 years
Occasional	7%	11%	20%	22%
Frequent	0%	0%	1%	8%

Etiology of CMD

There is a tendency that CMD are associated, although to a small extent, with functional malocclusion (occlusal interferences) and some morphologic malocclusions as crossbite, frontal open bite, distal and mesial occlusion. Impaired general health, poor social conditions or psychological traits as anxiety and even "stress" are probably some important factors in creating muscular hyperactivity and mandibular dysfunction. Most authors believe that bruxism and muscular hyperactivity play an important role in the development of CMD during childhood.

Prevalence of CMD

The most common clinical signs of CMD in children and adolescents are clicking (10-30%) and muscle tenderness on palpation (20-60%), often increasing with age. Such clinical signs as reduced opening capacity, tenderness of TMJ on palpation, or pain on movement are relatively infrequent in children. A standardized clinical dysfunction index(4) illustrates the signs of dysfunction at different ages (Fig. 16-25).

Such symptoms of CMD as fatigue of the jaws and face and difficulties in mouth opening are reported to occur only occasionally in young children and in up to every fifth adolescent. Table 16-7 shows

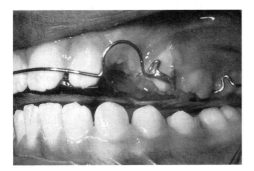

Fig. 16-26. Clasp-splint with full coverage plateaux.

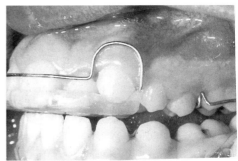

Fig. 16-27. Clasp-splint with anterior plateaux.

how TMJ sounds change with age. Symptoms are still increasing during growth, but
as spontaneous fluctuations are common,
there seems to be no consistent pattern in
the development of either subjective symptoms or clinical signs of CMD.

Headache is common among children
and the prevalence increases with age.
About 10-20% report recurrent headaches
(once a week or more). The prevalence of
headache is higher in girls than boys. Many
patients, especially children and adolescents, are not aware of the connection between headache, bruxism, hyperactivity of
jaw muscles and mandibular dysfunction.
Thus, the dentist must be extra observant of
this possible association.

Parafunctional habits such as bruxism or
tooth grinding and tooth clenching are very
common in children, although only 15% of
children or parents are aware of it.

Functional examination

Children with subjective symptoms and
those starting orthodontic treatment should
undergo a functional examination of the
stomatognathic system. The examination
consists of assessment of the occlusion
(functional and morphologic), dental wear,
mandibular mobility, TMJ function and palpation of the TMJ and jaw muscles. A thorough past history is also important, though

too time consuming to perform at annual
dental visits. However, one clinical symptom has proved more valid than others for
disclosing the presence of CMD: reduced
opening capacity of the mandible. If maximal opening, including the overbite, in
children older than 10 years is less than 40
mm, it is most often a sign of impaired
function of the masticatory system (average
maximal opening is 55 mm). Questions
about the occurrence and nature of recurrent headache are also important in this
context.

Treatment of CMD

Although the prevalence of CMD symptoms in childhood is relatively high, only a
few children with recurrent headache and
frequent stomatognathic symptoms need
treatment. Extreme tooth wear in children
may also be an indication for treatment.
Treatment principles used in adults with
CMD may, in general, be applied to children. However, the dynamic changes in occlusion in connection with tooth eruption
and facial growth should be taken into consideration.

The prevailing treatment in children and
adolescents is activators and/or splints.

A conventional stabilization splint to the
upper jaw can be used in adolescents.
Splints designed with clasps, facial bow and

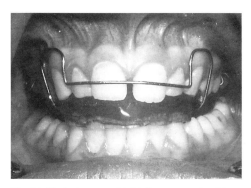

Fig. 16-28. Activator with high construction bite.

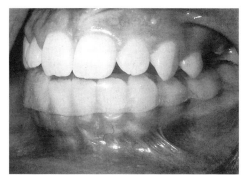

Fig. 16-29. Soft acrylic splint.

plateaux anteriorly and posteriorly are more useful in younger children (Fig. 16-26). The splint can easily be adjusted for erupting teeth, and it can be used for relatively long periods.

Another type of splint (corresponding to a relaxation splint) has anterior plateaux with contact only on the incisors (Fig. 16-27). This splint is considered useful for patients with headache and/or migraine. Note the adverse orthodontic effect of bite-opening which may occur in connection with long-term use of a splint of this type. During childhood a stabilization clasp-splint or an activator (often passive) is commonly used, and has proved effective in bruxism, for example. The activator should be designed with clasps in the upper jaw to secure retention and with extended wings lingually in the lower jaw.

In patients with obvious clicking and/or occasional locking, the therapy of choice is an activator or clasp-splint with a bite opening sufficient to unload the TMJ (Fig. 16-28). In the young an activator, passive and jumped enough to achieve translation, may have a good effect. A clasp-splint with a high plateau covering all occlusal surfaces is preferable in teenagers in order to diminish or to get rid of TMJ symptoms.

A soft acrylic splint is easy to produce and may be a good device for short-term use (Fig. 16-29).

Occlusal adjustment of primary teeth by grinding is common. Grinding of permanent teeth to establish occlusal stability in connection with mandibular dysfunction should not be undertaken in children, since most occlusal displacement in growing individuals will change with time. Selective occlusal grinding in young adults can be performed when a causal connection between interference and mandibular dysfunction is strongly suspected.

Jaw exercises may be useful in adults with CMD, but it may be difficult to motivate children and adolescents for such programs. However, training of one or two movements against resistance is usually accepted and performed.

In conclusion, it can be stated that although epidemiologic studies show high prevalence of signs and symptoms of CMD in children, only a few need treatment. Children with reduced maximal opening capacity of the mouth, and children suffering from recurrent headache and from juvenile rheumatoid arthritis require special attention.

Background literature

Egermark-Eriksson I. Mandibular dysfunction in children and in individuals with dual bite. *Swed Dent J* 1982; suppl 10.

Helm S. Prevalence of malocclusion in relation to development of the dentition. *Acta Odontol Scand* 1970; **28**: Suppl. 58.

Myllärniemi S. Malocclusion in Finnish rural children. An epidemiological study of different stages of dental development. *Proc Finn Dent Soc* 1970; **66**: 221-74.

Møller E, Bakke M, Rasmussen, O C. *Bidfunktionslære*. København: Odontologisk Boghandels Forlag, 1986.

Nilner M. Epidemiology of functional disturbances and diseases in the stomatognathic system. *Swed Dent J* 1983; suppl 17.

Solow B. The dento-alveolar compensatory mechanism: background and clinical implications. *Bri J Orthod* 1980; **7**: 145-61.

Thilander B, Rönning O. *Introduction to orthodontics*. Stockholm: Tandläkarförlaget, 1985.

Van der Linden FPGM. *Facial growth and facial orthopedics*. Quintessenz Verlags-GmbH, 1986.

Wänman A. Craniomandibular disorders in adolescents. A longitudinal study in an urban Swedish population. *Swed Dent J* 1987; Suppl. 44.

References

1. Björk A. The face in profile . An anthropological x-ray investigation on Swedish children and conscripts. *Svensk Tandläkartidskrift* 1947; 40, Suppl.

2. Björk A, Krebs Aa, Solow B. A method for epidemiological registration of malocclusion. *Acta Odontol Scand* 1964; **22**: 27-41.

3. Björk A, Skieller V. Facial development and tooth eruption. An implant study at the age of puberty. *Am J Dent* 1972; **62**: 339-83.

4. Helkimo M. Studies on function and dysfunction of the masticatory system II Index for anamnestic and clinical dysfunction and occlusal state. *Swed Dent J* 1974; **67**: 101-21.

5. Helm S. Prevalence of malocclusion in relation to development of the dentition. *Acta Odontol Scand* 1970; **28**: Suppl. 58.

6. Helm S. Indikation og behov for ortodontisk behandling. *Tandlægebladet* 1980; **84**: 175-85.

7. Ingervall B, Seeman L, Thilander B. Frequency of malocclusion and need of orthodontic treatment in 10-year old children in Gothenburg. *Swed Dent J* 1972; **65**: 7-21.

8. Järvinen S, Lehtinen L. Malocclusion in 3-year old Finnish children. *Proc Finn Dent Soc* 1977; **73**: 162-6.

9. Magnusson TE. *Maturation and malocclusion in Iceland*. An epidemiological study of malocclusion and of dental skeletal and sexual maturation in Icelandic school children. 1979 Thesis (Reykjavik).

10. Rasmussen I, Helm S. Forekomsten af tandstillingsfejl i det primære tandsæt. *Tandlægebladet* 1975; **79**: 383-8.

11. Ravn JJ, Nielsen LA, Nielsson B. *Småbørnstandpleje*. Københavns Tandlægehøjskole 1990 (in press).

12. Telle ES. A study of the frequency of malocclusion in the County of Hedmark, Norway. *Trans Eur Othod Soc* 1951; **25**: 192-8.

CHAPTER 17

ORAL PATHOLOGY AND SURGERY

Lesions of the oral mucosa

Bone lesions

Cysts

Tumors and tumor-like lesions

Pain control in oral surgery

Extraction of teeth

Surgical removal of impacted teeth

Surgical orthodontic treatment of impacted teeth

Autotransplantation of teeth

Treatment of soft tissue lesions and abnormalities

Postoperative considerations

Children present a variety of oral pathological conditions. Knowledge of such changes is a prerequisite for correct diagnosis and adequate treatment. This chapter will deal with some of the most frequent oral pathological conditions found in children. For further information the reader is referred to textbooks of oral pathology.

LESIONS OF THE ORAL MUCOSA

Impetigo contagiosa is more common in children than adults. It is caused by streptococci and staphylococci and often affects the perioral area. The infection causes inflammatory vesiculobullous lesions which rupture leaving secreting or crust-covered lesions (Fig. 17-1). As the disease is contagious it can spread within the family and also in connection with dental treatment. In most cases the lesions heal without complications, but in severe cases antibiotics are recommended.

Streptococcal gingivitis is usually preceded by tonsilitis and fever. The gingiva shows swelling, bleeding and is painful. Improved oral hygiene and antibiotics is the therapy of choice. Before prescription of antibiotics a microbiological diagnosis should be made.

Scarlet fever is a common disease in childhood caused by beta hemolytic streptococci. The general symptoms are fever, tonsilitis, lymphadenitis and a papular red skin rash. The most characteristic oral manifestation is

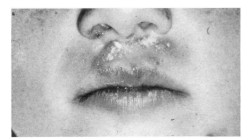

Fig. 17-1. Impetigo contagiosa in 7-year-old girl.

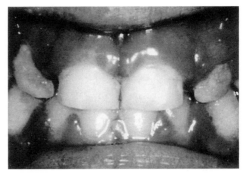

Fig. 17-2. General gingivitis as a result of herpes simplex infection.

the gradual change of the appearance of the tongue from a "strawberry" to a "raspberry" character. Initially the white-coated tongue shows a scattered pattern of hyperemic fungiform papillae. Later this coating is lost and the red edematous fungiform papillae dominate the clinical picture.

Herpes simplex virus infection is common in children. The incubation period is 3-5 days. The symptoms of a primary herpetic infection can vary widely and may proceed subclinically. The primary infection is often manifested as an acute herpetic gingivo-stomatitis where the entire gingiva is red, edematous and heavily inflamed (Fig. 17-2). The general symptoms are fever, headache, malaise and vomiting. After 1 or 2 days small vesicles develop (Fig. 17-3) on the oral mucosa. They quickly rupture, leaving painful ulcers with a diameter of 1-3 mm. The HSV is transmitted by personal contact and studies have found antibodies to HSV in 40-90% of the population. The incidence of primary herpes simplex infection increases from the age of 6 months and reaches its peak at the age of 2-4 years. It has been shown that recurrent herpes simplex infection originates from a reactivation of HSV, which remains dormant in nerve tissue between periods of excitation. Reactivation may be caused by injuries such as overexposure to sunlight, exposure to acid in fruit, or dental manipulations. Recurrent herpetic infection will develop in the same

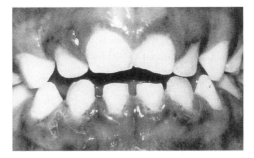

Fig. 17-3. Herpes lesions spread over the oral mucosa.

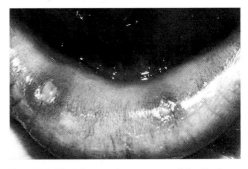

Fig. 17-4. Vesicles on the mucosa of the lip in a child with varicella.

location at every excitation, and usually has a less dramatic symptomatology than the primary.

Even though the use of antiviral agents has been tested during recent years, treatment still is primarily supportive, such as paracetamol for the fever and fluid to maintain sufficient hydration. If the lesions are too painful to permit eating, topical anesthetics may be used. Primary herpes simplex infection is selflimiting and the patient will recover within a 10-day period.

Varicella is a viral disease mostly seen in children. The general symptoms are fever, pharyngitis and vesicular lesions on the skin. The oral manifestations are whitish vesicles surrounded by a red halo found mostly on the mucosa of the lips, bucca and tongue (Fig. 17-4).

Mumps is a viral infection affecting the salivary glands. The general symptoms are fever and pain from the infected glands. In cases where the parotitis is unilateral difficulties in distinguishing the condition from a swelling of odontogenic origin may arise (Fig. 17-5).

Mononucleosis infectiosa is caused by the Epstein-Barr virus and is found mostly in children and young adults. The general clinical manifestations are a sore throat, fever and lymphadenopathy. The specific oral symptoms are stomatitis, oral membrane formation (tonsils) and petecciae on the palatal mucosa. Recovery from the disease is often prolonged.

Coxsackie virus infections often start with low-grade fever and oral vesicles, which rupture after 1-2 days, forming small ulcers. The most common infections of this type in children are herpangina and hand-foot-and-mouth disease. The infections often occur in epidemics. In herpangina the vesicles are restricted to the palate and posterior pharynx while in hand-foot-and-mouth disease the lesions are more widely spread all over the mucosa, and vesicles on the hand and feet are also found. The clinical symptoms are usually milder than those of herpes simplex virus infections.

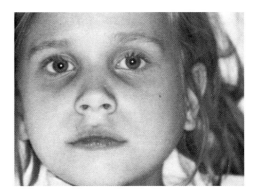

Fig. 17-5. Unilateral parotitis (mumps).

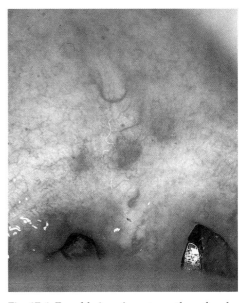

Fig. 17-6. Forschheimer's spots on the soft palate in rubella.

Supportive treatment including fluid control and, if necessary, topical anesthetics is recommended. The diseases are self-limiting and the child will recover within a 10-day period.

Rubella is a virus infection characterized by light red macules on the skin. Occasionally, macules are also found on the soft palate, Forschheimer's spots (Fig. 17-6).

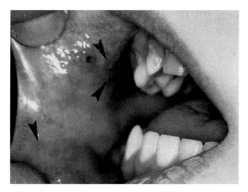

Fig. 17-7. Koplik's spots in measles.

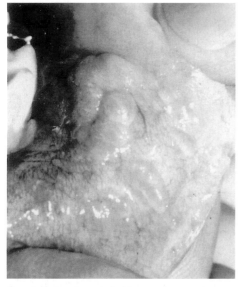

Fig. 17-8. Focal epithelial hyperplasia in lower lip mucosa.

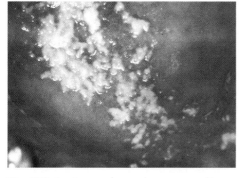

Fig. 17-9. Acute pseudomembranous candidiasis lesion in cheek mucosa.

Measles is a paramyxovirus disease affecting most children. After an incubation time of 10-12 days the child will have a cough, fever and photophobia. The oral manifestations, Koplik's spots, occur on the buccal mucosa as prodromal greyish-white macules surrounded by a slightly erythematous zone some days before eruption of the skin lesions (Fig. 17-7).

Focal epithelial hyperplasia (Heck's disease) is a virus-induced lesion located in areas which are exposed to mechanical irritation, such as lips, cheeks and tongue. The lesions are flattened, slightly raised papules with normal mucosal colour (Fig. 17-8). No treatment is usually required, and the lesions may disappear spontaneously.

Oral candidiasis is caused by the fungus *Candida albicans*, normally found in the oral flora in 30-50% of the population. It invades the mucosa only when there is a change in the oral environment or state of resistance. Such changes can be brought about by the administration of antibiotics, xerostomia or systemic diseases for example.

Acute pseudomembranous candidiasis (thrush) is the most common mucosal fungal infection in newborn children. It is characterized by raised, pearly-white patches (Fig. 17-9) which can be rubbed off leaving an erythematous surface. New-born babies have been found to have a relatively high frequency of thrush starting during the first 2 weeks of life, probably caused by maternal vaginal candidosis. A low pH in the oral cavity due to sparse secretion of saliva promotes the growth of *Candida albicans*.

Acute atrophic and chronic forms can also occur. Chronic atrophic candidiasis, here represented by angular cheilosis, is not rare in children (Fig. 17-10). In the Candida-endocrinopathy syndrome occurring in children with hypoparathyroidism and/or Addison's disease, the infection might affect the nails (Fig. 17-11) as well as the oral

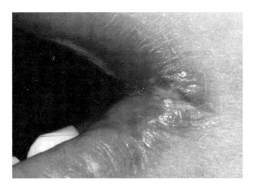

Fig. 17-10. Angular cheilitis.

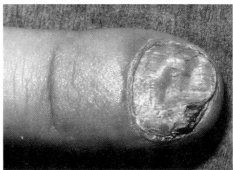

Fig. 17-11. Candida infection of the nails in a boy with hypoparathyroidism.

mucosa. It has been recommended to screen children with unexplained chronic candidiasis for metabolic or endocrine abnormalities since the infection often precedes such conditions. The diagnosis candidiasis is made from the clinical picture and detection of candida hyphae in smears.

For treatment, the use of antifungal agents such as nystatin, amphotericin B or miconazol are preferred. Mouthrinses, sucking tablets or topically applied gels containing these preparations will prove helpful in most cases. In severe infections the medication has to be extended over a period of months. In addition, predisposing factors should be checked.

Recurrent aphthous ulcer is more common after the age of 10 years. The lesion starts as a small white papule which gradually ulcerates. The ulcers are 0.2-1 cm in diameter with the central part covered with a yellow-grey coating, and a crateriform base with raised reddened margins. The surrounding tissue shows a light swelling. The ulcers are extremely painful and may be present varying in size and number, predominantly localized to the buccal and labial mucosa and the tongue (Fig. 17-12). The interval between recurrent episodes may vary from a week to several months. Reactions to antigen of oral streptococci (*S. sanguis* 2A) from an immunological crossreaction, re-

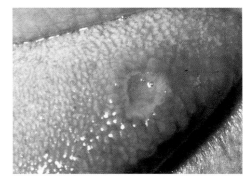

Fig. 17-12. Aphthous ulcer on the tongue.

sulting in deterioration of the epithelium, have been claimed as a releasing factor of aphthous ulcers. In severe cases, the child might be examined for Crohn's disease and coeliaki.

A varity of treatments have been suggested but most of them have proved failures. In mild cases slight etching solutions or topical anesthetics may keep the pain under control. If the lesions are more extensive, local corticosteroid treatment may shorten the healing time. In some cases mouth rinses with tetracyclin (especially Aureomycin®) solutions have been sucessful, but the risks of side-effects are not negligible.

Erythema multiforme is a dermatologic disease, which may also develop oral le-

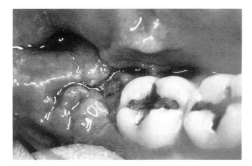

Fig. 17-13. Oral lesion in a boy with Crohn's disease.

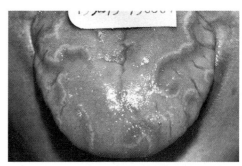

Fig. 17-14. Geographic tongue.

sions, or in which the oral lesions are the only symptom of the disease. The onset is very rapid. In 24 hours a child may develop extensive lesions of the skin and/or mucosa. The skin lesions are asymptomatic erythematous macules or papules, mostly affecting hands and feet. In the generalized vesiculobullous erythema multiforme even the eyes and genitals are involved (Stevens-Johnson's syndrome). Initially the oral lesion has the character of vesicles or bullae, which rapidly burst, forming ulcers. Compared with viral lesions the ulcers are larger, deeper and often bleed. Involvement of the lips is most common. After some days the ulcers will crust and healing takes place within 2 weeks. In cases where the lips and oral mucosa are severely affected the patient has great difficulties in eating and drinking. The diagnosis is based on the total clinical view.

Erythema is not regarded as a specific disease, but as a general reaction to a series of independent precipitating factors such as food or drug allergy, infection, radiotheraphy or general disease.

In mild cases topical anesthetics might be the only treatment. In severe cases systemic treatment with corticosteriods and antibiotics can be justified.

Crohn's disease is commonly associated with oral lesions and the lesions may also precede symptoms of bowel disease. The most common oral pathological findings in Crohn's disease are aphthous ulcers, areas of inflammatory hyperplasia including mucosal fissuring and indurated "tag-like" lesions on the retromolar area (Fig. 17-13). The lesions tend to run a remitting course.

Geographic tongue or benign migratory glossitis occurs in children in 1-3%. Clinical manifestation is pinkish red irregular depapillated areas surrounded by a well-defined, slightly raised, whitish border. Affected areas vary from day to day and the appearance can be described as a continuously changing map (Fig. 17-14).

Occasionally, other parts of the oral mucosa are affected (*stomatitis migrans*). There is a hereditary tendency, but the etiology is unknown. Some children will experience discomfort and a burning sensation from the lesions. In severe cases topical anesthetics are recommended during the acute phase.

Cheek-biting and other traumatic irritations of the mucosa are seen now and then in children. The mucosa involved often shows a whitish surface in the vicinity of the occlusal plane, sometimes interfoliated by desquamated areas or small ulcerations. The typical clinical appearance and the history make the diagnosis simple. Sometimes

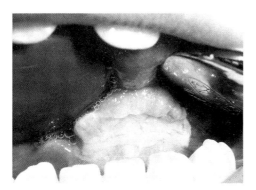

Fig. 17-15. Self mutilation of the tongue mucosa caused by the lower incisors.

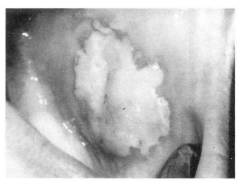

Fig. 17-16. Lesion in the cheek mucosa caused by bites in connection with local anesthesia.

the sharp edges of carious or fractured teeth irritate the oral mucosa so that chronic decubital ulcers develop with a hyperkeratotic whitish appearance - frictional keratosis. The treatment is to eliminate patient's habit or to remove the irritant.

Self-mutilation of the mucosa might sometimes be seen in handicapped children with uncontrolled tongue movements. The irritation of the mucosa is caused when the child forces the tongue out of the mouth and thereby injures it against the lower incisors (Fig. 17-15). In such cases hyperkeratotic areas develop rapidly. In one particular case, to make the lesion heal, and to prevent recurrence, a smooth acrylic onlay was cemented onto the incisors.

Traumatic injuries, e.g. cheek or lip bites after dental local anesthesia, can result in considerable swelling and bleeding. The clinical appearance is often a large white mucous lesion (Fig. 17-16). This lesion is self-limiting and will heal within a week.

Burns, either thermal, chemical or electric, of the oral mucosa will cause painful white lesions with coagulation and sloughing of the superficial mucosa. The most severe cases occur when etching solutions are accidentally taken in. Fig. 17-17 shows a 2-year-old boy who ingested concentrated caustic soda, which resulted in extensive

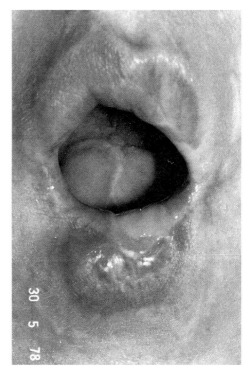

Fig. 17-17. Chemical burn of the lips of a 2-year-old boy caused by ingestion of caustic soda.

burns with scarred healing of the lips and tongue. The diagnosis of burns of the oral mucosa is made on the basis of the history, the clinical view and the fact that the coagulum can easily be removed. Burns are

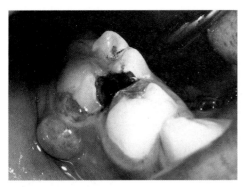

Fig. 17-18. Fluctuating abscess localized in the alveolar sulcus area.

treated by the rapid removal of the causative agent followed by symptomatic treatment. Most lesions will heal without complications, but in severe lip burns an extended acrylic splint may be used during healing to prevent contraction.

Pigmented lesions are mostly caused by melanin. Ephelis, or freckles, which are a form of endogenous pigmentation, are often found on the lips. Melanin macules may also be seen intraorally. Children of dark-skinned races show a diffuse and wide-spread pigmentation of the oral mucosa, especially on the attached gingiva.

Pigmented nevi can be found intraorally in exceptional cases. They are brownish, sometimes slightly raised above the mucosa and are distinctly demarcated from the surrounding mucosa. As there is a risk, however minimal, of an intraoral pigmented nevus developing into malignant melanoma it is recommended that the child be referred for removal of the lesion, and that histological analysis be performed.

Endogenous pigmentation of the oral mucosa might also be a symptom of systemic diseases as in Addison's disease and Peutz-Jeghers syndrome.

Exposure to bismuth, lead, mercury, silver, gold or arsenic may lead to deposition of metal salts in the gingival tissues.

Leukoplakia or extensive hyperkeratotic lesions are extremely rare in children. The only cases with a tendency to more severe hyperkeratosis in children are those that occur in combination with long-standing trauma of the mucosa (frictional keratosis) and in patients with a habit of holding snuff in a local area of the mucosa. Most of these changes in children will cease after elimination of their causes.

BONE LESIONS

Most of the bone lesions found in the jaws in children are infectious in origin. There are a great number of other conditions resulting in bone lesions such as periodontitis, cysts and tumors or tumor-like conditions. These are presented in their respective sections.

Periapical osteitis (apical periodontitis), abscess formation and cellulitis are frequent in children. One of the most common reactions caused by periapical infection of necrotic teeth is abscess formation. Sometimes the periapical lesion of the necrotic tooth will result in a more diffuse type of infection involving the soft tissues and causing considerable swelling. This situation is diagnosed as cellulitis and is more common among children than adults. Infection in the jaws of children may spread rapidly due to the comparatively wide marrow spaces.

An abscess is usually found as a localized or more diffuse swelling of the mucosa in the alveolar-sulcus area adjacent to the infected tooth. The inflammation in the periapical area will perforate the bone plate and reach the periosteum. The abscess develops from a relatively hard and diffuse subperiostal swelling into a more localized fluctuating lesion (Fig. 17-18). Spontaneous rupture may occur, or a fistula develop and the pus formed is then forced into the oral cavity. The early stages can be seen radiographically as a widened periodontal contour, but

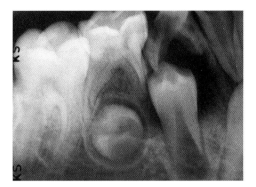

Fig. 17-19. Bone destruction caused by infection from necrotic primary teeth.

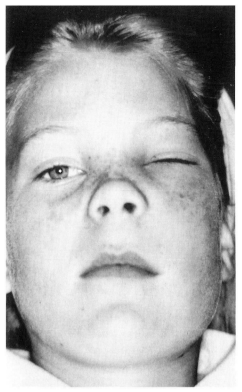

Fig. 17-20. Cellulitis in the upper jaw.

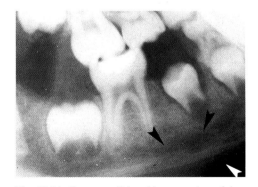

Fig. 17-21. Osteomyelitis with expansion of the periosteum at the lower border of the mandible. Note also the radioluscent areas in the mandible.

in more advanced stages a radiolucency involving the periapical and interradicular areas can be found (Fig. 17-19). Often the tooth is sensitive to movement, percussion and heat. The first sub-periostal stage of abscess formation is often accompanied by considerable pain.

Cellulitis will often result in considerable swelling of the face or neck (Fig. 17-20). X-ray results are the same as for an abscess. Patients often have a high fever, considerable pain, difficulty in opening the mouth and feel acutely ill.

In the acute stages of an abscess and cellulitis the most important treatment is to establish drainage and, in cases with affected general condition, to combine this with the use of antibiotics. Drainage is obtained by opening the pulp chamber of the affected tooth, by incision or extraction. The acute symptoms usually subside within a few days.

The most common microorganism associated with periapical lesions is *Streptococcus viridans*. This microorganism is susceptible to most antibiotics.

Chronic sclerosing osteomyelitis (Garré) is much more common in the lower than the upper jaw. It usually starts as a dull tooth-ache and fever. Radiographic signs may be diffuse or lacking.

Gradually, a bony swelling occurs caused by an expansion of the juvenile periosteum.

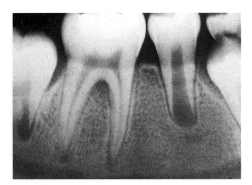

Fig. 17-22. "Orange-peel" appearance of bone some years after first symptoms of osteomyelitis (same patient as in Fig. 17-21).

On x-rays this is seen as an onion-like bone formation (Fig. 17-21). At this stage, the extraoral swelling becomes more accentuated and radiolucent areas develop in the bone indicating necrotic or sclerotic conditions. Treatment with antibiotics for periods of months, often in combination with surgical intervention, has proved successful in some cases, but recurrences are frequent, even during periods of medication with broad spectrum antibiotics. Short-term treatment with corticosteroids at the time of recurrence has proved successful with prompt effect.

During healing the bone gradually takes on a more "orange-peel" appearance (Fig. 17-22). The etiology of chronic sclerosing osteomyelitis in children is not fully understood and the prognosis in young children is questionable.

CYSTS

Cysts are often described as a cavity in the tissues containing fluid or gas and frequently lined with epithelium. The following cysts which occur reasonably frequently in children will be discussed:

Epithelial cysts of the jaw

Developmental odontogenic cysts
Odontogenic keratocyst
Gingival cyst of the newborn
Dentigerous (follicular) cyst
Eruption cyst
Paradental cyst

Non-odontogenic cysts
Nasopalatine duct cyst
Globulomaxillary cyst

Inflammatory cysts
Radicular cyst

Non-epithelial cysts of the jaw

"Traumatic" bone cyst

Soft tissue cysts

Mucocele
Ranula

Odontogenic keratocysts (primordial cysts) are thought to develop from enamel organ epithelium of tooth germs. Often the epithelium of the cyst is keratinized. The cysts can be found in children, but are more frequent after the age of 20. The most frequent site is the mandible. The cyst may extend considerably without causing the patient any pain or swelling of the jaw. It often appears on x-ray as unilocular, well-demarcated radiolucency. Keratocysts in close contact with non-erupted teeth may be mistaken for true dentigerous cysts. The treatment of a keratocyst is careful extirpation, as the cyst has a tendency to recur. Keratocysts may recur after periods as long as 10 years.

Gingival cysts of the newborn occur with high frequency up to the age of 3 months. Multiple whitish cysts, about 2-3 mm across, may be found in the buccal or lingual areas of the dental ridge, Bohn's nodules (Fig. 17-23), or at the midpalatine raphe at the borderline between the hard and soft palates (Epstein's pearls). Gingival cysts in the new-born, which are sometimes misinterpreted as early erupting primary teeth, will quickly disintegrate and no treatment is needed.

Dentigerous (follicular) cysts involve the crown of unerupted teeth and are attached to the enamel-cementum border. This cyst is the most common in children. However, it has to be distinguished from the dilated follicle often seen in the pre-eruptive phase, which is a normal condition unless the pericoronal width exceeds 3-4 mm.

The teeth most frequently affected are the premolars. The cysts may grow to a consid-

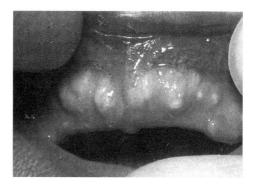

Fig. 17-23. Bohn's nodules in a new-born.

erable size (Fig. 17-24a) and cause swelling and sometimes pain. They grow slowly and there is often displacement of the teeth involved.

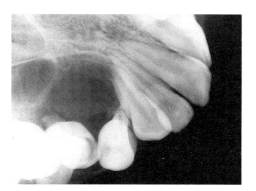

Fig. 17-24a. Dentigerous cyst in the upper jaw. Note the displaced premolar.

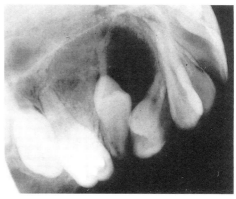

Fig. 17-24b. The cyst 5 months later and after treatment with obturator and daily rinsing of the cyst with saline.

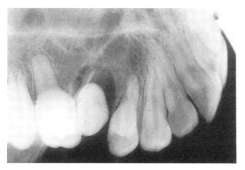

Fig. 17-24c. Another 5 months later.

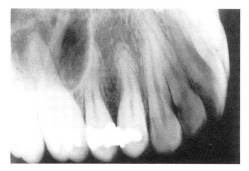

Fig. 17-24d. After 2 years. The cyst is completely healed and the teeth in the right position.

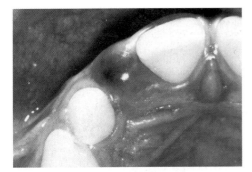

Fig. 17-25. Eruption cyst.

The etiologic factor is believed to be accumulation of fluid between the reduced dental epithelium and the enamel caused by a disturbance in the venous outflow. The infected root of a primary tooth may also be an etiologic factor.

Large cysts may be treated by marsupialization and, thereafter, daily rinses with saline. Following this treatment even extensive cysts will be healed within a short period of time (Figs. 17-24 b-d). Small dentigerous cysts may be treated by extirpation.

Eruption cysts may be defined as dentigerous cysts located in the soft tissues. If there is a bleeding in the cyst it is classified as an eruption hematoma. The cyst can occur in very young children, but is more commonly found in connection with tooth eruption. Usually, there is a small, smooth swelling in the gingival tissues at the site of the erupting tooth (Fig. 17-25). If treatment is indicated, marsupialization is the treatment of choice. The tooth will then erupt rapidly.

Paradental cysts often develop in the lower jaw in combination with erupting molars. The child will have a swelling of the jaw and often pain due to secondary infection. Clinical examination frequently reveals a deep bone pocket formation buccally to the affected tooth. X-rays show a radiolucent area extending apically from the margin (Fig. 17-26a). Periostal reaction including expansion is frequently observed (Fig. 17-26b).

In young children it seems reasonable to believe that the cyst arises from an idiopatic stimulation of epithelial cell remnants in the periodontium. When the tooth erupts the cyst will be left in the jaw in close contact with the root surface. Careful extirpation is recommended, if the results are to be successful.

Non-odontogenic cysts include series of developmental cysts caused by epithelial remnants enclosed in fusion lines of the embryonic processes, e.g. the *nasopalatine duct cyst* and the *globulomaxillary cyst*. The

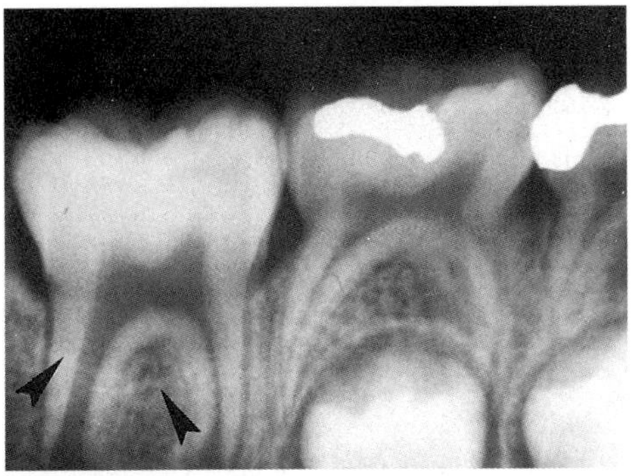

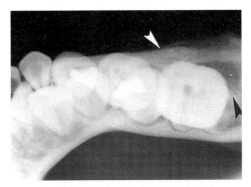

Fig. 17-26a. Paradental cyst buccally 46 in a 6-year-old girl.

Fig. 17-26b. Same patient as in 17-28a. Note the expanded periosteum.

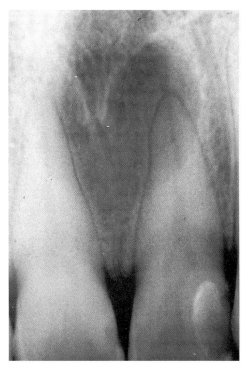

Fig. 17-27. Nasopalatinal duct cyst (courtesy Dr. S. Ericson).

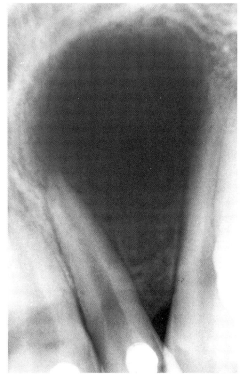

Fig. 17-28. Globulomaxillary cyst (courtesy Dr. S. Ericson).

frequency of these cysts in children is relatively low. Clinically, they may result in considerable swelling of the labial aspects of the alveolar ridge and palatum.

On x-ray, the nasopalatinal duct cyst is situated in the midline (Fig. 17-27) and the globulomaxillary cyst between the upper lateral and canine (Fig. 17-28). The recommended treatment is surgical excision.

Radicular cysts develop from epithelial remnants in the periodontium and are caused by an inflammation from a non-vital tooth. Such a cyst is often symptomless and grows slowly. Root deviation and considerable swelling of the bone are sometimes found. On x-ray there is often a well-circumscribed radiolucence at the apex of the affected tooth, surrounded by a lamina dura. Radiocular cysts are rare in primary dentition, but more common in young per-

manent dentition in combination with extensively carious teeth, invaginations and traumatic injuries. In primary dentition the affected tooth is extracted and the cyst extirpated. In the permanent dentition endodontic treatment, often in combination with surgical removal of the cyst, is an accepted therapy. A radicular cyst left behind in the jaw when the affected tooth is extracted is named a *residual cyst*.

"Traumatic" bone cyst is a single cyst without epithelial lining, found mostly in the lower jaw in young patients. It may contain fluid, but mostly is apparently empty. Swelling is only occasionally present. The teeth in the area are vital. X-rays show an irregular border often with a slight cortication and there is no root deviation (Fig. 17-29a). The etiology is unknown, but some

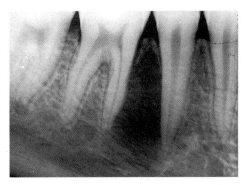

Fig. 17-29a. Traumatic cyst in a 15-year-old boy.

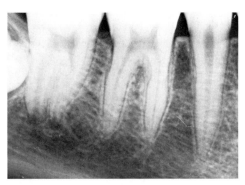

Fig. 17-29b. Healing of the cyst (17-29a) 3 months after surgical opening.

authors claim a traumatic history. Surgical opening of the cyst cavity and provocation of bleeding has been recommended, but as spontaneous healing is often seen, surgical treatment has been questioned (Fig. 17-29b).

Mucocele may be divided into two entities: a) mucous extravasation cysts, where mucus is forced into the connective tissues and where no epithelial lining is present, and b) mucous retention cysts where there is an epithelial lining. Mucocele occurs frequently in childen mostly in the lower lip. It may develop very quickly and then drain spontaneously. The swelling is often round and smooth, and the size varies from 1-15 mm in diameter. Mucocele is painless and may recur.

Is is believed that mucous extravasation cysts are caused by traumatic rupture of the salivary duct from the gland. An obstruction of the excretory duct can lead to formation of a lined mucocele, a mucous retention cyst. The treatment is removal of the cyst and associated salivary glands (Figs. 17-30 a-c). Marsupialization often leads to recurrence.

Ranula is a mucocele in the floor of the mouth. Due to extravasation or retention of mucus from excretory ducts of sublingual glands caused by trauma or infection, ex-

tensive translucent swellings may occur in the floor of the mouth, often unilaterally. The first choice of treatment is marsupialization, but if recurrences do occur, surgical removal of the entire gland is recommended.

TUMORS AND TUMOR-LIKE LESIONS

Tumors and tumor-like lesions of the head and neck are recognized even in very young children. Fortunately, most of these lesions are benign tumors and the frequency of malignant neoplasms is very low. However, about 25% of all malignant neoplasms in children develop in the head and neck area. Many of the tumors in the oral region are to be regarded as hamartomas. Due to the disproportionality of the tissues in hamartomas, they can expand the surrounding tissues. Normally, growth stops when it has reached a certain stage. Examples of hamartomas are hemangioma, lymphangioma and some odontogenic tumors.

It is important that all tumors and tumor-like lesions in the oral region are properly diagnosed and handled. If a lesion looks suspicious and the diagnosis is uncertain, the child should be referred to a specialist.

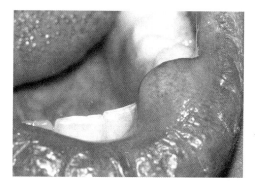

Fig. 17-30a. Mucous retention cyst in the lower lip.

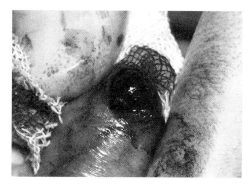

Fig. 17-30b. Surgical removal.

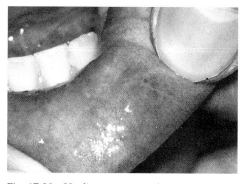

Fig. 17-30c. Healing.

When tumors or tumor-like lesions are excised all material removed should be sent for histological analysis in order to verify the diagnosis. Tumors deriving from odontogenic tissues are generally benign.

In the following, only tumors with a considerable frequency in children will be discussed. For other lesions and for more detailed information about the tumors presented, the reader is referred to textbooks on oral pathology.

Tumors from odontogenic tissues

Ameloblastoma
Adenomatoid odontogenic tumor
Ameloblastic fibroma
Myxoma
Benign cementoblastoma
Odontomas

Ameloblastoma is a slowly growing, destructive neoplasm with a capacity for local invasion, mostly located in the molar region of the mandible where it can reach a considerable size. Metastasis has been reported. Radiographically it resembles an expanding uni- or multilocular cyst. Histologically, there is a fibrous stroma with proliferating odontogenic epithelium. The treatment is excision with good margin as the tumor has a tendency to recur. The ameloblastomas are rare in children except for unicystic ameloblastomas which have a low incidence of recurrence.

Adenomatoid odontogenic tumor is surrounded by a capsule and is mostly located in the anterior region of the maxilla. Histologically, duct-like or adenomatoid structures of columnar epithelial cells cross the tumor mass. Slight amorphous calcification may occur.

Ameloblastic fibroma is a slowly growing, expansive encapsulated neoplasm, predominantly found in children. It is composed of odontogenic epithelium in cellular mesodermal tissue with the character of dental papillae. It resembles an ameloblastoma on x-ray.

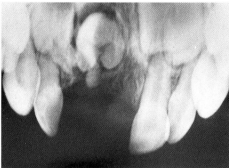

Fig. 17-31a. Complex odontoma in a 2-year-old girl as a result of trauma.

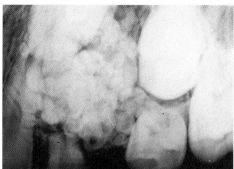

Fig. 17-31b. X-ray of compound odontoma.

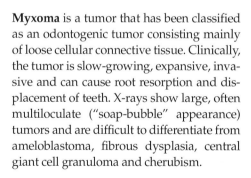

Fig. 17-31c. Compound odontoma in Fig. 31b after removal showing about 80 small tooth-like formations.

Myxoma is a tumor that has been classified as an odontogenic tumor consisting mainly of loose cellular connective tissue. Clinically, the tumor is slow-growing, expansive, invasive and can cause root resorption and displacement of teeth. X-rays show large, often multiloculate ("soap-bubble" appearance) tumors and are difficult to differentiate from ameloblastoma, fibrous dysplasia, central giant cell granuloma and cherubism.

Benign cementoblastoma is a well-circumscribed tumor consisting of fibrous tissue with varying amounts of mineralized cementum or cementoid tissue often in connection with the roots of the teeth. The hard tissue may be fused to the root. On x-ray, the tumor may resemble a periapical cyst, but differentiation is based on a sensitivity test.

Odontomas are tumors of a hamartomatous character. They vary in size and are often revealed in x-rays of children with late tooth eruption or retentions. Complex odontoma is a more or less homogeneous mixture of different calcified dental tissues. Compound odontoma is a tumor consisting of a varying number of tooth-like formations where the different dental hard tissues can be distinguished clearly (Figs. 17-31 a-c). Odontomas are often well-encapsulated and surgical removal is uncomplicated.

Tumors related to osteogenic tissues

Central ossifying fibroma
Central giant cell tumor
Familial fibrous dysplasia (cherubism)
Juvenile monostotic fibrous dysplasia
Malignant tumors

Central ossifying fibroma is a benign tumor very similar to central cementifying fibroma. The tumor can grow considerably and cause cortical expansion.

Central giant cell tumor is a benign tumor consisting of giant cell tissue with a capacity to destroy bone. Clinically, the child has swelling, expansion of the cortical plates of the jaw, and tooth mobility. The tumor is often located in the anterior part of the jaws and also spreads over the midline. Radio-lucency is seen with resorption and displacement of teeth. The condition might be difficult to differentiate from cherubism and juvenile fibrous dysplasia. Excision is recommended. All patients with diagnosed giant cell tumor should be referred for further examination concerning hyperparathyroidism, as this disease might be connected with giant cell tumor.

Familial fibrous dysplasia (cherubism) is a bilateral enlargement of the mandible starting at an early age and resulting in a cherubic appearance. A great number of multilocular radiolucent areas are found spread all over the jaw. The upper jaw is also sometimes affected. Histologically, multinucleate giant cells are found in the areas of destruction. Spontaneous loss of teeth may occur. As the child grows older the lesions seem to become more fibrous and new bone formation has even been found. Excision of the lesions is recommended if the lesions are not too widespread.

Juvenile monostotic fibrous dysplasia is a benign tumor, which often starts early in childhood. The lesion is restricted to one bone, usually the maxilla. During growth it may expand and cases have been reported where the tumor has extended into the floor of the orbit and has also produced severe malocclusion. Extraorally, a clear swelling of the maxilla is recognizable.

Histological findings resemble other fibro-osseous lesions and it may be difficult to diffentiate them from such other changes as central ossifying fibroma, central cementifying fibroma and chronic sclerosing osteomyelitis. X-rays of the affected area often show a fine granular "orange-peel" pattern and the lesion is not surrounded by a radiolucent area, indicating a capsule (Fig. 17-32). The tumor often ceases to grow after puberty. The decision to operate is therefore postponed until this age, unless the growth

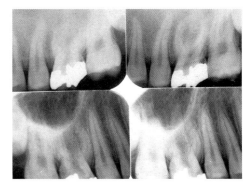

Fig. 17-32. 15-year-old boy with fibrous dysplasia. Note the granular appearance of the bone on the affected side.

of the tumor causes unacceptable complications.

Fibrous dysplasia might also occur in a polystotic form involving multiple bones, and accompanied by other developmental changes (Albright's syndrome).

Malignant tumors of osseous origin are rare in children. However, cases of fibrosarcoma, osteogenic sarcoma, chondrosarcoma and Ewing's sarcoma are a reality in children's dentistry. It is therefore important to recognize the early signs and make a correct diagnosis.

The following clinical and radiographic symptoms may indicate malignancy:

– rapid swelling and expansion of the cortical plate

– loosening of teeth

– simultaneous engagement of the soft tissue

– pain

– paresthesia

– enlarged regional lymph nodes

– x-ray: ragged margins of the lesion, erosions of cortex, root resorption, widening of periodontal membrane.

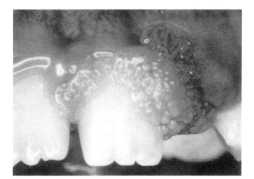

Fig. 17-33. Papilloma.

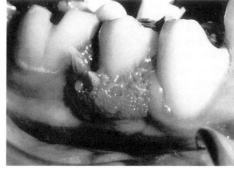

Fig. 17-34. Wart.

Tumors from soft tissues

Papilloma
Fibroma
Epulide
Hemangioma
Lymphangioma
Neurofibroma
Pleomorphic adenoma
Malignant tumors

Papilloma is a common benign tumor which occurs even in young children. Clinically, papillomas are rather small, showing "finger-like" projections and may develop at any site on the oral mucosa (Fig. 17-33). The tumor closely resembles the common wart (*verruca vulgaris*), which can also occur on the oral mucosa, especially in children with warts on their hands (Fig. 17-34). Excision is recommended.

Fibroma is a characteristic tissue change. It has a smooth surface and a normal color. It is sessile or pedunculate, the size varies up to a centimeter and its consistency is usually firm. The tumor can be found at any site in the oral mucosa and is often the result of a long-standing trauma (reactive hyperplasia). Excision is recommended.

Epulides are a group of tumors caused by a local irritation and are, by definition, found on the gingiva. The size may vary up to several centimeters. *Pyogenic granuloma, peripheral calcifying granuloma* and *peripheral giant cell granuloma*, when found on the gingiva, can be included in this group. Pyogenic granuloma is often soft, red and ulcerated (Fig. 17-35). Histologically, proliferating granulation tissue is found. Peripheral calcifying granuloma (Fig. 17-36) is firmer than the pyogenic granulomas. Diffuse calcification in the stroma of connective tissue is found. Peripheral giant cell granuloma (Fig. 17-37) is relatively firm and has a characteristic bluish-reddish color. Resorption of adjacent bone may occur. The treatment of the epulides is excision.

Hemangioma is a relatively common hamartomatous tumor in children. Most of the lesions are present at birth. the most common location is the tongue, followed by the lips and buccal mucosa. Clinically, two different forms can be distinguished: the *capillary hemangioma* and the *cavernous hemangioma*. The former consists of a proliferation of tiny capillaries, often manifest as red birthmarks on the skin and oral mucosa (Fig. 17-38). The cavernous form is frequently situated more deeply and consists of large cavernous blood-filled vessels. The tumor often causes a compressible swelling of the tissue affected and the color is frequently

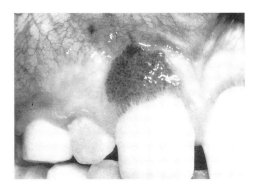

Fig. 17-35. Pyogenic granuloma.

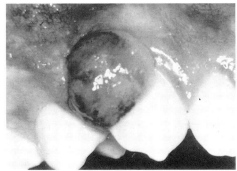

Fig. 17-36. Peripheral calcifying granuloma.

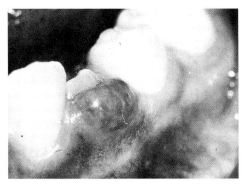

Fig. 17-37. Peripheral giant cell granuloma.

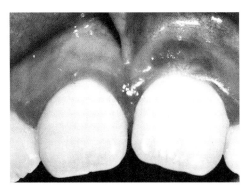

Fig. 17-38. Capillary hemangioma.

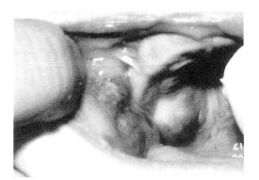

Fig. 17-39. Cavernous hemangioma in the palate of a newborn. Note also the capillary hemangioma in the cheek.

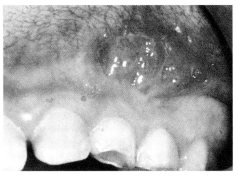

Fig. 17-40. Lymphangioma.

more bluish than the capillary hemangioma
(Fig. 17-39). Hemangioma can also occur as
a central tumor of the maxilla and mandible. This condition is difficult to distinguish on x-ray from other osteolytic tumors
and cysts.

The treatment of hemangioma is always
complicated because of the risk of uncon-

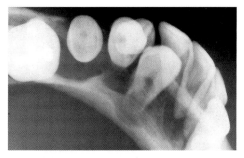

Fig. 17-41. 9-year-old boy with acute lympho-blastic leukemia in combination with lympho-sarcoma (courtesy Dr. S. Ericson).

trolled bleeding. Fortunately, many congenital hemangiomas undergo spontaneous regression.

Lymphangioma is mostly a congenital tumor and resembles hemangioma, but the vessels contain lymph fluid instead of blood. The most common location is the tongue, but the buccal mucosa and the lips are often involved. When it affects the tongue it is one of the causes of congenital macroglossia. Lymphangioma has a tendency to spread in the spaces of the soft tissues. Clinically, there is a firm swelling and the mucous lesion shows a nodular enlargement of the same color as the surrounding mucosa (Fig. 17-40). Surgical treatment is only performed in cases with functional disturbances or extensive disfiguration.

Neurofibroma is a hamartomatous tumor arising from nerve sheath and perineural fibroblasts. The tumors are found as solitary lesions or, in the case of the syndrome of von Recklinghausen's neurofibromatosis, as multiple lesions. Clinically, there are solitary or multiple smooth-surfaced nodules spread over the skin and mucosa. Histologically, the tumor is encapsulate and contains connective tissue and axons, sometimes with a myelin sheath. The tumor can also occur as a central neurofibroma of the jaws,

predominantly in the mandible. Radiographically the lesion resembles a well-demarcated cyst. Solitary lesions in the mucosa, as well as in the bone, are removed surgically. The high frequency of sarcomatous transformation in patients with extensive neufibromas has to be noted.

Pleomorphic adenoma is the most common tumor of salivary glands in children. The parotid gland is the one most affected. The first sign is swelling, sometimes even pain and in severe cases a tendency to facial paralysis occur. The histological examination reveals a connective tissue stroma with hyaline cartilage-like areas and epithelial cells. It has beeen recommended to assume pleomorphic adenomas are adenocarcinomas because of the risk of malignant transformation. Here, sialography is a valuable diagnostic aid in distinguishing these conditions from other swellings occurring in the region in question.

Malignant tumors derived from the soft tissues in children are mainly malignant lymphoma and rhabdomyosarcoma. Carcinoma in the oral region is extremely rare in children.

Malignant lymphoma affects even very young children. It often begins as a swelling of solitary lymph nodes in the neck region. the affected nodes have a firm rubbery consistency and the changes are mostly unilateral. The lymphoma may also involve the lymphoid tissue in the oral cavity and from here rapidly invade the soft tissue and the jaws. Biopsy is strongly recommended to verify the diagnosis. Malignant lymphoma covers a group of conditions among which lymphosarcoma and Hodgkin's disease are included (Fig. 17-41).

Rhabdomyosarcoma is a malignant tumor of striated muscle masses. The tumor, which is often of the embryonal type and occurs predominantly in young children, may develop in the oral mucosa starting as a rapidly growing painless mass. Location is often the tongue or soft palate. The tumor will ulcerate and more or less fill the oral cavity resulting in dysphagia and pain. The prognosis is poor.

PAIN CONTROL IN ORAL SURGERY

The most important prerequisite for performing surgery, not only on children, but in principle on everybody, is effective pain control, the ability to remove or reduce pain and discomfort before, during, and following surgery.

It is important that the patient understands that you will do your utmost to achieve effective pain control, and that you explain to the patient how this is achieved.

Modern pain control encompasses:

– information to the patient

– premedication with sedatives, analgesics, antibiotics, anti-inflammatory agents, etc.

– local analgesia

– conscious sedation (nitrous oxide)

– general anesthesia, when indicated

– analgesics postoperatively

– physical methods (heat, cold, TENS, laser)

For further details, see Chapter 7. To supplement this, the following guidelines are recommended:

Premedication

The term premedication just means that some kind of medication is administered before a certain act. However, most clinicians relate the meaning of premedication to the administration of a relaxing agent to the nervous patient.

Antibiotics

Antibiotics can be used either prophylactically (simultaneous therapy) or curatively. The prophylactic indication can be either systematic or local. Three types of antibiotics attract interest in dental practice, i.e. phenoxymethylpenicillin (penicillin V), metronidazole, and erythromycin. Penicillin is still the drug of choice in almost all situations, and is actually only contraindicated in case of genuine allergy. Metronidazole, which is very active against anerobic bacteria, has become increasingly popular recently, as it has been discovered that the anerobic flora are an integral part of most oral infections. Metronidazole is contraindicated only for pregnant women, and can even be given to small children (dosage 20 mg/kg 24h in three daily dosages).

If surgery is performed at an acute stage, penicillin should be administered p.o. 1 hour preoperatively (1 mill.U. = 0.6 g to children 1-6 yrs, and 2 mill.U. = 1.2 g to older children). For other dosages, see local reference guides.

Anti-inflammatory agents

As most acute traumatic (= surgical) pain actually is inflammatory in origin, any anti-inflammatory treatment administered preoperatively will decrease the inflammatory response, and, thus, the pain and swelling postoperatively.

The most effective drugs in this respect are the glucocorticosteroids, i.e. dexamethasone 4 mg injected into an oral region, where local analgesia has already been applied. It is used only preoperatively as a one-time dosage. The only contraindication is acute infection.

Analgesics postoperatively

As previously noted, either paracetamol or antirheumatics (NSAIDs) are recommended for pain control postoperatively in children. However, children rarely experience as much pain and discomfort as adults.

Physical methods

Cold packs (ice packs) can with advantage be placed on the skin over the operated area for 10-15 min, 2-3 times on the day of operation. The cold will most likely activate temperature-sensitive receptors in the skin, which will help close the "pain-gate". Infrared heat is recommended for the following days, 10-15 min. 2-3 times a day.

Soft laser therapy and TENS (transcutaneous electric nerve stimulation) are new, very interesting and promising methods for treating pain and swelling postoperatively. These methods, which require special knowledge, can easily be applied in pedodontic practice.

The key-point in modern pain control is to be ahead of the pain, instead of waiting for the pain to establish itself!

EXTRACTION OF TEETH

In some cases a seemingly simple easy extraction can turn into a difficult surgical removal, so it is wise never to tell the patient beforehand that this is going to be an easy procedure.

Extraction procedure involves:

– application of forceps and/or an elevator

– loosening of the tooth by rotation and/or luxation

– removal of the tooth from the socket.

At extraction of deciduous teeth the amount of physiologic resorption of the roots, and the position of the permanent successors in relation to the roots of the deciduous teeth have to be taken into account. In some cases the developing crown of the permanent tooth is more or less encircled by the root of a primary molar, and will follow this tooth out (Fig. 17-42). Should it happen, the permanent tooth should immediately, but carefully be replaced in the socket in correct position.

Extraction or surgical removal of teeth may be indicated in the following situations:

– extensive caries

– nonvital pulps where endodontic treatment is not indicated or impossible to perform

– serious marginal periodontitis with extensive bone loss

– apical periodontitis where endodontic treatment or apicoectomy is not possible

– axial root fracture (corrosion of post)

– root fracture in coronal $\frac{1}{3}$ of root

– teeth interfering with normal bite functioning or restorative dentistry

– semi-impacted or impacted teeth with symptoms or signs of pathology

– supernumerary teeth blocking eruption for normal teeth

– lack of space (orthodontic indication)

– ectopic position or eruption pattern

– teeth traumatizing soft tissues

– non-healthy teeth in line of irradiation.

Many of these indications are absolute, others are relative. It is important that the dentist performs a thorough clinical and x-ray examination before putting the results to the patient in order to make a treatment plan. If the patient, or the parents of a patient, refuse to accept or agree upon a treatment plan proposed by the dentist, it is

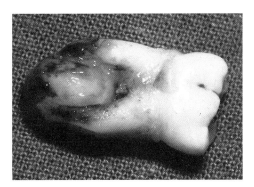

Fig. 17-42. Permanent tooth bud accidentally avulsed at extraction of a primary molar.

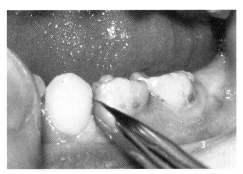

Fig. 17-43. An elevator is first used to loosen the primary molar carefully.

their right - and their own responsibility. The treatment plan and its refusal should be carefully noted in the records.

Contraindications or warnings of precaution against extraction of teeth are:

Local
– acute infections in gingiva, pericoronally or periapically

– recent irradiation of the area

– acute sinusitis when extracting upper premolars and molars

Systemic
– blood dyscrasias

– leukemia

– hemorrhagic disorders

– platelet deficiencies anti-coagulation

– immune apparatus deficiencies (incl. glucocorticosteroid therapy)

– cardiac diseases

– previous valve operations

– previous endocarditis

– juvenile diabetes mellitus

As far as extractions or operations in areas of acute infection are concerned, it is reasonable to look at the extent of proposed surgery. If an infected tooth is simple to remove, it is fair to do this during the acute phase, provided that the patient is covered sufficiently with antibiotic before the procedure, i.e. small children: 1 mill. U. of penicillin V, and larger children 2 mill. U. of penicillin V, administered ½-1 hour before. If the general condition of the patient is poor, antibiotic administration should be continued for 2 days postoperatively.

If the proposed surgery on the infected tooth is deemed to be difficult, then the infection should be treated first, and the tooth extraction delayed until after the infection has cleared.

In cases of such previous cardiac disease as valve operations, valve replacement, or endocarditis, the patient should always be covered with antibiotics before extraction or other operations. The drug of choice is amoxicillin: adults 3 g and children 50 mg/kg p.o. 1 hour before surgery as a single dosage. In case of penicillin allergy, clindamycin 300-600 mg p.o. 1 hour before surgery, is recommended.

Extraction procedure

After sufficient analgesia has been obtained, the gingiva around the tooth to be extracted is carefully loosened with a periosteal elevator or a straight elevator (Fig. 17-43). The

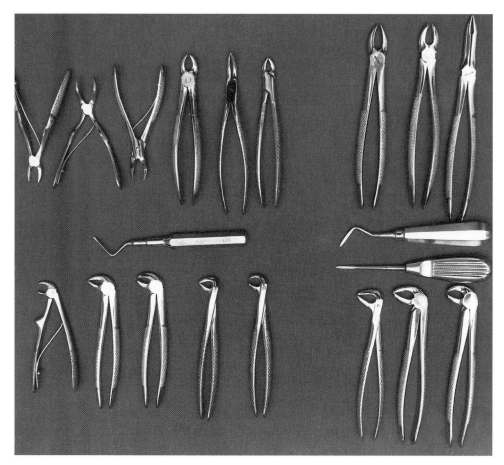

Fig. 17-44. To the left a set of forceps and elevators for primary dentition and to the right for permanent dentition.

latter instrument is also used to luxate the tooth by applying pressure on all surfaces. Watch out for pressure against neighbouring teeth, especially if they are root open, as they can unintentionally be traumatized or loosened. Extraction forceps of good quality and suited for the tooth to be extracted are selected (Fig. 17-44). Apply the working branches around the crown and the neck of the tooth, and begin the extraction movements slowly and carefully in order not to scare the patient (Fig. 17-45). Prepare the patient for the sounds and movement that follow this procedure. When doing extraction or operation in the lower jaw, a bite block to support the mandible is recom-

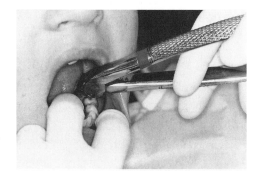

Fig. 17-45. Forceps are used to extract the tooth.

mended. Watch out for the soft tissues, so they are not unduly traumatized.

If a root tip fractures, the best treatment is probably to leave it, unless:

– infected,

– it will interfere with eruption of a succeding tooth,

– it will interfere with orthodontic treatment.

If you decide to remove the fractured root tip of a deciduous tooth, consideration should always be given to the permanent successor. To prevent root fractures it is an advantage to cut a deciduous molar into two halves with a diamond burr before extraction (Figs. 17-46 a, b).

After the extraction, the oral cavity is cleansed with water spray and suction, and a gauze pad is placed over the extraction socket, and the patient is asked to keep pressure on the gauze pad for 15 minutes. Instructions should be given both to the child and any accompanying adults, and preferably both verbal and written.

SURGICAL REMOVAL OF IMPACTED TEETH

The incision should be carefully planned, and right away carried through to bone. The most common error seen, is a too-small incision. After periosteal elevation, bone can be removed with a round burr under sterile saline irrigation. In order to remove the tooth easily it is often preferable to divide it with a tungsten fissure burr, and then split with a sharp straight elevator.

After tooth removal, the follicle is taken out with a round-ended bone rongeur, and the sharp bony edges are smoothed with a large round burr. Before closing, the wound should be thoroughly irrigated with saline, and inspected. Suturing is done with 4-0 silk or a resorbable suture on a semicircular, reverse cutting needle. Approximal sutur-

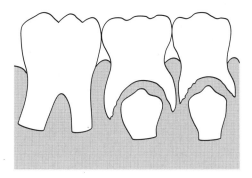

Fig. 17-46a. Primary molar encircling the permanent bud.

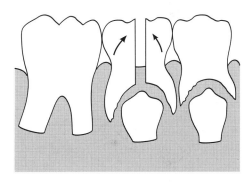

Fig. 17-46b. Primary molar cut into two halves before extraction.

ing is best achieved with a small straight needle.

If a regular, impacted tooth, placed in the middle of the alveolar process has to be removed, e.g. a second premolar, it can be very helpful to open up both the buccal and lingual aspects. The bone is removed on the buccal side, the tooth is divided at the collum area, and through an opening on the lingual aspect, the fragments can be pressed out in a buccal direction.

If a tooth fragment is loose, but caught by bone or neighbouring roots, "a two-instru-

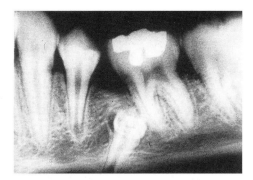

Fig. 17-47. Impacted lower second molar that should not be removed.

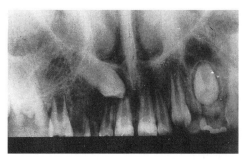

Fig. 17-48a. Impacted upper cuspid in close relation to apices of central and lateral incisors.

ment" procedure can be performed. Use a thin elevator as a chute and lift the tooth or the fragment along the chute with a small elevator or a pointed instrument.

If a regular tooth is deeply impacted without any signs of pathology, and not interfering with other teeth or planned orthodontic treatment, the patient is probably better off with the tooth in place than removed (Fig. 17-47). Before an operation is decided upon, there should always be a serious evaluation of indications for surgery. If the decision to leave the tooth is made, the patient should be told, and the tooth followed by regular x-ray checks. If in doubt about possible resorption damage to neighbouring roots, the impacted tooth should be removed, or if the damage has already taken place, it might be a better idea to extract the resorbed tooth, and guide the impacted tooth into correct position. This consideration holds especially true for the impacted upper canine (Figs. 17-48 a, b).

Regular, permanent teeth most likely to impact are, in decreasing order of frequency: $M_{3inf.}$, $M_{3sup.}$, C_{sup}, $P_{2inf.}$, and $P_{2sup.}$.

Third molars should be removed in children around the age of 12 years, if they will interfere with an orthodontic treatment or demonstrate pathology. Otherwise, the decision to remove third molars should be postponed, until 16-18 years of age.

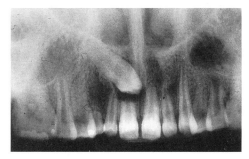

Fig. 17-48b. Impacted cuspid has caused resorption of root of central incisor in just 1 year.

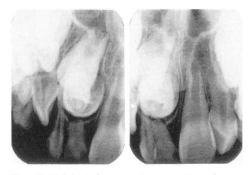

Fig. 17-49. Mesiodens causing retention of upper right central incisor.

Supernumerary teeth causing retention should be removed (Fig. 17-49). It is important to follow the eruption pattern of teeth, and if an asymmetrical development takes place, the reason for this should be investi-

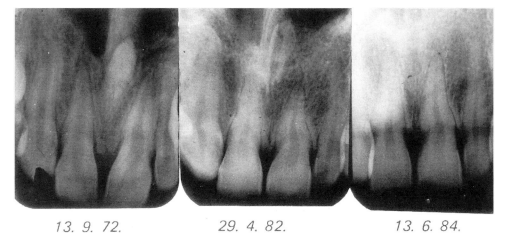

13. 9. 72.   29. 4. 82.   13. 6. 84.

Fig. 17-50. Mesiodens disappearing due to resorption during 12 years.

gated in order that optimal treatment is not surpassed.

However, if a supernumerary tooth is incidentally discovered on a routine x-ray, and there is no pathology and it has not interfered with normal eruption of teeth in the region, the best treatment is to leave it. Studies have shown that many supernumerary teeth will resorb in adulthood without causing any problems (Fig. 17-50). If orthodontic treatment is to take place in a region with supernumerary teeth, they should be removed, before the orthodontic treatment is initiated.

SURGICAL ORTHODONTIC TREATMENT OF IMPACTED TEETH

Surgical orthodontic treatment of impacted teeth will usually consist of a denudation and in most cases, orthodontic treatment to guide the impacted tooth into its proper location. In certain cases, when dealing with erupting teeth that are caught just below the approximal contact point, the teeth can,

sometimes, be forcefully guided or pressured into place with a straight elevator. This is called "redressement force", and can typically be applied to upper cuspids or second molars.

Denudation

If the eruption path for a tooth is blocked, the hinderance should be removed at the latest, when the erupting tooth root is ⅔ formed. If the procedure for some reason is postponed, there is always the risk of bending of the root tip in close relation to the floor, nasal cavity, maxillary sinus, or mandibular canal.

Bone superficial to the impacted tooth is carefully removed with a round burr, taking care not to touch the cervical or the root surface, as this can damage the periodontal ligament, and cause anchylosis and resorption. As much bone as possible, in the direction of the future movement of the tooth, should be removed, of course taking into consideration the neighbouring roots. Ideally, a bracket should be attached to the denuded crown after acid etching with composite, but, usually, it is not possible to get the area sufficiently dry for this procedure,

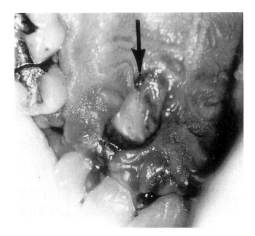

Fig. 17-51. Impacted cuspid in palate position is denuded.

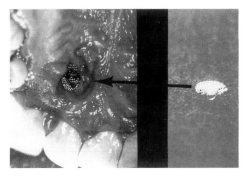

Fig. 17-52. Bracket is attached to denuded cuspid.

so it has to be postponed until later. In the meantime, the denuded crown is covered with surgical paste that is secured with a cross-suture on top of it for one week. At the time of paste removal, the bracket can normally be attached (Figs. 17-51, 52).

If the tooth is placed very deeply, a small-bore canal can be drilled in a cusp or in the marginal crest of the crown, and a 0.25 mm soft wire passed through this canal and a small hook be placed in the canal. After the eruption the canal or hole can easily be covered with composites.

Previously, the placement of a collum ligature has been advocated, but studies have shown that this might damage the periodontal ligament in this region, resulting in a denuded root surface after eruption.

Sometimes, a "window" has to be cut in the covering soft tissues in order to facilitate the eruption.

Redressement forcé

This procedure is best performed, when the tooth is still root-open, and the proposed movement is small, more like a rotation around the apical region, so the pulpal blood supply is disturbed least. If necessary, the "replaced" tooth can be fixed with composite to the neighbour tooth.

AUTO-TRANSPLANTATION OF TEETH

Autotransplantation of teeth is in the same person, while transplantating from one human to the other is called allotransplantation. The latter does not have a good long-term prognosis, while autotransplantation under optimal conditions will succeed in almost 100% of cases. Today, the most common indication for autotransplantation is a premolar transplantation to a premolar region with aplasia.

Requirements for the transplant:

– it should be root-open,

– the root should be between ½ to ⅔ formed,

– it should be placed in such a position that it is possible to get it out intact and undamaged on the root surface

Requirements for the recipient site:

– free of infection,

– large enough in all dimensions to accomodate the transplant,

– enough bone in height and width to harbor the transplant

Requirements for the surgical procedure:

– should be atraumatic

– the transplant is not allowed to dry

– the preparation of the new alveolar socket should be under constant saline irrigation with sharp burrs using slow speed,

– the patient should be treated with antibiotics starting just prior to surgery and continuing for one week.

Dosage of penicillin is typically 2 Mill. U (= 1.2 g) preoperatively, followed by 1 Mill. U (= 0.6 g) twice daily for one week.

Previously, the transplant was fixed tightly for 6-8 weeks, but studies have shown that this will increase the risk for anchylosis. It is better to employ a loose fixation for one to two weeks, i.e. a cross-suture of silk. The tooth should be placed in a slight infraocclusion. Any traumatic occlusion should be corrected.

If a pulp necrosis develops, endodontic treatment should be undertaken, and the root canal temporarily filled with calcium hydroxide for 6-9 months, before a final root filling is performed.

More rare indications for autotransplantation are upper third molars to the front region in case incisors are lost traumatically. Also, in cases with multiple aplasia, the indications for autotransplantation are wider in order to create natural supports for bridge reconstruction.

A particular form of autotransplantation is cases with tilted or inverted permanent anlage. This means to turn or erect the developing tooth into a correct position. This procedure is termed "autotransplantation *in situ*" in contrast to "autotransplantation *ad regionem*".

Autotransplantation of fully developed teeth

If a fully developed tooth is transplanted, it is likely that the pulp will undergo necrosis, as the possibilities for revascularization through the apical foramen are far less than in the root-open tooth. The transplant should, therefore, be endontically treated with calcium hydroxide, preferably before removal if possible; or 2-3 weeks after the surgical procedure.

TREATMENT OF SOFT TISSUE LESIONS AND ABNORMALITIES

Frenuloplasty

A large and vertically placed frenulum that attaches close to the gingiva, or even to the lingual aspect should be extirpated or apically repositioned. If interfering with the closing of a diastema mediale, the fibrous band between the two maxillary processes should be removed at the same time. The principle of frenuloplasty is to cut fibrous tissue in the submucosa without disturbing the periosteum (Figs. 17-53 a-f).

If a lingual frenulum is frequently traumatized by the lower incisors, or interferes with nourishment or speech development or hygiene procedures, it should be cut. Two structures are of vital importance to

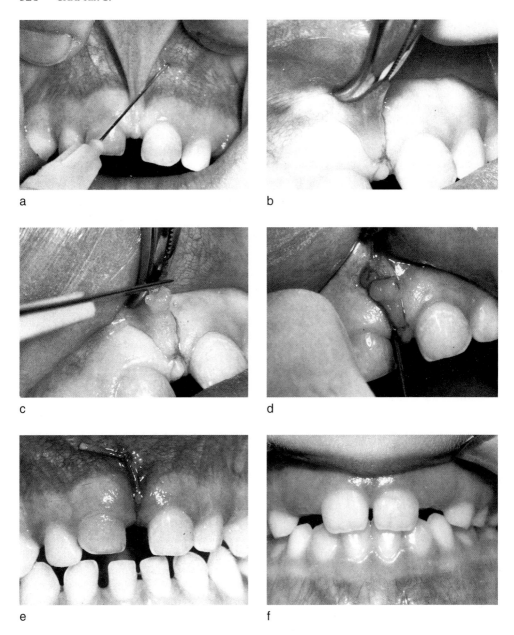

Fig. 17-53a-f. Labial frenuloplasty: a) local anesthesia of labial frenum; b) curved hemostat placed close to the lip; c) frenum is cut along the hemostat; d) lateral incisions; e) healing after 2 days; f) three years after operation.

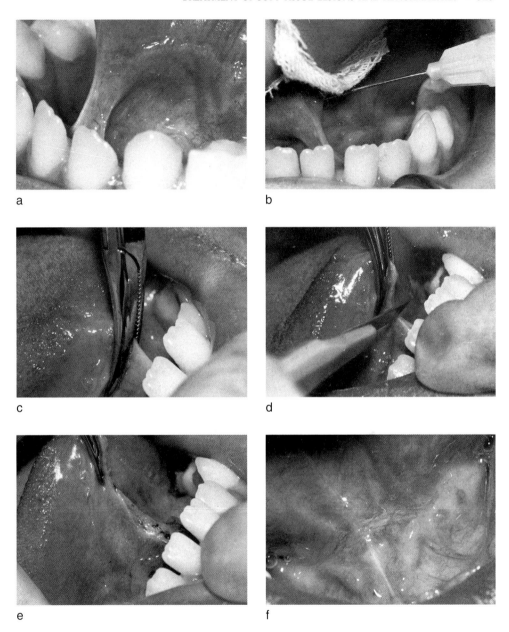

Fig. 17-54a-f. Lingual frenuloplasty: a) lingual frenum restricting the movements of the tongue; b) local anesthesia; c) curved hemostat is placed close to the tongue; d,e) frenulum is out; f) healing after 10 days.

avoid in this region, the submandibular duct and the sublingual vein. The dissecting cut is best made lingually to the caruncles, parallel to the undersurface of the tongue, taking care not to go too deep (Figs. 17-54 a-f).

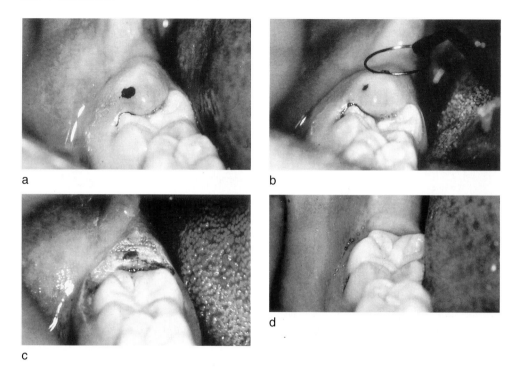

a

b

c

d

Fig. 17-55a-d. Removal of operculum: a) soft tissue covering first molar; b) flap removed with electrosurgery loop; c) immediately after removal; d) healing after 1 week.

Soft tissue flap over erupting tooth

A soft tissue flap (operculum) over a normally erupting tooth can sometimes give
rise to irritation. It can be treated by irrigation beneath the flap with saline or 0.2%
chlorhexidine solution. Removal of the flap
is sometimes indicated. This is easily done
with a loop electrode of electrosurgery or by
conventional surgery (Figs. 17-55 a-d).

Epulis

Epulis means a local extended growth on the gingiva, and can occur along the free gingival margin. Most often, it is hyperplastic tissue that can be curetted or removed with electrosurgery, especially if attached to the gingiva by a small stalk.

POSTOPERATIVE CONSIDERATIONS

The patient and the parents should be given careful verbal and written instructions about surgical procedures. Preferably, these instructions should be given preoperatively, so preparations can be made as far as the postoperative course is concerned.

Some important considerations:

– information about duration of local analgesia, and about care not to traumatize anesthetized tissue

– information about expected bleeding, and what to do in case of extended or excessive hemorrhage. Gauze pads should be handed out with the instructions, and the patient instructed in how to place the gauze pads correctly in order to offer sufficient compression of the surgical site

– information about postoperative pain control

– information about food and liquid intake. To many patients, this point is actually the most important

– information about restricted physical activities during the first 1-2 days postoperatively

– information about suture removal or any other postoperative precautions to be taken, drugs to be taken, next appointments, etc.

The dentist should never forget that the procedure might be a minor one and routine to the dentist, but to the patient it is *always* a major intervention.

Background literature

Pindborg JJ. *Atlas of diseases of the oral mucosa.* Copenhagen: Munksgaard, 1985.

Pindborg JJ, Kramer JRH, Torloni H. *Histological typing of odontogenic tumors, jaw cysts and allied lesions.* Geneva: World Health Organization, 1971.

Shafer WG, Hine MK, Levy BN. *A textbook of oral pathology.* Philadelphia: WB Saunders, 1983.

Shear M. Cyst of jaws: recent advances. *J Oral Pathol* 1985; **14**: 43-59.

CHAPTER 18

MEDICALLY COMPROMISED CHILDREN

Cardiac diseases

Renal disorders

Endocrine disorders

Chronic inflammatory intestinal diseases

Malabsorptions

Cystic fibrosis

Immunologic diseases

Bleeding disorders

Malignant tumors

Leukemia

Convulsive disorders

Skeletal diseases

Chromosomal aberrations

The incidence of chronic diseases in children has been relatively stable in recent decades. Due to early diagnosis and more effective medical treatment, an increasing number of children with chronic diseases survive. In such conditions as cystic fibrosis, Down's syndrome and acute lymphatic leukemia a dramatic increase in life expectancy and quality of life has occurred. As a consequence, the demand for specialised dental treatment of chronically sick children is increasing.

These children constitute a group where special knowledge is required to make dental care as optimal as possible. Not only is knowledge of the disease *per se* necessary, but also knowledge about management of the oral complications that may accompany the various diseases.

Daily life is more or less affected for children with a chronic disease, either by the disease itself, or by medication and treatment. For some children it may mean that a special diet has to be followed, or that staying away from preschool or school for shorter or longer periods becomes necessary. Daily oral hygiene may be difficult to perform and dental examinations can be irregular. Sick children are often in special need of support and professional help with tooth cleaning and individual preventive programs to keep mouth and teeth healthy. It is important that these aspects are taken into consideration in the planning of dental care for the individual child.

The pedodontist is responsible for the oral health of children with chronic diseases as one member of a multiprofessional group with various skills and capacities needed to care for the sick child. In addition to the pediatrician and the medical nurses, this group may include a physiotherapist, speech therapist, dietician, etc. In the planning of dental treatment, continuous contact with the pediatrician is of utmost importance.

Knowledge and ability to give the child the best possible oral care is necessary during all phases of a disease. Adequate information to child and parents about the oral complications that may appear as side effects of disease or medication and how they can best be avoided should be given at an early stage, also to very sick children.

One of the problems that may be difficult to deal with, is the over-compensation that children naturally experience from parents, friends and relatives when they become ill. During their stay in hospital as well as at home, the consumption of sweets, cakes, soft drinks, etc tend to increase. There is no need to interfere if this applies to a short period only, but if it seems to become a habit it should be discussed with the parents, although with understanding of the special situation.

Only a few of many chronic diseases will be discussed in this chapter. The main reasons for inclusion have been either that the disease itself induces oral manifestations or a decreased host resistance or that medication and other treatment induce side effects in the oral cavity and/or masticatory system. Other diseases included are those where altered diet and oral hygiene habits may make the child more prone to dental disease.

CARDIAC DISEASES

Cardiac diseases can be congenital or acquired. In children they are almost always congenital, while the acquired, rheumatic heart disease, hypertension and atherosclerosis, are very rare.

Congenital cardiac disease

The etiology is in most cases unknown, but genetic factors, teratogenic agents (viral diseases, drugs, alcohol) may be causal. Children with chromosomal aberrations (Down's syndrome) often have congenital heart conditions.

Pathology – The congenital cardiac defects can be classified into cyanotic and noncyanotic.

In the cyanotic cardiac disease, blood is shunted from right-to-left within the heart due to a cardiac defect. The most common is the tetralogy of Fallot, a ventricular septal defect in combination with pulmonary stenosis, right ventricular hypertrophy and dextrorotation of the aorta. Transposition of great vessels, pulmonary stenosis with patent foramen ovale and pulmonary atresia are other cyanotic cardiac failures.

In the non-cyanotic cardiac defects, there is no shunting or a shunting from left-to-right in the heart. The most common form is the ventricular septal defect (VSD). Aortic valve stenosis, atrial septal defects (ASD), patent *ductus arteriosus*, pulmonary valve stenosis and coarctation of aorta are other forms of non-cyanotic heart diseases.

Frequency – The total incidence of cardiac failure in children is a little less than 1%.

Pathology – Congenital cardiac defects are diagnosed early and decisions for operation can also be taken early. Surgery is carried

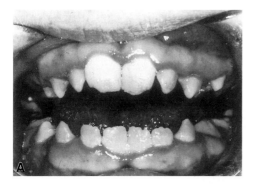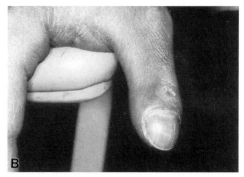

Fig. 18-1. 19-year-old boy with Down's syndrome and a cyanotic cardiac disease showing (left) cyanotic gingival margin and (right) typical changes of finger nails in cyanotic patients.

out more frequently than previously, usually during the first or second year and with good prognosis.

Minor cardiac failures may remain without symptoms for many years while more severe defects may reduce the physical capacity of the child significantly. Common features in the more severe cases are retarded physical growth and reduced resistance to infections, dyspnoea and cyanosis during physical exertion. In addition to medical care, children with disabling cardiac failure, as well as their parents, are often in need of psychological and sociomedical support.

Bacterial endocarditis

Children with congenital and acquired cardiac disease are at high risk to develop bacterial endocarditis. As dental procedures are very likely to be causative, antibiotic prophylaxis is required for any dental treatment which may cause gingival bleeding and a subsequent bacteremia. The proposed prophylaxis for children below 12 years is amoxicillin 50 mg/kg body weight given as a single dose one hour before or within two hours after dental treatment. For adolescents 3 g is given as a single dose as above. In children oversensitive to penicillin, erythromycin or clindamycin can be prescribed.

Oral manifestations – Oral manifestations of cardiac disease are relatively few. In cyanotic children, the teeth have a paperwhite appearance against a background of cyanotic mucosa, lips and tongue (Fig. 18-1). This tooth-colour is related to mineralization disturbances, reported to be more prevalent in these children than in healthy children. The low oxygenation of the blood predisposes for gingival and periodontal infections. Individualized preventive programs should be instituted to reduce the risk of dental disease. Special attention should be given to children on sucrose-containing medication. If treatment becomes necessary, it should always be carried out in close cooperation with the physician. Abnormal bleeding following surgery, e.g. extractions are a risk in some children with congenital cardiac defects due to abnormalities in the coagulation system. Pain control is necessary, and local anesthesia with epinephrin can be used in adequate dosages. Preoperative sedation might be valuable to reduce fear and apprehension and minimize the risk of blood pressure rise, but must never be administered without prior consultation with the child's physician.

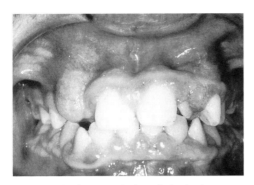

Fig. 18-2. Cyclosporin-induced gingival overgrowth and enamel hypomineralisation of the central incisors in a 13-year-old girl treated with renal transplantation.

RENAL DISORDERS

Chronic renal failure

Chronic renal failure (CRF) results from progressive and irreversible renal damage, as indicated by a reduced glomerular filtration rate. The causes of CRF include chronic glomerulonephritis, chronic pyelonephritis, congenital renal anomalies, hypersensitivity disease and diabetes. Early in the course of the disease a secondary or compensatory hyperparathyroidism develops due to the steady decline in the levels of serum calcium. CRF is initially managed by a low protein diet as the kidneys cannot efficiently excrete nitrogen wastes. Large amounts of carbohydrates are therefore needed to provide energy. If renal function deteriorates, hemodialysis should be followed, when appropriate and possible, by renal transplantation is the treatment of choice.

Frequency – About 0.04‰ of children in Sweden suffer from chronic renal failure.

Oral manifestations – Children with an early onset of the disease exhibit growth retardation and retarded tooth development. Eruption is generally not severely affected. In children with a very low glomerular filtration rate, approximately 50% show mineralization disturbances. Despite the high and frequent consumption of carbohydrates and a reduced salivary secretion rate, caries prevalence is not higher in CFR children than in healthy controls. The reasons for this may be the increased concentration of urea in saliva and a high salivary pH.

Children with CRF exhibit significantly less gingivitis than healthy children. This may be explained by the immunosuppression that leads to an inadequate inflammatory response in the gingival tissues. In children treated with renal transplantation, azathioprine and cyclosporin are the two main immunosuppressive drugs, used together with steroids to prevent graft rejection. About 30% of patients on cyclosporin develop gingival overgrowth, which is correlated to dose (Fig. 18-2). As in all immunosuppressed patients oral candidiasis may be persistent.

A triad of x-ray features of CRF children includes:

– total or partial loss of lamina dura,

– demineralization of bone and

– localized radiolucent cyst-like lesions in the jaws.

ENDOCRINE DISORDERS

Thyroid gland disorders

The main function of the thyroid gland is to synthesize thyroxine (T4) and 3,5,3,'- triiodothyronine (T3). The thyroid hormones increase oxygen consumption, stimulate protein synthesis, influence growth and dif-

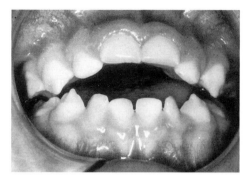

Fig. 18-3. Enamel hypoplasias in primary canines in a 3.5-year-old girl with hypopituitarism where hypothyroidism is a major feature.

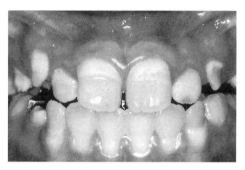

Fig. 18-4. Enamel hypoplasia in a 13-year-old girl with hypoparathyroidism.

ferentiation, and affect carbohydrate-, lipid- and vitamin-metabolism.

A disturbed function of the thyroid gland is the most common metabolic disturbance in children and young people next to diabetes. It is more common in girls than in boys.

Hypothyroidism

Hypothyroidism results from a deficient production of thyroid hormone. Congenital hypothyroidism occurs with an incidence of 1 per 3,800 - 4,000. Diagnosis is made early nowadays, due to neonatal screening programs. In juvenile hypothyroidism the deficiency may become manifest during periods of rapid growth.

Oral manifestations – Hypothyroidism results in a prolonged retention of the primary dentition and a retarded eruption of the permanent dentition. A skeletal open bite characterized by a short posterior face height and a retruded maxilla in relation to the mandible is present. An increased prevalence of enamel hypoplasia in both dentitions has been reported (Fig. 18-3).

Disorders of the parathyroid gland – When serum levels of calcium falls, secretion of parathyroid hormone (PTH) is stimulated. Production of vitamin D-metabolites increases as well as calcium absorption. PTH mobilises calcium by direct enhancement of bone resorption.

Hypoparathyroidism

Congenital aplasia or hypoplasia of the parathyroid glands or unresponsiveness of the tissues to parathyroid hormone (pseudohypoparathyroidism) leads to hypocalcemia. Muscular pain and seizures are early manifestations of hypoparathyroidism.

Oral manifestations – Enamel hypoplasia is considered to be the most characteristic oral sign of hypoparathyroid disease (Fig. 18-4). The enamel hypoplasias are often seen as narrow horizontal bands of pits and grooves transversing the crowns of the affected teeth. Delayed eruption or impaction of teeth are observed in almost all patients. Blunting of the root apices or shortened roots is another sign seen in the majority of hypoparathyroid patients.

Hyperparathyroidism

The increased production of PTH is often compensatory, aimed at correcting hypocalcemic states of diverse origins. At all ages the clinical manifestations of hypercalcemia of any cause include muscular weakness, anorexia and fever.

Oral manifestations – Withdrawal of calcium from the bones produces a triad of x-ray features:

– total or partial loss of lamina dura which is considered a pathognomonic sign of hyperparathyroidism;

– demineralization of bone with alterations in the normal trabecular pattern creating a "ground-glass" appearance, and in severe cases;

– localized radiolucent cyst-like lesions in the jaws and in the long bones.

Diabetes mellitus

This is a chronic metabolic disturbance, characterized by a decreased insulin production. There are various forms of this disease. The one that has its onset in infancy, childhood or adolescence is referred to as juvenile diabetes or Type I diabetes.

Frequency – Diabetes mellitus is a common chronic disease in childhood. Its incidence below the age of 18 varies between 1 and 3.5 per 1,000, depending on the population surveyed. In the Nordic countries, the incidence is among the highest in the world. It is somewhat more common in boys than in girls.

Etiology – More than 90% of the children with diabetes mellitus have Type I diabetes, which is insulin dependent. There is a strong genetic background to the disease, but auto-immune, as well as endocrinological factors have been discussed. Virus-infections have been mentioned as exogenous etiologic factors, but may rather act as a releasing factor of a diabetes that has been latent for some time.

Pathology – The result of the reduced or altered insulin activity leads to a rise in blood levels of glucose due to a decreased active transport of glucose across cell membranes, and a decreased conversion of glucose to its storage form in the liver. Glucosuria, due to incomplete reabsorption of glucose from the renal tubules is another effect, as well as ketonuria. The patient has a variety of symptoms including excess thirst and excess urine. Muscular weakness and weight loss are other symptoms. If untreated, the child can get into a diabetic coma.

Therapy – The treatment is mainly aimed at normalising the blood level of glucose. This is achieved by 1) insulin treatment, 2) regulation of the diet and 3) an adaption of diet and insulin treatment to the child's exercise habits.

Most children have insulin injections 3-4 times daily. The diet of the diabetic child is recommendedly low in fat and rich in fibre. The proportion of refined sugars should be low. Three main meals and 2-3 between-meals is the recommended meal pattern.

Oral complications – Several studies have shown that children with diabetes have lower salivary secretion rate and higher glucose content of saliva and gingival exsudate than healthy children. These factors are caries promoting. In spite of this, diabetic children have been shown to have a lower caries prevalence than healthy children. This is most likely an effect of the low intake of refined carbohydrates. Children with poorly controlled diabetes, a low ability to follow dietary restrictions, and a large variation in their level of blood glucose should, as a consequence, be considered at risk for dental caries.

Diabetic children with poor metabolic control have been shown to have increased gingivitis prevalence. The prevalence of periodontitis has also been shown to be higher in diabetics, with an onset in early puberty. Recent studies indicate, however, that periodontal disease in diabetic children

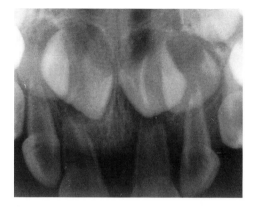

A

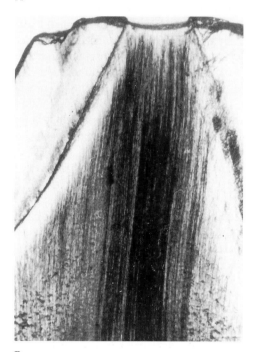

B

Fig. 18-5. 3-year-old boy with vitamin-D resistant rickets.
A. Radiograph showing large pulp chambers of upper primary incisors.
B. Microradiogram of a caries free primary molar, extracted due to apical infection. Disturbed dentine formation, large amounts of globular dentine, and tracts of giant tubules extending from pulp to enamel-dentine border. After enamel attrition, the pulp is easily infected.

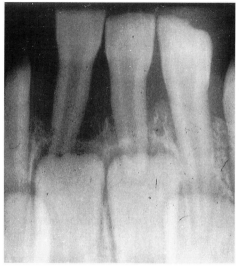

Fig. 18-6. Radiograph showing premature exfoliation of 81 in a 3-year-old boy with hypophosphatasia.

and adolescents nowadays approaches the level of healthy controls. The etiologic factor is, of course, dental plaque, but decreased resistance due to reduced chemotactic ability of the PMN-cells of the diabetic adolescent may be a contributing factor. Extra prophylaxis, including professional tooth-cleaning and a close control of periodontal health as soon as the child reaches puberty, is recommended, especially in children with a poorly controlled diabetes.

Appointments for dental treatment should be set together with parents of young children, as they know the time of the day when the blood sugar level is stable. This is often during the morning hours.

Vitamin D-resistant rickets

Vitamin D-resistant rickets (VDRR) is an inherited x-linked dominant disease, the most common form of rickets in the developed countries today, but even so very uncommon. The pathogenesis of VDRR results from a selective disorder of the trans-epithelial transport of phosphate in the kidney, leading to decreased tubular reabsorption of phosphate and persistent hypophosphatemia which, in turn, induces defective calcification.

Oral manifestations – In patients with VDRR, characteristic multiple "spontaneous" dental abscesses are frequently found. They are a result of pulp exposure which easily occurs due to the large pulp chambers usually evident on dental x-rays of these patients. An increased prevalence of enamel hypoplasia has also been observed. Histological studies often show abnormal dentine calcification (Figs. 18-5 A, B).

Hypophosphatasia

Hypophosphatasia is a rare inborn error of metabolism with a prevalence of 1 per 100,000 live births. The condition is characterized by inadequate production of serum alkaline phosphatase, elevation of phosphoethanolamine in urine, leading to defective formation of calcified tissue.

Oral manifestations – Premature exfoliation of primary teeth is found in 75% of patients with hypophosphatasia. Affected teeth are mainly incisors, where the roots show hypoplasia or aplasia of cementum (Fig. 18-6).

CHRONIC INFLAMMATORY INTESTINAL DISEASES

The two most common chronic inflammatory dieases of the intestines are Crohn's disease and ulcerative colitis. Both diseases have recently also been found in children, however rarely in preschool children.

Frequency – About 2 in 10,000 adolescents in Sweden are affected by Crohn's disease and by ulcerative colitis, respectively. The incidence of Crohn's disease was increasing up to the end of the 1970's, but is now decreasing.

Etiology – The etiology of both diseases is unknown, but there seems to be a familial disposition. Immunologic reactions of tissue-destructive type have also been mentioned.

Pathology – The diseases are characterized by a long-standing inflammation of the intestines and/or rectum. Both diseases are characterized by active phases interrupted by periods of remission. The most common symptoms are diarrhoea and abdominal pain, followed by reduced weight, fever and rectal bleeding. In more severe cases growth and development may be retarded.

Therapy – Patients with chronic inflammatory intestinal disease are recommended a high-energy diet, sometimes enriched with iron and vitamins and reduced in fat. Many patients prefer a diet free from milk-products. Anti-inflammatory drugs may be prescribed. In more severe cases, resection of part of the intestines can become necessary.

Oral complications – Patients with Crohn's disease have been shown to have a high consumption of sugar, even before the disease is diagnosed. Less milk in the diet may enhance the risk of consumption of sucrose-containing drinks as a substitute, and reduction of fat may make carbohydrate intake high. A high fibre content is sometimes negative. Abdominal pain is often relieved by small and frequent food intakes, which may increase the risk of dental caries.

An individualized program of prevention is often necessary for patients with Crohn's disease. In cooperation with the dietician and the doctor, adequate dietary advice should be given, on how to reduce the risk of dental caries without disturbing the dietary regime. Intense topical fluoride treatment should be used.

Recurrent aphtous ulcers are often seen in patients with chronic inflammatory disease and may even constitute an early sign.

MALABSORPTIONS

In malabsorption, absorption of one or more nutrients from the intestines is reduced. It appears as nutritional deficiencies or as gastro-intestinal disturbances. Examples of malabsorbtions are coeliac disease which is a general malabsorption and lactose-intolerance, a specific malabsorption. Cow milk protein intolerance is a reaction against one or more proteins in milk.

Coeliac disease

Frequency – About 1 child in 800 in Sweden and in 1,500 in Denmark and Finland are affected by coeliac disease.

Etiology – The etiology is not entirely known, but a certain heredity has been shown.

Pathology – Due to damage of the mucosa of the small intestines by gluten – the germ protein of wheat, rye, barley and oats – absorption is disturbed. The mucosa becomes swollen and the intestinal villi destroyed. The symptoms appear when the child starts to eat flour-containing food. Voluminous loose stools, diarrhoea, vomiting, irritability and failure to thrive are the classical symptoms. If no treatment is instituted, such nutritional deficiencies as anemia, rickets and bleeding follow.

Therapy – Removal of gluten from the diet leads to a complete remission of the disease, and gluten challenge will again provoke abnormal small intestinal mucosa. With adequate diet, the child starts to recover after 4-5 weeks, and after about 2 years clinical status is normalized.

Oral complications – Coeliac disease has been shown to induce mineralization disturbances of permanent teeth because of malabsorption. If the disease is diagnosed at an early age, and dietary recommendations followed, these complications will be less frequent. An association between recurrent oral ulceration (ROU) and coeliac disease has been shown, and screening for coeliac disease in patients with ROU has been suggested.

Lactose-intolerance

Malabsorption of lactose due to lack or shortage of the lactase-enzyme is more or less normal in children over the age of 5 in many parts of the world. It is becoming increasingly common in Scandinavia.

Pathology – The common symptoms are stomach pain and loose stools after intake of milk.

Therapy – Milk should be partially or completely excluded from the diet.

Oral complications – If milk is substituted with soft drinks, dietary advice should be given to avoid dental caries.

CYSTIC FIBROSIS

Cystic fibrosis (CF) is a congenital disorder with many different symptoms, caused by an abnormal viscous secretion from most exocrine glands.

Frequency – The incidence of CF is about 1 in 2,000 births. It is the most common genetic lethal disease.

Etiology – CF is genetically determined, with an autosomal recessive inheritance pattern. Normally, both parents are unaffected carriers, and the risk for any of their children developing the disease is 25%.

Pathology – The pathogenic mechanism is so far not completely understood, but believed to be mediated through an enzyme deficiency. The viscous secretion may obstruct ducts and passages in the lungs, pancreatic gland, etc. The main problems are respiratory distress with frequent airway infections and serious lung complications. Obstruction of pancreatic ducts result in enzyme deficiency and malabsorption causing reduced physical growth, vitamin deficiency and recurrent intestinal obstruction.

Therapy – No causal therapy is available, but the clearance of bronchial mucus is helped by physiotherapy and medication, while pancreatic enzyme replacement therapy and diets will improve the absorption. Therapeutic measures have, in 10 years, increased the average life span from 7.5 to 18 years.

Oral implications – Changes in salivary excretion, chronic medication and a diet rich in carbohydrates may predispose to caries, but antibiotic coverage is often frequent and children with CF have not been shown to have a higher caries prevalence than healthy children. Mouth breathing and bad oxygenation of peripheral blood may cause gingivitis. An increased prevalence of enamel disturbances has been reported, especially on incisors and first permanent molars.

IMMUNOLOGIC DISEASES

The ability of a child to resist infections is influenced by a variety of factors, specific as well as inspecific. Defects of the immune system are rare. They can be classified into primary or congenital deficiencies, secondary or acquired deficiencies and autoimmune disorders. They are all characterized by chronic or recurrent inability of the child to respond adequately to infections.

Congenital or primary immune deficiencies are due to a congenital disturbance in the differentiation of the cells that are responsible for the formation of antibodies during fetal life. Agammaglobulinemia, thymus hypoplasia and Wiscott-Aldrich's syndrome are examples of this group of diseases. Selective IgA deficiency has an incidence of 1 per 600. This deficiency is related to severe chronic diseases. Children with congenital immunodeficiencies have a greater risk of contracting auto-immune disorders.

Acquired or secondary immune deficiencies may be caused by treatment with cytotoxic drugs. It is also seen in malignant disease of the lymphoid system or after severe protein-loss, for example in the nephrotic syndrome or after severe burns.

AIDS (acquired immune deficiency syndrome)

Children are also reported as being infected with the HIV-virus, most frequently through blood transfusions (children with hemophilia A). Some have also been born with the disease. In this disease that disrupts the T-cells, the cellbound immunity is seriously diminished and the patients die of opportunistic infections.

Oral manifestations of immunologic disorders. The oral symptoms in patients with immune deficiencies, either primary or secondary, may vary. In general they have a high prevalence of bacterial, viral or fungal

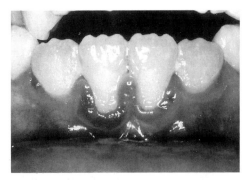

Fig. 18-7. Ulcerations in the marginal gingiva in a 7-year-old boy with an IgA-deficiency.

infections, as well as ulcerations of the oral mucosa (Fig. 18-7). As in children treated with cytotoxic drugs, the primary and most important aim is to prevent oral infection.

All kinds of dental treatment should be carried out in close cooperation with the physician. Gammaglobulin therapy might be necessary. The oral mucosa is vulnerable, and careful, but meticulous, oral hygiene is essential.

Auto-immune disorders

Auto-immune disorders include asthma/ allergy, juvenile rheumatoid arthritis (JRA), *lupus erythematosus disseminatus* (LED) and dermatomyositis. Auto-immunity is the production of antibodies that react with normal cells in the tissues in response to mutation, neoplasm or organism-tissue cross-reaction.

Asthma /allergy
Allergy is by far the most common type of immunologically mediated disease and affects about 10% of all children.

Asthma
Asthma is generally defined as a condition characterized by constriction of the bronchial muscles, edema of the bronchial mucosa and increased secretion within the airways. Extrinsic or allergic asthma is the type most commonly seen in children and young adults.

Frequency – The prevalence is about 1.5%.

Pathology – In asthma in children, allergic hypersensitivity is the main etiologic factor. The interaction between the antigen and the IgE antibodies leads to the release of such humoral mediators as histamine.

Therapy – Adrenergic β2-receptor stimulants (salbutamol, terbutaline, fenoterol) and theophyllamine are the most important drugs in the treatment of asthma. These agents with a β2-selectivity are given locally as inhalers and provide an effective bronchodilatation. Sodium cromoglycate is used for prophylaxis and inhibits release of inflammatory mediators from mast cells. The effect of corticosteroids is mediated by specific proteins inhibiting the prostaglandin synthesis.

Oral manifestations – Asthmatic children have been shown to have a reduced salivary secretion rate compared with healthy children. Recent studies have compared caries prevalence in asthmatic children and healthy controls, but the results are contradictory. Asthmatic children treated with corticosteroids have an increased prevalence of gingivitis compared with healthy children. The use of corticosteroid inhalers has also been shown to predispose to the development of oropharyngeal infection with *Candida albicans*.

Due to the frequent use of various drugs and the reduced salivary flow rate, children with asthma should be given individualized programs of prevention.

Juvenile rheumatoid arthritis
Rheumatic diseases are caused by an autoimmune reaction. The process is started when a genetically predisposed individual is exposed to an environmental factor, most

often an infection or a virus. The rheumatic diseases affect joints, tendons, muscles and sometimes also internal organs, skin and mucosa.

When rheumatoid arthritis is present in a child below the age of 16, it is referred to as the juvenile form (JRA). It differs in many respects from rheumatoid arthritis seen in adults and the manifestations also vary in children.

Frequency – The incidence of the disease is 10-15 per 100,000 children.

Pathology – The etiologic factors are not known, but as mentioned above, JRA is an auto-immune disorder, more common in children with a congenital deficiency of IgA and IgG.

If pain, swelling and edema in a joint persists for more than 3 months, arthritis should be suspected. A positive rheuma-factor is not always found in the blood. There are various forms of the disease, depending upon the presence of the various symptoms and how many joints are involved. In some children, iridocyclitis (inflammation of the iris and uvea) is present, and growth disturbances may be seen, particularly in the affected joints.

Therapy – With adequate treatment, 50% of JRA patients can recover completely without any permanent marks, and another 30-40% can recover with only a slight handicap. The treatment is, however, extremely important, and is usually a combination of physiotherapy, pharmacology and, in rare cases, surgery. Pharmacological treatment is usually started with salicylates, and if these fail, corticosteroids or, in severe cases, cytotoxic drugs are given. Physiotherapy with training of the joints and strengthening of the muscles can give good results.

Oral manifestations – Children with JRA have a higher risk of developing mandibu-

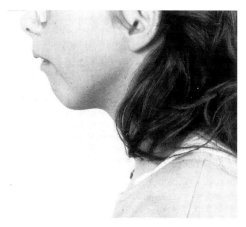

Fig. 18-8. Profile of a 13-year-old girl with juvenile rheumatoid arthritis since the age of 6.

lar dysfunction than healthy children. Common symptoms are clickings and crepitation in the TM joints and difficulties in opening the mouth wide. This may make tooth cleaning more difficult. If the hands are affected by the disease, special aids may be needed (Chapter 19). The prevalence of postnormal occlusion and frontal open bite is higher than in healthy children, due to a rotational change of the corpus (Fig. 18-8).

The treatment includes occlusal adjustment and therapeutic exercises. Treatment with functional appliances has also been recommended.

BLEEDING DISORDERS

Bleeding disorders are caused by a disturbance in normal hemostasis. They can be seen as coagulation disorders or disorders of the platelets, either as thrombocytopenia or as platelet dysfunction. The coagulation disorders are caused by a congenital or acquired lack of one or more of the coagulation factors known today. The most common forms are hemophilia A and B and von Willebrand's disease.

Hemophilia A and B.
von Willebrand's disease

Frequency – About 1 child per 10,000 in Sweden suffers from a coagulation disorder.

Etiology – Hemophilia A and hemophilia B are caused by a lack of Factor VIII and Factor IX respectively. Both are genetically determined and the inheritance pattern is X-linked recessive. Thus, the children of a woman who is a carrier of the disease will get the disease in 50% of cases if they are boys, while 50% of the daughters will be carriers. The children of a man with the disease will be healthy, while all his daughters will be carriers.

Von Willebrand's disease is characterized by a deficiency or defect in the plasma protein, von Willebrand Factor, that together with Factor VIII is necessary for normal thrombocyte-function and coagulation. It is usually transmitted as an autosomal dominant trait, and can thus be inherited by 50% of the children, boys and girls alike, of an affected parent. It is often a moderately severe hemorrhagic disorder.

Pathology – There are severe, moderate and mild forms of hemophilia, representing a factor content in plasma of < 1%, 1-4% and 5-25%. Children with the mild form only suffer from prolonged bleeding after surgery or major trauma, while the other forms are increasingly severe.

The tendency to bleed often becomes obvious by the end of the first year of life, as these children bruise easily. External bleeding from trauma to the skin or mucosa are less of a problem, but bleedings in the mouth or in the nose may be difficult to stop. A far greater problem is internal bleeding in the muscles or joints, where particularly the latter may cause deformities later in life. Intracranial hemorrhage can cause a life-threatening situation.

Therapy – Bleeding can be treated or prevented by intravenous infusion of factor concentrate once or more per week. Exercise programs and physiotherapy aim at minimizing joint damage.

Oral complications – The bleeding disorders in themselves do not affect dental health, but it is of utmost importance that oral tissues are kept healthy to minimize the need for invasive dental procedures. Preventive programs should therefore be instituted early and carefully supervised. Brushing with a soft toothbrush and careful flossing will result in firm, healthy gingiva and reduce episodes of spontaneous bleeding.

Supragingival scaling can usually be carried out without factor replacement, but deep scaling and the use of local anesthetics requires consultation with the physician. Surgery, e.g. tooth extraction, requires careful planning and should always be referred to a specialist; screening of the present bleeding status is advocated. Today, it can often be safely undertaken with no or very little Factor VIII substitution, provided that strict attention is paid to local hemostatic measures, systemic anti-fibrinolytic treatment and prevention of infection.

Platelet disorders

Platelets are necessary for blood coagulation and for clot formation. Qualitative defects in the function of the platelets are rare in children. Thrombocytopenia caused by a lack of platelets is rather common in children, most often appearing before the age of 12. The most common form is acute thrombocytopenia that often appears after an infection, and is most likely due to an immunologic disturbance. The prognosis is good, with recovery within about 3 months, even without any therapy.

Chronic idiopathic thrombocytopenic purpura is a rare disease, that may last

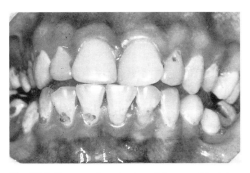

Fig. 18-9. Rampant caries in a 16-year-old girl treated with irradiation against the right side of the neck. No precautions were taken to prevent dental decay during treatment.

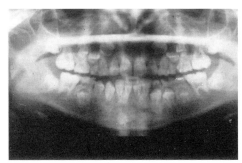

Fig. 18-10. Disturbances in dental development in an 8-year-old girl treated with 10 Gy total body irradiation at 2 years of age. Note short v-shaped roots.

throughout life. Like acute thrombocytopenia, it is characterized by a short life span of the platelets.

Pathology – When the platelet count drops below 20-30,000 x 10^9 per litre, bleeding may occur, predominantly in the skin, as ecchymoses and petechiae.

Therapy – Treatment with corticosteroids is the most common therapy.

Oral complications – Oral findings include petechiae and ecchymoses, and bleeding if the disease is severe. In children with acute thrombocytopenia, operative treatment should, if possible, be postponed until after recovery. In children with the chronic form, platelet transfusions may be used in an acute situation, but usually efforts should be made to increase the platelet level by corticosteroid treatment preoperatively.

MALIGNANT TUMORS

Cancer is the most common lethal disease in children. Malignant tumors constitute two thirds of cancer cases and leukemia the rest. About 1 per 600 children below the age of 15 is affected by malignant tumors each year. Tumors of the CNS, tumors in the kidneys and malignant lymphomas are the dominating forms, but also bone tumors like osteogenic sarcoma, Ewing's sarcoma and eosinophilic granuloma are found in children.

Malignant tumors in children are most common during the first five years of life, with the exception of bone tumors that are more often seen after the age of 10.

The etiology is nearly always unknown, but brothers and sisters of a child with cancer are more at risk.

Children with cancer are treated with chemotherapy sometimes in combination with surgery and/or radiation therapy. If irradiation is directed against head or neck, destruction of the salivary glands can give pathological oral conditions with an extreme reduction of salivary secretion, and an increased risk for dental caries (Fig. 18-9). If irradiation is given to children with developing teeth, these may become affected resulting in short V-shaped roots, enamel hypoplasias etc (Fig. 18-10). Use of irradiation in children is now greatly reduced.

Other oral complications, like ulceration and oral infections are similar in patients with leukemia and other malignancies, as are the principles for treatment.

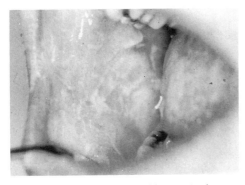

Fig. 18-11. Atrophic lichenoid lesions in the buccal mucosa of a 16-year-old boy with a severe graft-versus-host disease after allogeneic bone marrow transplantation.

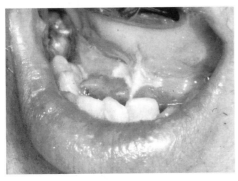

Fig. 18-12. Methotrexate-induced sublingual ulceration in a 19-year-old boy with acute lymphoblastic leukemia.

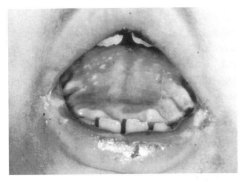

Fig. 18-13. Radiation-induced mucositis and angular cheilitis in a 7-year-old boy with acute lymphoblastic leukemia.

LEUKEMIA

Leukemia is characterized by an uncontrolled proliferation of the leukocytes and their precursors in bone marrow, blood and reticuloendothelial tissues, that are invaded by immature blood cells. It is the most common form of malignant disease in children below the age of 15. Acute lymphoblastic leukemia (ALL) is the dominating form, accounting for more than 75-80% of the cases. Also acute myelogenous leukemia (AML) is seen in children.

Frequency – Each year, about 60-70 children in Sweden get leukemia. The majority are between 1 and 5 years of age.

Etiology – The etiology of the disease is unknown, but viral, as well as genetic factors have been discussed.

Pathology – The symptoms of the disease include anemia, weakness and fatigue and sometimes fever. Petechiae, ecchymoses and bruises even after minor traumas can be seen due to thrombocytopenia. The granulocytopenia causes an increased tendency to infections. Pain in legs and arms due to leukemic infiltrations in the skeleton are not uncommon. If no treatment is instituted, death occurs in about four months, due to bleeding or infection.

Therapy – Leukemia is treated with cytotoxic drugs in various combinations, with steroids and sometimes with irradiation. The goal is to eliminate leukemic cells from the body. Various drugs, routes of administration and protocols have been tried and are currently under evaluation. With this treatment, the long-term survival rate may be 55 to 60% in children with ALL.

Cytotoxic drugs not only affect leukemic cells, but also such rapidly dividing cells as those in the bone marrow, gastro-intestinal tract and hair follicles. The treatment causes

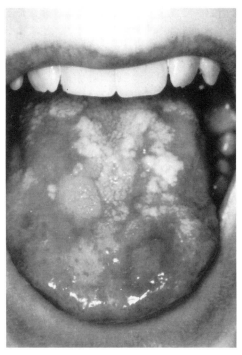

Fig. 18-14. Oral candidiasis and reactivation of herpes simplex virus infection in a 13-year-old boy with acute lymphoblastic leukemia treated with chemotherapy.

thrombocytopenia, as well as granulocytopenia and, as a consequence, a great risk of infection, the risk being highest when the granulocyte count decreases below 1,000 per ml. Under certain conditions, bone marrow transplantation can be performed when the child has an HLA-identical sibling (Fig. 18-11).

Oral complications – A child with leukemia can have early symtoms from the oral cavity, with mucosal pallor as a sign of anemia, petechiae and ecchymoses as signs of thrombocytopenia and leukemic infiltrations seen as hypertrophy of the gingiva. Fungal infections can be present.

When the treatment with cytotoxic drugs starts, these have a direct toxic effect on the oral mucosa. Painful ulcerations in the buc-cae, under and on the tongue, on the lips and in the palate may appear. Petechiae and ecchymoses are often present, and angular cheilitis can be seen. Candidiasis and reactivation of herpes simplex virus infections are frequently found (Figs. 18-12, 13, 14).

Extremely careful oral hygiene is important to avoid infection. Before treatment with cytotoxic drugs is instituted, the child should be seen by a dentist, a thorough clinical and x-ray examination should be performed, and necessary dental treatment accomplished. Fillings and teeth should be carefully polished, as even a minor trauma can give rise to painful ulcers, due to the extreme vulnerability of the oral mucosa during cytotoxic treatment.

The patient should brush carefully with an extra soft toothbrush, and food like crispbread should be avoided. Rinses with chlorhexidine should only be used when all other forms of oral hygiene are impossible, as chlorhexidine may change the ecology of the oral cavity, favouring pathogenic microorganisms.

Children treated with chemotherapy during periods of tooth development have a higher risk of tooth developmental disturbances, like enamel hypoplasias or disturbances of tooth morphology.

CONVULSIVE DISORDERS

Convulsions are among the most common acute and potentially life-threatening events encountered in infants and children. About 5% of children have had one or more convulsions by the time they reach maturity.

Epilepsy

Epilepsy refers to recurrent seizures either of unknown etiology (idiopathic) or due to congenital or acquired brain lesions (secondary). Epileptic seizures reflect abnormal

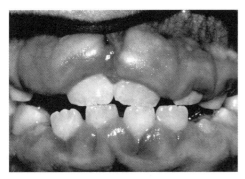

Fig. 18-15. Phenytoin-induced gingival overgrowth in a 9-year-old girl with epilepsy.

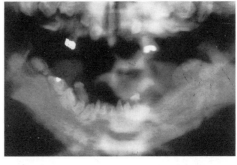

Fig. 18-16. Panoramic radiograph of a 13-year-old girl with osteopetrosis. The tooth-germs are severely defect. The mandible shows signs of osteomyelitis.

electrical activity in cerebral neurons. The normal balance between excitatory and inhibitory influences on the activity of nerve cells seems to be disrupted.

Frequency – The incidence of idiopathic epilepsy ranges from 2-6 per 1,000.

Pathology – The manifestations of epilepsy range from short absences or petit mal epilepsy to grand mal epilepsy. In petit mal epilepsy, the absences are often so short that they go unnoticed by the patient. In grand mal epilepsy, seizures are generalized, the patient becomes unconscious and muscle spasms occur. Grand mal epilepsy may have its onset at any age from infancy to early adult life. In the young child, the first convulsions are often triggered by fever. In some instances, seizures may be triggered by such specific activities as reading or exposure to a specific sound pattern.

Therapy – The treatment of epilepsy is long term anticonvulsant drug therapy. Four major preparations are available: phenobarbitol, phenytoin, carbamazepine and valproic acid. In grand mal epilepsy, phenytoin and carbamazepine are the drugs of choice.

Oral manifestations – Most patients on phenytoin medication exhibits gingival overgrowth of varying degree. The clinical appearance varies between a minor increase of the marginal gingiva to severe overgrowth with gingival tissue covering the whole clinical crown of the tooth (Fig. 18-15).

Treatment – The development of phenytoin-induced gingival overgrowth can be minimized and sometimes nearly totally prevented by plaque control. This program should be instituted before the start of phenytoin medication, and then individualised depending on the degree of gingival overgrowth that may develop. In mentally retarded children where oral hygiene is not optimal, a rather conservative approach to surgical removal of gingival overgrowth is recommended because of the high risk of reoccurrence.

SKELETAL DISEASES

Skeletal diseases are a heterogenous group of disorders comprising malformations of bones as well as abnormalities and diseases of bone tissue. The etiology includes genetic factors, endocrinologic factors, nutritional deficiencies, intoxications, infections and neoplasms.

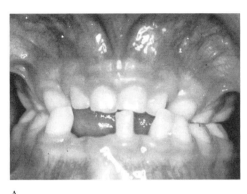
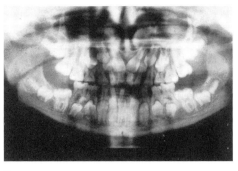

A

B

Fig. 18-17. An 11-year-old girl with cleidocranial dysostosis A) clinical appearance B) panoramic radiograph showing lack of eruption of permanent teeth and presence of supernumerary teeth in regio 35 and 45.

Malformations of bones

Developmental disturbances in bone morphology may affect all bones. In most cases the etiology is unknown. Of special odontological interest are the cranial anomalies, which are often part of a syndrome. These anomalies may be mediated through early closure of cranial sutures (e.g. oxycephalus), increased size of the brain (e.g. hydrocephalus) or reduced size of the brain case (e.g. cerebral hypoplasia).

Abnormalities and diseases of bone tissues

These disorders comprise quantitative (e.g. osteoporosis, osteopetrosis, Paget's disease) or qualitative aberrations in bone matrix production (e.g. osteogenesis imperfecta) or mineralization (e.g. rickets). Some of the disorders with oral implications will be shortly described.

Osteopetrosis

Osteopetrosis is characterized by a general increase in bone density due to a defect in bone resorption. The patients may suffer

from bone pain, fractures and osteomyelitis. In severe cases cranial neuropathias are seen (e.g. optic atrophy). There is bone marrow replacement and anemia. Treatment may include corticosteroids and bone marrow transplants.

Oral complications – Tooth eruption is strongly disturbed and also retarded (Fig. 18-16). The risk of osteomyelitis and fractures are complicating factors in tooth extractions. These patients also suffer from trigeminal and facial neuropathias.

Osteogenesis imperfecta

Osteogenesis imperfecta is a group of autosomal dominantly inherited disorders of the connective tissue, usually involving the skeleton, sclera, ligaments, tendons and ear. Dentinogenesis imperfecta (Types II/III) may be simultaneously present. A more detailed description of osteogenesis imperfecta is given in Chapter 19.

Cleidocranial dysostosis

This disease is an example of genetically determined bone disorders. It is a defect mainly of membrane bone formation, often inherited as an autosomal dominant trait, and involving mainly the skull and clavicles. The middle facial third is hypoplastic, leading to a relative mandibular protrusion. The clavicles are absent or defect. There may be persistence of primary teeth and unerupted permanent teeth, in addition to many supernumerary teeth (Figs. 18-17 A, B).

CHROMOSOMAL ABERRATIONS

Chromosomal aberrations are deviations in numbers of chromosomes (hyper-/hypoploidy) or in their gross morphology (deletions, duplications, translocations).

Etiology – Chromosomal aberrations arise during meiotic division in egg formation. Prevalences increase with the age of the mother. Radiation and other teratogenic agents are known to cause chromosomal aberrations.

Pathology – Lack, surplus or ectopic location of a genetic material in the genome seem to have a profound influence on the developing fetus. Thus, they are a common cause of spontaneous abortions and of early neonatal death. Sex chromosome anomalies are ususaly compatible with life and rarely associated with severe physical disability, while the autosomal abnormalities often are lethal. However, anomalies of the smaller chromosomes may be compatible with life, but cause multiple handicaps. Most important are the mental retardations and the heart failures.

Down's syndrome

Down's syndrome, mongolism, is the most prevalent of the chromosomal aberrations. In 95% of cases there is a free extra chromosome (trisomy 21). The rest have the additional chromosome attached to another chromosome (translocation). Patients with Down's syndrome have several aberrant features as reduced height, small head, short neck, round flat face, short hands etc. There is a muscle hypotonia and a hypermobility of the joints. Death at an early age is common, often caused by congenital cardiac failure or respiratory tract infection. Patients with Down's syndrome also have a low resistance to infections and a high incidence of leukemia. The syndrome is associated with mild to severe mental retardation.

Oral manifestations – Children with Down's syndrome may have an underdeveloped maxilla, which contributes to a relative mandibular protrusion, an anterior open bite and posterior crossbite (Figs. 18-18 A, B). Due to low muscle tone of the lips, they may have an open mouth posture and a protruding tongue. Drooling is sometimes a problem. Hypodontia and a tooth morphology characterized by a small mesio-distal crown diameter resulting in dental spacing, may account for the low caries prevalence seen in children with Down's syndrome compared to healthy children. A delay in tooth eruption may also contribute to the difference noted in caries prevalence between children with Down's syndrome and healthy children.

An early onset of periodontal disease is associated with the syndrome, sometimes evident already in the primary dentition. The disease is severe with a rapid progression, and often localized to the lower incisor region. Many factors have been claimed to be responsible. Besides the common exogenous factors like plaque and calculus, an altered constitution of the connective tissue, functional defects of the granulocytes and monocytes have been mentioned. In combination with a poor oral hygiene, these factors may be responsible for the early onset

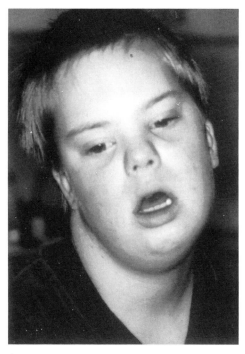

A

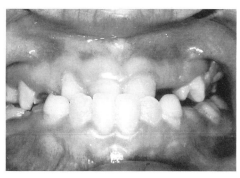

B

Fig. 18-18. A) An 11-year-old boy with Down's syndrome, and B) anterior and posterior cross-bite.

and rapid progression of periodontal disease in Down's syndrome.

To keep the periodontal tissues as healthy as possible, individualized programs of prevention should be instituted.

The most prevalent of the chromosomal aberrations are:

Autosomal aberrations:

Trisomy 21 (Down)	1/700
Trisomy 18 (Edward)	1/8,000

Sex chromosome aberrations:

XYY	1/1,000
XXY (Klinefelter)	1/1,000
XO (Turner)	1/10,000
XXX	1/1,000

Viral hepatitis

Hepatitis B virus (HBV) infection is increasing in prevalence and can present an infective risk in dental practice.

The hepatitis non-A, non-B viruses are the most common cause of post-transfusion hepatitis and high risk carriers are the same as in HBV.

Spread is mainly parenterally (via blood or blood products), sexually, and perinatally. HBV antigens have also been identified in saliva, but the infectivity is generally low because of low antigen titers. Most patients who have been affected by hepatitis recover completely, but about 5% are infectious. Children born to mothers with active infection remain infectious.

TABLE **18-1**

Hepatitis B high risk groups:

Patients requiring blood transfusions;
Patients with a recent history of jaundice;
Patients in institutions for mentally
    retarded;
Certain groups of immigrants from
    the Third World;
Intravenous drug abusers;
Homosexual males.

Frequency – Less than 1% of the general population in Western Europe are positive for hepatitis B surface antigen, compared with 15-20% in South-East Asia, or even higher in some of these countries.

Infectivity – Several patient and population-groups considered to be at high risk of carrying HBV have been identified, among them certain groups of immigrant children and adopted children from the Middle East, Africa and South East Asia (Table 18-1). Children, who after arrival in Scandinavia have been shown to be HBV carriers, go to school and have no restrictions on their daily life.

Precautions should, however, always be taken in the dental treatment of these children, specially if invasive surgery is planned. As an indication of the degree of infectious risk, blood markers are used. These markers are antigens or antibodies, and to be able to evaluate the infectious risk, knowledge of the respective type is important. The main danger for the dentist comes from needle-stick injuries when treating an infected patient.

Background literature

Friis-Hansen B (ed). *Nordisk lærebog i pædiatri.* København: Munksgaard, 1985.

Scully C, Cawson RA. *Medical problems in dentistry.* Bristol: Wright, 1982.

Scully C. *The mouth and perioral tissues.* Clinical dentistry in health and disease. Series 2. Oxford: Heinemann Medical, 1989.

Thompson JS, Thomson MW. *Genetics in medicine.*, Philadelphia: Saunders, 1980.

Thornton JB, Wright JT. *Special and medically compromised patients in dentistry.* Massachusetts: PSG Publishing, 1989.

CHAPTER 19

DENTISTRY WITH HANDICAPPED CHILDREN

Epidemiology

Handicapped children in society

Risk factors

Neuropsychological disabilities

Sensory disabilities

Physical disabilities

Prevention

Children with chronic diseases or with congenital or acquired conditions interfering with normal physical and/or mental development are often defined as disabled or handicapped. While Chapter 18 has concentrated on children with chronic diseases this chapter will describe a number of other disabling conditions and the particular dental problems associated with them.

EPIDEMIOLOGY

The incidence of children with disabilities is unclear since there is a vague borderline between normal function and disability. It has been estimated that 3 to 3.5% of children in the Nordic countries aged 0-15 years have a chronic disease or a long-standing disability. In Sweden in 1981 the number of children aged 0-19 years who were severely disabled was estimated at 15:1000.

Handicap is a disadvantage for a given individual, resulting from an impairment or a disability that limits or prevents the fulfilment of a role that is normal for that individual. Disability is any restriction or lack of ability (resulting from an impairment) to perform an activity in the manner or within the range considered normal for a human being, whereas impairment is any loss or abnormality of psychological, physiological, or anatomical structure or function.

Hence disability represents a departure from the norm in terms of individual performance, whilst handicap is a social phenomenon, representing the social and environmental consequences for the individual stemming from the presence of *impairment and disability*(1).

The concepts can be integrated in the following manner:

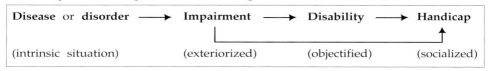

Disease or disorder ⟶	Impairment ⟶	Disability ⟶	Handicap
(intrinsic situation)	(exteriorized)	(objectified)	(socialized)

At any stage, medical, educational, social, psychological and dental intervention, can be utilized to minimize the disadvantage for the individual.

HANDICAPPED CHILDREN IN SOCIETY

When a disabled child is born into a family, or when a previously healthy child becomes chronically ill or disabled, the whole family is affected. Feelings of guilt, anger, remorse, grief, helplessness and uncertainty are all common in parents. Implications for family life vary with the actual condition, but in most cases there will be increased emotional and physical, as well as financial, strain. Many parents, mostly mothers, have to abandon or reduce their own professional aspirations because the disabled child needs more and longer-lasting care than a healthy child. The relationship between the parents and their behavior towards the disabled child's siblings, family and friends may be influenced in various ways. Parents of disabled children will often have little or no time for leisure and social activity. Whilst burdens of child caring decrease as healthy children become more independent, many disabled children demand more extensive care as they grow older.

Children with disabilities are aware from an early age of being different. Full understanding of their different life situation emerges around the age of 9-10 years. This can be recognized as mental depression in the disabled child, not normally seen in children of this age. During adolescence, disabled children may pass through periods of neglecting necessary treatment and reacting to being "different" in various ways. Lately it has been recognized that some disabled children need psychological assistance to be able to handle this developmental crisis.

Multiprofessional cooperation

A family with a disabled child may have to cooperate with many different health professionals (Fig. 19-1). Parents often experience lack of coordination between the different services so that they may have to make many separate visits for various kinds of examinations and treatment. Many parents have, therefore, expressed the need for coordination of services and better multiprofessional cooperation. Visits to the physiotherapist might be combined with consultation with the speech therapist and regular dental prophylaxis could perhaps be performed at the same time as a visit to the health nurse. In fact, dental health personnel could profit from closer cooperation with most of the agencies shown in Fig. 19-1.

Early contact is essential to prevent dental disease in most disabled children. Many agencies could refer patients to the dental team earlier if they had some knowledge of the oral problems in various disabling conditions. However, many health workers have little information about the dental health consequences of various conditions, treatments and medications. Therefore, few disabled children are ever referred to a dentist unless there is dental pain.

In the treatment of disabled children the dental team is one of many around the child and his/her family. Besides knowledge about special dental and general health problems associated with a certain condition, our own reactions to disability and disfigurement are important to understand. Therefore, therapy planning either in a multiprofessional group or within the group of dental personnel may include discussions concerning our attitudes as professional helpers.

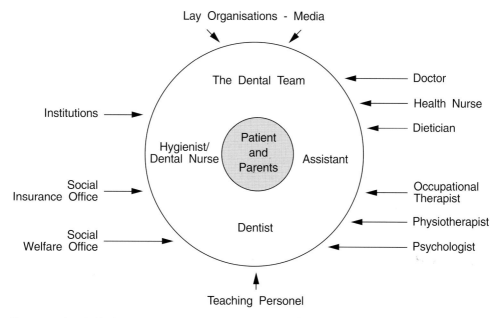

Fig. 19-1. The child, the dental team and possible co-workers.

RISK FACTORS

Certain factors may make disabled children more at risk for dental problems than healthy children.

Diet – Many parents experience difficulties feeding a child with sucking or chewing problems due to such conditions as congenital heart disease, facial clefts, oesophageal defects, generalized hypotonia, muscular dysfunction or mental retardation. Each meal may last an hour or more. Liquid or soft cariogenic foods are common. Food is often retained in the mouth for a long time before it is swallowed. Some children may also ruminate. In certain conditions, where a high calory diet is needed, frequent meals are recommended.

Many disabled children have chronic constipation or diarrhoea. Sweet remedies are often used to cure such conditions: prunes, or dried fruit in the former case, cola drinks and blueberry juice in the latter.

Frequent intake of beverages is often recommended for children on medication to avoid kidney damage. To make them drink enough, the parents often have to resort to sugar-containing drinks.

Muscular function – Hypotonia or pareses may influence salivation, cause drooling, chewing problems, retention of food and reduced self-cleaning of the oral cavity. It may also make tooth cleaning difficult.

Hyperfunction may result in extensive tooth wear due to grinding of teeth (bruxism). This is often seen in spastic cerebral palsy and in some children with mental retardation.

Oral hygiene problems may be experienced by parents of mentally retarded or autistic children in particular and also in many spastic patients.

Medication – Long-term use of sweetened medicines may represent a hazard to dental health. Various drugs may also reduce salivation and, thereby, increase susceptibility to caries.

NEUROPSYCHOLOGICAL DISABILITIES

Coping with conditions which interfere with a child's intellectual development are often a great challenge to the dental profession. The most common neuropsychological disabilities are described on the following pages.

Childhood autism

Autistic children are a very heterogeneous group and many different criteria have been used to describe them. It is usually not possible to confirm the diagnosis before the age of 1½ years. The symptoms are often first interpreted as sight or hearing impairment. Autistic children are frequently considered to be mentally retarded because of their lack of communication skills. However, the intellectual capacity of autistic children varies widely. An autistic child avoids contact, does not like to be fondled, does not look you in the eye. Self-stimulation, stereotype movements and repetitive words are frequent features of this condition. Any change in routines or surroundings may trigger fear and aggression. The following diagnostic criteria are internationally accepted: a) debut of symptoms before 2½ years of age; b) serious defect in ability to establish and keep social contact; c) problems with verbal communication; d) weird language, if any; e) absence of hallucinations.

Frequency – Childhood autism appears with a frequency of 2-5 in 10,000 children in Europe and North-America. There are more autistic boys than girls. The reasons for the condition are considered to be of organic/ biologic origin, but the mechanisms are hitherto unknown.

Special considerations for dental care – All children with autism may react negatively to new situations and abrupt changes in routines. Therefore, dental care should be planned longterm and in close cooperation with parents and teachers. Early introduction of toothcleaning routines, frequent visits (4-6 times per year) to the same dental office and minimal change of personnel are important factors for good cooperation with an autistic child.

Dental treatment may be very difficult to perform and sedation with benzodiazepines or nitrous oxide often has little effect. A careful recording of the child's special phobias (cotton rolls, strong smells, etc.) and favourite activities (music, playing with water, touching special fabrics) may make it easier to perform necessary preventive and curative treatment. General anesthesia for dental treatment should, if possible, be avoided as some parents have reported loss of elaborately acquired skills in their autistic child after general anesthesia.

Mental retardation

Mental retardation (MR) can be defined as a deficiency in theoretical intelligence which is congenital or acquired in early life. The consequences of MR depend on demands and conditions in the society. Hence, more persons may be considered lacking in intellectual ability in a complex industrialized society than in regions where life is "simpler".

Frequency – The incidence of MR in a country is, therefore, difficult to assess. If one accepts that it can be difficult to function in Nordic societies for a person with the intellectual ability of a child below 11 years of age, the prevalence of MR in the Nordic countries will be 1-3%.

Level of understanding

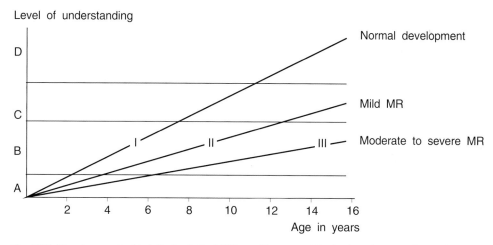

Fig. 19-2. Development of intellectual disabilities with age and limitations in mental retardation.

Etiology – Many different pre-, peri- and postnatal factors may lead to MR, but prenatal causes dominate (90%): a) dominant hereditary conditions which may comprise mental retardation are: myotonic dystrophy, neurofibromatosis, Sturge Weber's syndrome and tuberous sclerosis; b) recessive hereditary conditions may also cause MR, for example mucopolysaccharidoses and Fragile-X syndrome; c) chromosomal aberrations like Down's syndrome; d) infections (rubella, toxoplasmosis), intoxication (alcohol, drugs, pregnancy-intoxication), irradiation, malnutrition and trauma are other prenatal causes of MR.

Perinatal factors like trauma, lack of oxygen during birth or extreme prematurity comprise 5% of cases.

Postnatal factors like infections (meningitis, encephalitis), intoxication, trauma and tumours account for another 5%.

Levels of MR

Intellectual ability – Comparing the intellectual ability of a mentally retarded child with that of other children according to Kylén and co-workers(2,3), levels of understanding can be divided into four sections (Fig. 19-2): A, B, C and D. On Level A there is very limited understanding of pictures and words. On Level B there is a certain understanding of own experiences only. On Level C a more general, but limited, understanding of reality is achieved. On Level D the child starts developing more advanced theoretical abilities. The average child will function approximately on Level A until 2 years of age, on Level B until around 7 years, on Level C until 11 years and on Level D for the rest of his/her life. A child with mild mental retardation will remain on Level C all his life, while the more severely mentally retarded never will pass Level B.

Mild MR (Level C) may not be detected before school age. Such children can normally manage quite well in daily life, but will often have problems with school performance. There may also be behavioral disturbances.

The moderate to severe MR (Level B) will have symptoms of slow mental and motor development from an early age. Most children with Down's syndrome fall into this category.

Medical complications – Mentally retarded children may have cerebral palsy, epilepsy,

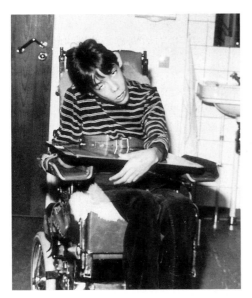

Fig. 19-3. Spastic CP-boy with severe motor handicap.

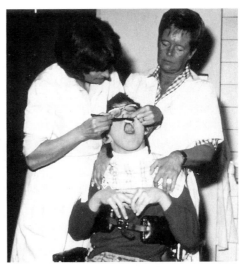

Fig. 19-4. Problems related to oral hygiene.

sensory defects and congenital deformities like heart-disease. There may also be severe speech difficulties and behavioral aberrations. Some mentally retarded children show "autistic tendencies" without being classified as autistic. In recent years, two mental retardation syndromes with behavior similar to children with autism have been described: Fragile-x syndrome which mainly affects boys and Rett syndrome where only girls are affected.

Special considerations for dental care – All new procedures should be started slowly and one should try to concentrate on communicating directly with the child, not through the accompanying adult. Although communication skills are limited, many are very sensitive to body language and voice sounds, and most will react positively to a warm and friendly atmosphere.

Oral manifestations – Many mentally retarded children will have hypomineralized teeth, malocclusion and hypodontia.

It is well documented that children with

Down's syndrome often have small teeth with short roots, hypodontia and Class III malocclusion (hypoplastic middle face with small maxilla). Rapid development of periodontal disease with loss of teeth at a young age due to reduced resistance to infections has also been reported (Chapters 13, 18).

Tooth grinding and drooling are problems reported frequently by parents of MR children. Feeding and toothbrushing difficulties are also common.

Cerebral palsy

Cerebral palsy (CP) is a chronic condition in the neuromuscular system resulting from early brain damage. The origin may be prenatal, perinatal or postnatal: before the CNS has reached relative maturity.

CP is characterized by spasticity (increased muscular tone), paresis (decreased muscular strength), dyskinesia or atethosis (involuntary movements), tremor (trembling) and/or rigidity (stiffness). A symptom can occur alone or in combination with one or several of the others.

Frequency – The incidence of CP in the Nordic countries is approximately 1.7:1000, and 85% of the patients are spastic. Half of all CP cases have a slight motor handicap, 25% have a medium motor handicap and will need some help in everyday living. The remaining 25% have a severe motor handicap which means that they need help with almost everything (Figs. 19-3, 19-4).

Medical complications – Severe mental retardation is seen in 15% and light to moderate mental retardation in 10% of children with CP. More than 30% have problems with speech. It is important to remember that defective speech is not synonymous with mental retardation.

The frequency of epilepsy in CP children is about 10%. Failing sight and other visual or auditory defects are seen in 6% of the cases. Drooling is a common complication, and eating and drinking problems occur.

Medical treatment – Treatment consists of physiotherapy, orthopaedic treatment and surgical procedures. Occupational therapy is very important, because correct use of special equipment like wheelchairs, eating appliances, and in some cases a computer for communicating, will make life much easier.

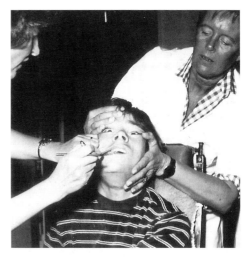

Fig. 19-5. Spastics may need help to hold the head in position during examination and treatment.

Oral manifestations – Mineralization defects and delayed eruption of permanent teeth have been reported in CP children.

Occlusal attrition can be extensive, especially in patients with athetosis. CP children have a lower DMFS score than healthy children.

Defective muscular function and coordination often reduces the possibility of maintaining an adequate oral hygiene (Fig. 19-5) and severely handicapped CP patients have a high frequency of gingivitis.

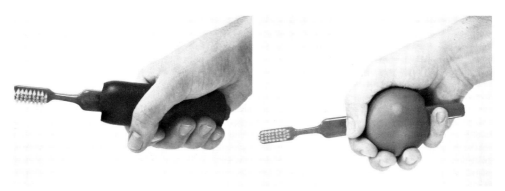

Fig. 19-6. To ensure a firm grip, the handle of the tooth brush may be modified by adding a foam rubber or isopore grip, or by a rubber ball.

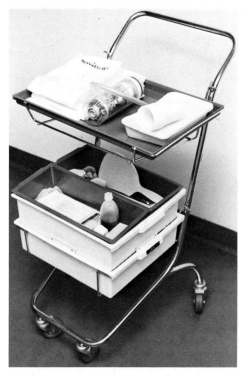

Fig. 19-7. A trolley for preventive dental care in hospitals and institutions.

Special considerations for dental care – For oral hygiene, toothbrushes with special handles or an electric toothbrush may be useful (Fig. 19-6). In the most severely affected patients, parents or other helpers will have to take responsibility for toothbrushing.

Generally, cooperation during dental treatment is good, but the lack of muscular control makes it difficult for patients with excessive involuntary movements. Various technical aids which may be useful in the treatment situation are shown in Figs. 19-7 to 10. Consultation with the patient's physiotherapist can be of great help.

Nitrous oxide or other sedatives may be used with good effect for some children with CP. General anesthesia should only be used if other forms of treatment prove impossible.

If the child has speech problems, the dentist must be patient and wait until the child has been able to express what he wants to say.

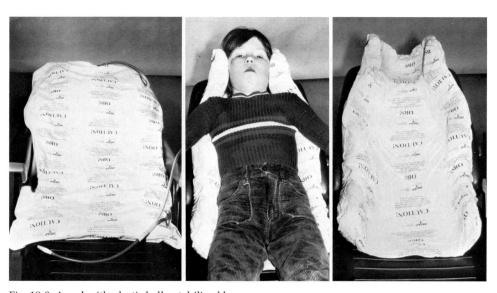

Fig. 19-8. A pad with plastic balls, stabilized by vacuum.

Minimal brain dysfunction

Minimal brain dysfunction (MBD) implies impaired cerebral function without a specific location in the brain. The syndrome includes several manifestations: concentration problems, hyperactivity, motor disturbances and deviant behavior. The impairment develops during fetal life or in connection with delivery. Genetic factors also play a role.

Frequency – In a study from Gothenburg, Sweden, the incidence was reported to be 1.2% for severe MBD and 3-6% for milder forms; boys are more frequently affected. The diagnosis is usually made at the age of 6-7 years and arises from teamwork of several professionals.

Medical treatment – Therapy includes family counselling and a dynamic education programme. Amphetamine derivatives to improve behavior and concentration may be used with good effect for some patients. From a neurobiological view MBD has a good prognosis, but a risk of psychiatric handicap in adulthood remains.

Special considerations for dental care – Cooperation in dental treatment is a major dental problem for children with MBD. Use eye contact when giving the child instructions, use few words and short sessions. N_2O/O_2-sedation may be of help.

SENSORY DISABILITIES

Children with sensory disabilities like blindness, deafness or deaf/blindness may have very different concepts and perspectives of reality than the rest of us. It is important to keep this in mind when we meet children with sensory disabilities.

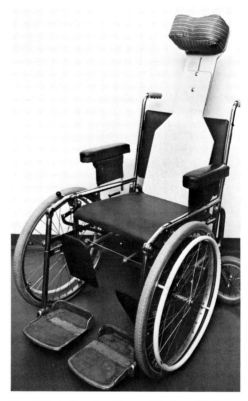

Fig. 19-9. A "head-rest" on a thin board helps to stabilize the head of a wheel-chair-bound patient.

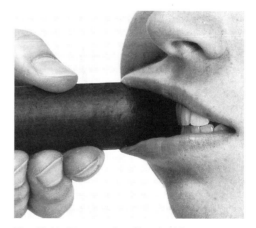

Fig. 19-10. Bite spatula of hard rubber.

Blindness

Blindness in children can be caused by prenatal insults such as infections in early pregnancy (rubella). Blindness may also be present as one of the symptoms of various syndromes. Postnatal causes of blindness may be prematurity, tumours, trauma or the consequence of certain medical conditions.

Special considerations for dental care – Since vision is restricted or absent, verbal communication must be extensive and comprehensive. The blind child must be allowed to touch with his hands and to smell objects so that he can become familiar with them without seeing. It is important to use time for explanation and familiarization before dental treatment starts. Remember that the tongue is a useful tool for feeling plaque and other structures in the oral cavity. Information material in Braille (point alphabet made for blind persons) is available in many countries. The associations for the blind can give information on available material.

In some cases the cause of blindness (infection, prematurity) may have affected tooth mineralization.

Due to the higher incidence of tooth anomalies and the possible initial problems with communication, frequent (bi-monthly) consultations for familiarization and prophylactic treatment, particularly in the early years may be useful.

Deafness

Deafness in children may be due to genetic disorders, infections, prematurity, blood incompatibilities or trauma. Approximately 50% of cases have a hereditary cause. Rubella alone accounts for around 20% of the cases of congenital deafness in some countries. Most deaf children will have delayed speech development. However, with the help of sign-language and lip-reading some deaf children may develop adequate communication abilities with time.

Frequency – The incidence of deafness in children varies in different countries. In the Nordic countries and in the United Kingdom 1-2 per 1,000 school children need hearing aids.

Special considerations for dental care – It is important to speak slowly and clearly with good lip-movements when communicating with a deaf child. Then the child will usually be able to understand what you say. Try to talk directly to the child, not through the parent. If you are going to have regular contact with one or more deaf children, it would be useful to learn a few signs to communicate better. Pictures are very useful tools for informing deaf children.

There are no specific dental problems associated with deafness alone. However, a higher incidence of hypodontia has been reported. If the child has a hearing-aid, it may be best to switch it off during noisy periods of dental treatment procedures (drilling, suction, etc.).

Deaf-blind children

A child with severely impaired vision combined with deafness will have serious problems with communication. Most blind people develop a particularly sensitive hearing skill to compensate for what they cannot see and deaf people use their eyes in the same way. When both these senses are defective or lacking, it may be extremely difficult to make sense of what is happening. Many deaf-blind children have other handicaps as well. Deaf-blindness is most frequently associated with rubella and prematurity. Certain syndromes also comprise deaf/blindness.

Special considerations for dental care – All deaf-blind individuals have severe communication problems. Some can hear a little with hearing aids or see enough to interpret sign language under optimal conditions (good light, contrasting colours and correct distance to the person communicating). In other cases communication can be made through signs in the palms of the deaf-blind person's hands. Although many deaf-blind will come to the dental office with an interpreter who can help with communication, direct contact through touching and feeling is still very important for establishing a trusting relationship between therapist and patient.

PHYSICAL DISABILITIES

Various hereditary or progressive conditions may lead to severe physical disability. Accidents also contribute to the group of physically disabled children.

Many muscular diseases cause physical disability and the most serious ones will be mentioned here:

Progressive spinal muscular atrophy

This disease is inherited autosomal recessive. Two different types are seen.

Type 1. Werdning-Hoffman's disease is the most severe. The symptoms start intrauterine or in the first year. The motor development is delayed. The disease progresses constantly and many of the children die in childhood often due to pneumonia.

Type 2. Proximal spinal muscular atrophy progresses slowly, but during puberty the progression may accelerate and some children become wheelchair-dependent. After puberty the disease is stationary.

Muscular dystrophy Duchenne

The disease is x-linked recessive, which means that mothers are carriers and patients are boys. Other recessive inherited muscle dystrophies similar to Duchenne are also seen and they may affect girls as well. The patients seem healthy in infancy although walking may be delayed. The disease may be diagnosed between 2 and 8 years of age.

The disease progresses rapidly and the child will be needing a wheelchair at 8-10 years of age. Heart insufficiency, pneumonia or infections are often causes of death. Most Duchenne boys die before 20 years of age.

Oral manifestations – In muscular diseases the cough reflexes may be reduced and the patient may not be able to clear his throat by coughing up any foreign material that falls to the back of the throat during dental procedures. Nitrous oxide sedation decreases the cough reflexes so nitrous oxide sedation is not recommended for this group of patients.

Special considerations for dental care – Due to the dystrophy of the muscles in the tongue, lips and cheeks, the self-cleansing mechanisms of the oral cavity may become insufficient in muscular dystrophy. Tooth cleaning ability may also be reduced, sometimes resulting in severe gingivitis. Open bite and lateral cross-bite may be present in patients with muscular diseases. Treatment of this is difficult and prolonged and the risk for recurrence is high. In serious progressive disorders (Duchenne), extensive orthodontic treatment is not adviceable.

Osteogenesis imperfecta

Osteogenesis imperfecta (OI) is a connective tissue defect involving bones and teeth, but also skin, ligaments, tendons, fasciae, sclerae and the small bones of the inner ear. The classic syndrome consists of brittle bones, clear or blue sclerae, loose ligaments, alter-

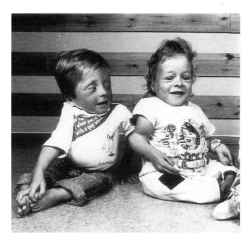

Fig. 19-11. OI-congenita. Girl aged 13 and boy aged 8 years.

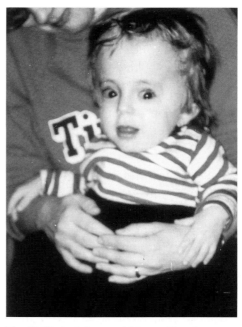

Fig. 19-12. A. A 4-year-old-boy with osteogenesis imperfecta handicapped by multiple fractures of long bones.

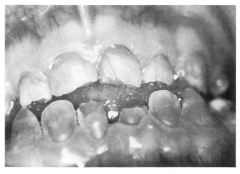

Fig. 19-12.B. Dentinogenesis imperfecta Type I involving the primary dentition at 5 years of age.

ations in teeth, and short stature and reduced hearing in adults. Functionally, the most important defects are brittle bones. Two types of OI are recognized: OI congenita (Fig. 19-11), where the child may be stillborn or die early in childhood. In this type of OI intrauterine fractures may be numerous. The child with the congenital type is a severely handicapped person who often is not even able to sit up.

OI tarda manifests itself later, may be crippling but not fatal. The syndrome is inherited as an autosomal dominant condition, but many cases are new mutations.

Patients with OI tarda have a motor handicap, but most of them are able to walk, some with the help of a stick.

Oral manifestations – OI-patients may suffer prolonged bleeding after tooth extraction. As mentioned earlier some of these patients have dentinogenesis imperfecta (Fig. 19-12): 15-20% (see Chapter 15). OI-patients without dentinogenesis imperfecta may have increased tendency to root canal obliteration and tooth fracture. A Class III malocclusion is more commonly found in OI-patients than in healthy individuals.

Spina bifida

Spina bifida is a congenital abnormality of the spinal cord and can be divided into three different forms: spina bifida occulta, where the spinal cord in a segment is uncovered by bone, meningocele which is a cystic lesion in the midline containing only meninges and myelomeningocele (MMC) in which the cystic lesion contains meninges, nerve roots and immature spinal cord. In MMC several disabilities may develop like paralysis or muscular hypotonia of legs, urinary bladder and/or rectum. Seventy per cent of these children develop hydrocephalus and need operations with a ventriculo-jugular shunt.

Frequency – The incidence of spina bifida varies widely from 1 in 1,500 newborn in Sweden to 7-8 in 1,500 in Scotland and Wales. The etiology is so far unclear. Most children with MMC have to undergo several examinations and operations during early childhood.

Special considerations for dental care – Dental infections should be avoided in children with a shunt, as bacteraemia may cause bacterial growth and clogging of the shunt.

Hypoplastic teeth and high caries activity has been reported in children with spina bifida.

Accident victims

When accidents give rise to a disability most often the brain or spinal cord are injured. Injury to the lower part of the cervical spinal cord may cause tetraplegia. The degree of disability depends on what part of the nervous system is injured.

Special considerations for dental care – In cerebral injuries disturbance in oral motor coordination may develop with e.g. eating problems and development of malocclusion. The patient's ability to perform tooth cleaning may also be limited and an electric toothbrush is often useful (Fig. 19-13). Severely disabled accident victims may need professional tooth-cleaning and preventive treatment as often as every two weeks.

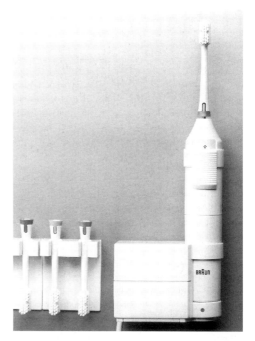

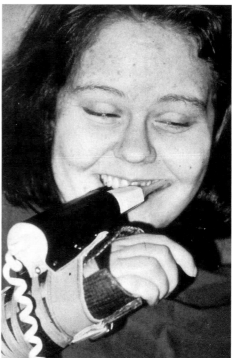

Fig. 19-13. Electric toothbrush. To be used by an accident victim.

PREVENTION

Children with handicap may have an increased need for preventive dental care. (For general rules for prevention of caries and periodontal disease (Chapters 9, 13). Persons with certain disabilities may also develop oral mucosal lesions which need special preventive programmes.

Recommendations for a dental care programme are not only intended for the disabled child (and parents), but can also be made for other health professionals, teachers, kitchen personnel in institutions, relatives and lay organizations.

It is important to establish good contact between medical and dental personnel. Dentist and dental hygienist may, for instance, make regular visits to paediatric wards in hospitals (Fig. 19-14) and long-stay institutions to promote oral hygiene and to give preventive treatment to patients.

Intervals

In practical work it has proved effective to have certain routines for check-up intervals for disabled children:

Routine A – An appointment with the dental hygienist/prophylactic nurse once every 6 months and with the dentist once a year. (For children with slight disabilities without oral or medical implications)

Routine B – An appointment with the dental hygienist/prophylactic nurse once every 3 months and with the dentist once a year. (Recommended for children with a moderate disability and problems with daily hygiene)

Routine C – An appointment with the dental hygienist/prophylactic nurse once every 3 months and with the dentist once every 6 months. (Recommended for children where development of dental disease should be followed more closely (congenital heart disease, haemophilia, progressive disorders)

Routine D – An appointment with the dental hygienist/prophylactic nurse once a month and with the dentist once every 6 months. (Recommended in cases where daily oral hygiene is very difficult to perform, and during treatment with cytostatic drugs, for example).

For many disabled patients Routine B is recommended during childhood and adolescence. During periods of intensive medical treatment Routine D performed in the hospital may be necessary.

Diet

The basic dietary principles are the same for all children whether they are healthy or disabled. In patients with reduced salivary secretion or impaired self-cleansing mechanisms of the oral cavity, the parents/caretakers have to be especially attentive to the diet. Certain restrictions are necessary, but parents and caretakers should be advised that total prohibition is meaningless. Sweetened medicines and drinks are a major problem for many sick children. If sweetened medicines cannot be replaced by sugar-free synonymous drugs, one should recommend that medicines are taken with meals. Parents may have been told that a child should drink a lot to prevent dehydration and/or kidney damage due to medication. If water is not acceptable for the child, sugar-free beverages should be recommended for drinks between meals.

Children with impaired muscular function may retain food in the mouth for a long time after meals. A glass of water after each meal should be recommended in such cases.

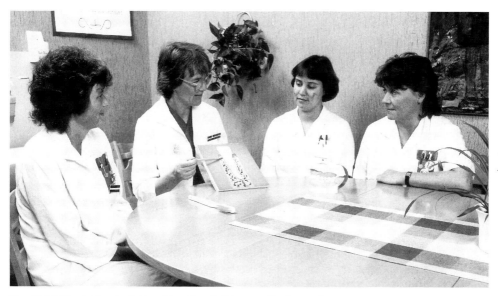

Fig. 19-14. Dental hygienist teaching the staff in a pediatric ward.

Fluorides

Children with hypomineralized teeth, reduced salivary secretion, a cariogenic diet or impaired muscular function may need an intensive fluoride program (see Chapter 9).

Chemical plaque control

In cases where oral hygiene is very difficult to perform, and when dental disease should be avoided for medical reasons, chemical plaque control with chlorhexidine or other agents with similar properties should be recommended:

Such agents can be used daily during periods of certain medical treatment procedures (irradiation to the head and neck,

cytostatic drugs, etc). Daily use for 7-10 days prior to dental treatment can be recommended for patients when bleeding or bacteraemia caused by treatment should be minimized (haemophilia, cardiac disease, immunedeficiency). For some children, continuous use of chlorhexidine should be considered during cyclosporine or diphenylhydantion medication when adequate oral hygiene cannot be obtained by mechanical means, and for children with progressive lethal conditions where oral hygiene is difficult to perform.

Chlorhexidine can be applied on a tooth brush, by the help of cotton sticks (Q-tips), or as gel in individual trays.

Background literature

Almer Nielsen L. Den generelle fysiske, psykiske og sociale situation hos patienter med cerebral parese. *Tandlægebladet* 1988; **92**: 717-21.

Almer Nielsen L. Den odontologiske status hos børn med cerebral parese vurdert ut fra oplysninger i Sundhedsstyrelsens centrale odontologiske register. *Tandlægebladet* 1988; **92**: 722-7.

Alborn B, Hallonsten AL. *Handikapptandvård.* Stockholm: Invest-Odont, 1986.

Friis-Hansen B (ed). *Nordisk lærebog i pædiatri.* Chapters 32-41. Copenhagen: Munksgaard, 1985.

Gillberg C, Rasmussen P, Carlström G, Svensson B, Waldenström E. Perceptual and attentional deficits in six-year-old children. Epidemiological aspects. *J Child Psychol Psychiatry* 1982; **23**: 131-44.

Nordisk Klinisk Odontologi, Chap 26. Handikapptandvård. København: Forlaget for Faglitteratur, 1980.

Storhaug K (ed). *Tannpleie for funksjonshemmede og kronisk syke.* Oslo: Den norske tannlegeforening/-NKI-forlaget, 1991.

Storhaug K. Caries experience in disabled preschool children. *Acta Odontol Scand* 1985; **43**: 241-8.

Storhaug K, Holst D. Caries experience of disabled school-age children. *Community Dent Oral Epidemiol* 1987; **15**: 144-9.

Literature cited

1. World Health Organization. *International classification of impairments, disabilities and handicaps.* Geneva: WHO 1980.

2. Göransson K, Kylén G. Begåvningshandikappades verklighetsuppfatning. *Socialmedicinsk tidsskrift* 1986; **4**: 152-6.

3. Kylén C, Göransson K. Begåvning och begåvningshandikapp. *Socialmedicinsk tidsskrift* 1986; **1-2**: 17-20.

INDEX